Hands of Love

Seven Steps to the Miracle of Birth

New Dawn Publishing

Layout Design King Elder
Cover Art Alec Syme
Cover & Text Photography Dr. Carol Phillips
Content Editors Jody Peterson Lodge
Wendy Phillips Piret
Rena Croft
Copy Editor Lori McLaughlin

First American Edition, 2001
24681097531

Published in the United States by
New Dawn Publishing
P.O. Box 16539
St. Paul, MN. 55116
NewDawnPublish@cs.com

Text and photographs copyright © 2001 by Carol J. Phillips. All rights reserved. No part of this publication may be reproduced, stored in a retrieval system, or transmitted in any form or by any means, electronic, mechanical, photocopying, recording, or otherwise, without the prior written permission of the copyright owner.

This book is not intended to be a substitute for professional medical advice or care, and any user of this book should always consult a licensed physician and chiropractor before adopting any particular course of treatment.

Library of Congress Catalog Card Number: 99-93496
Phillips, Carol J.
Hands of Love, Seven Steps to the Miracle of Birth/ Dr. Carol J. Phillips
p. cm.

ISBN 0-9673942-0-1
1. Pregnancy. 2. Prenatal care 3. Childbirth

Printed in China

Hands of Love

Seven Steps to the Miracle of Birth

Dr. Carol J. Phillips

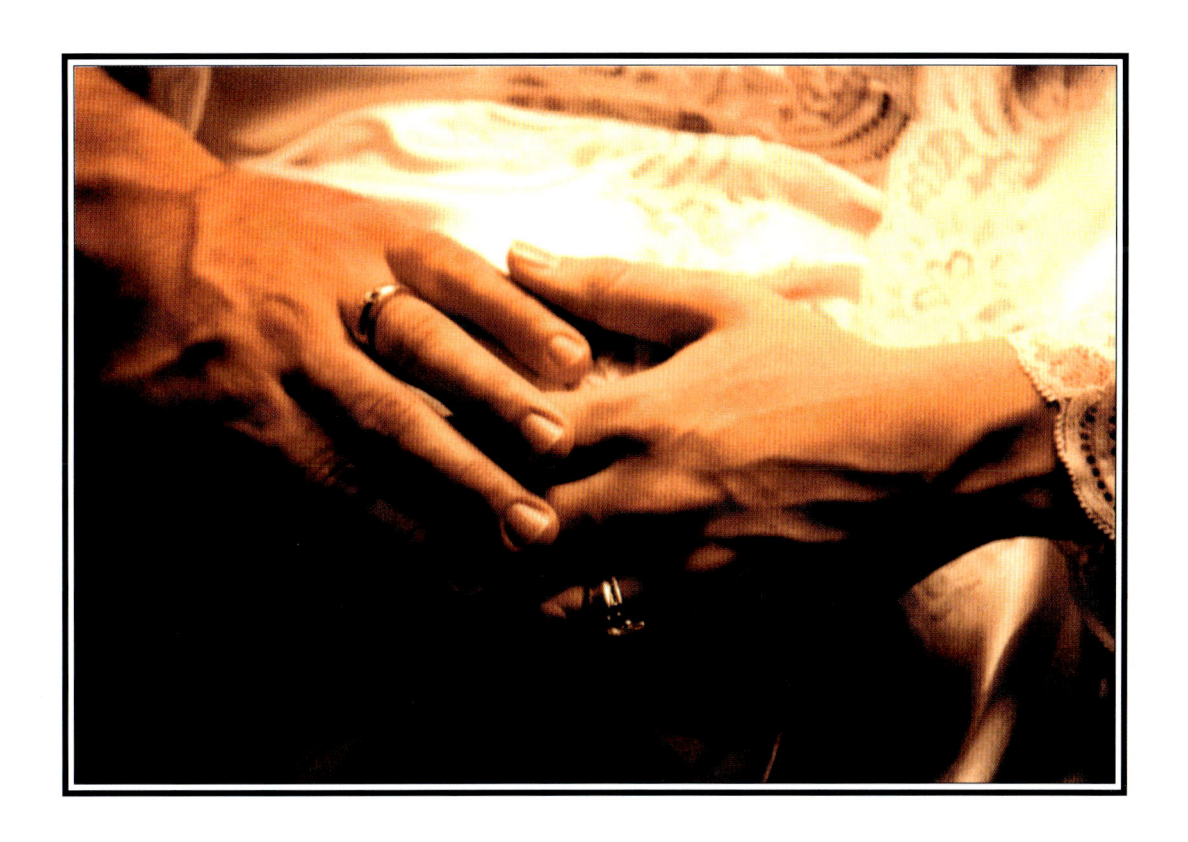

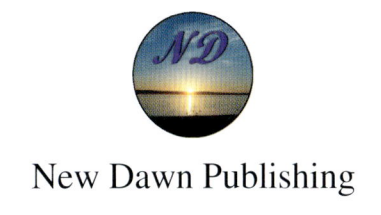

New Dawn Publishing

Hands of Love
Seven Steps to the Miracle of Birth

STEP 1

Pg 15: Decide on a Birth Model that Supports Your Belief System

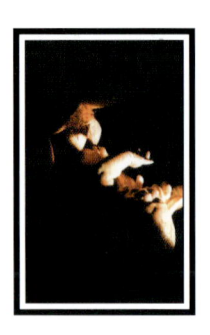

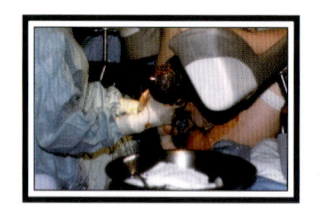

STEP 2

Pg 33: Choose A Birth Attendant

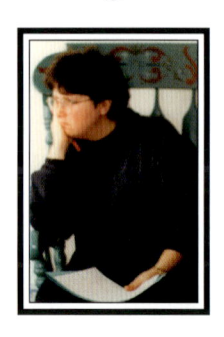

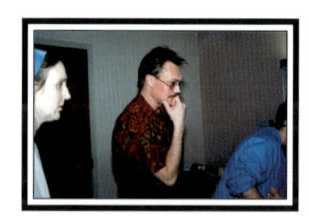

STEP 3

Pg 55: Create a Birth Team

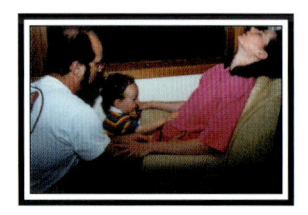

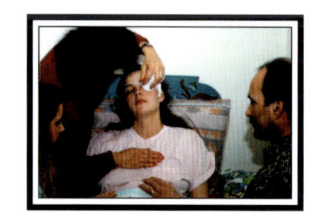

STEP 4
Pg 97: Seek Relief for the Discomforts of Pregnancy and Birth

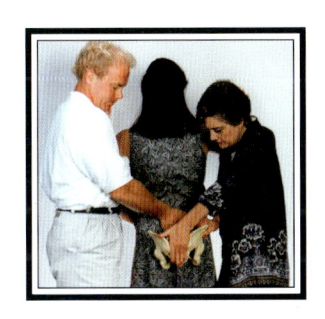

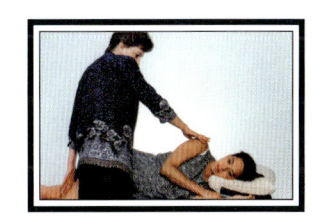

STEP 5
Pg 139: Be Prepared in the Event of a Cesarean Delivery

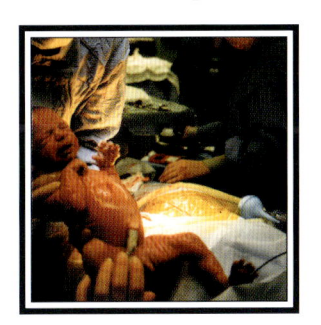

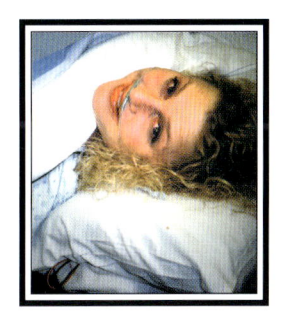

STEP 6
Pg 159: Accept the Dual Reality of Human Existence

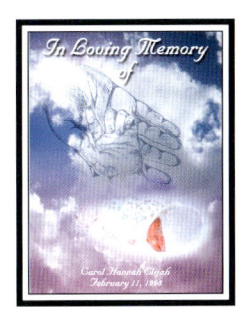

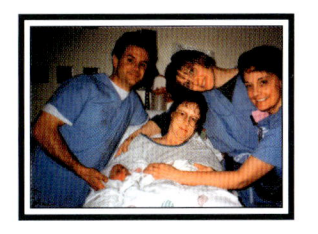

STEP 7
Pg 173: Follow Your Instincts and Trust Your Inner Voice

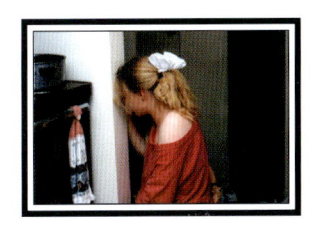

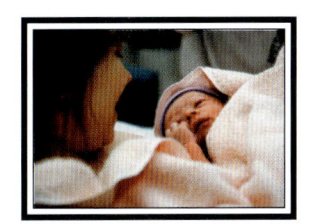

Stories of a Miracle

Part One: Peace of Mind

Pg 16   Angel's Birth

Pg 20   The Joy of Birth: *A mother maintains control despite chaos*

Pg 24   A Family Conquers Their Fear of Birth: *A successful VBAC at home*

Pg 37   My First Birth Educator: *A humanistic homebirth with a midwife*

Pg 49   A Father Catches the Baby: *A humanistic hospital birth with an obstetrician*

Pg 58   A Mother's Intuition: *A grandmother rocks her daughter through contractions*

Pg 60   A Father Knows Best: *A grandfather teaches me to be a better doula*

Pg 66   Luke: *A two-year-old helps his mother during her water birth*

Pg 68   Kevin: *A three-year-old giggles through the home delivery*

Pg 69   Sarah: *A five-year-old steps in with a foot massage*

Pg 71   Gretta and Luke: *Siblings voice their appreciation for being included in the delivery*

Pg 72   Alex: *A seven-year-old videotapes the hospital delivery*

Pg 78   Birth Is a Family Affair: *Parents, siblings, friends, doulas, and midwives all assist in this family-centered homebirth*

Part Two: Respect for the Human Body

Pg 99   Pebbles and BamBam: *Chiropractic care helps a mother of twins*

Pg 112   A Chance to Grow: *Craniosacral therapy prevents an early birth*

Pg 114   The Chiropractic Advantage: *A mother learns how to stop premature contractions with a simple, non-invasive maneuver*

Pg 129   Marie's Birth Story: *The structural cause of back-labor is addressed and a birth is complete*

Pg 140   Becky's Birth Story: *A surprise breech presentation leads to a planned cesarean delivery*

Pg 148   Julia's Birth Story: *An operating room is transformed into a spiritual place of welcoming for a newborn with cord complications*

Pg 152   Sharilyn's Birth Story: *A mother's wish is honored and she is allowed to touch and bond with her newborn within seconds of her cesarean section*

Part Three: Reverence for the Spirit

Pg 161   A Spirit Returns: *Two parents face grief head-on as they work together to give their child's body a graceful birth*

Pg 169   One Year Later: *Life goes on and another child is born into the family*

Pg 174   A Mother's Wisdom: *A mother follows her instincts and saves her baby*

Pg 181   A World of Choice: *A mother listens to her inner voice and abandons her dream of a homebirth for her firstborn child*

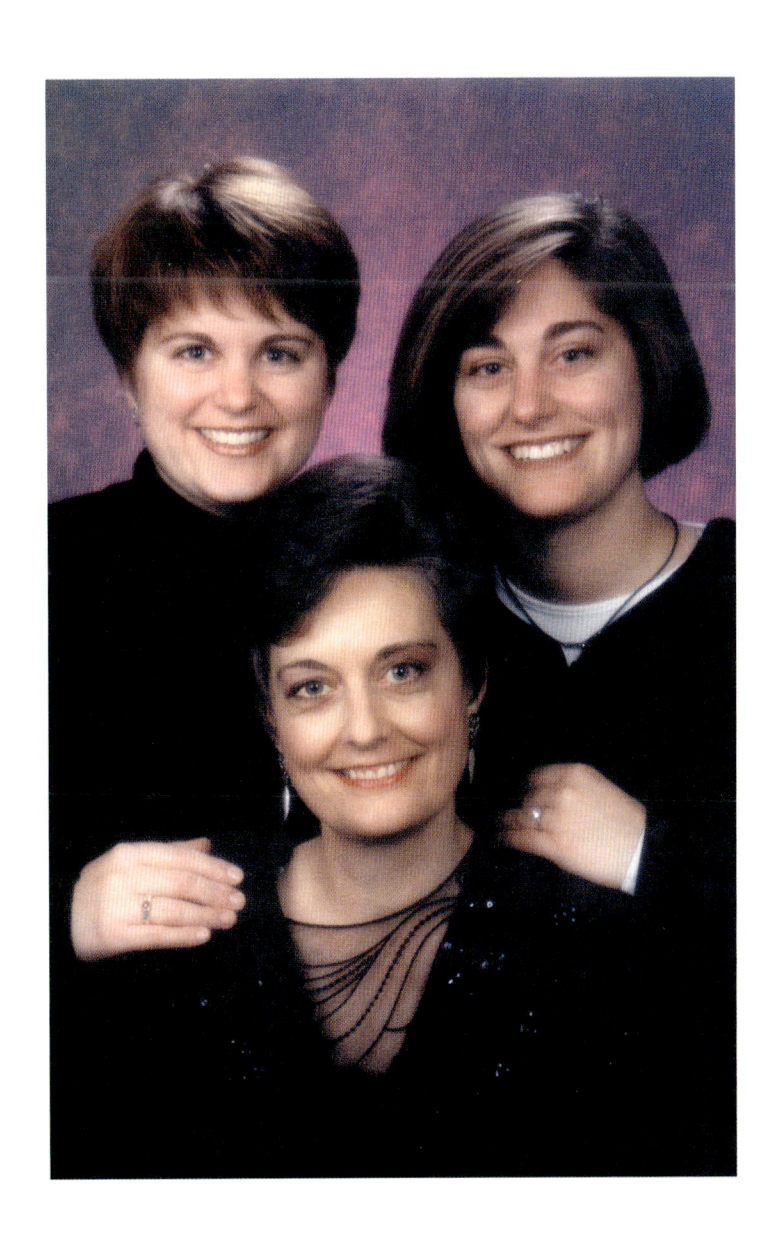

This book is dedicated to my girls,
Angel and Wendy

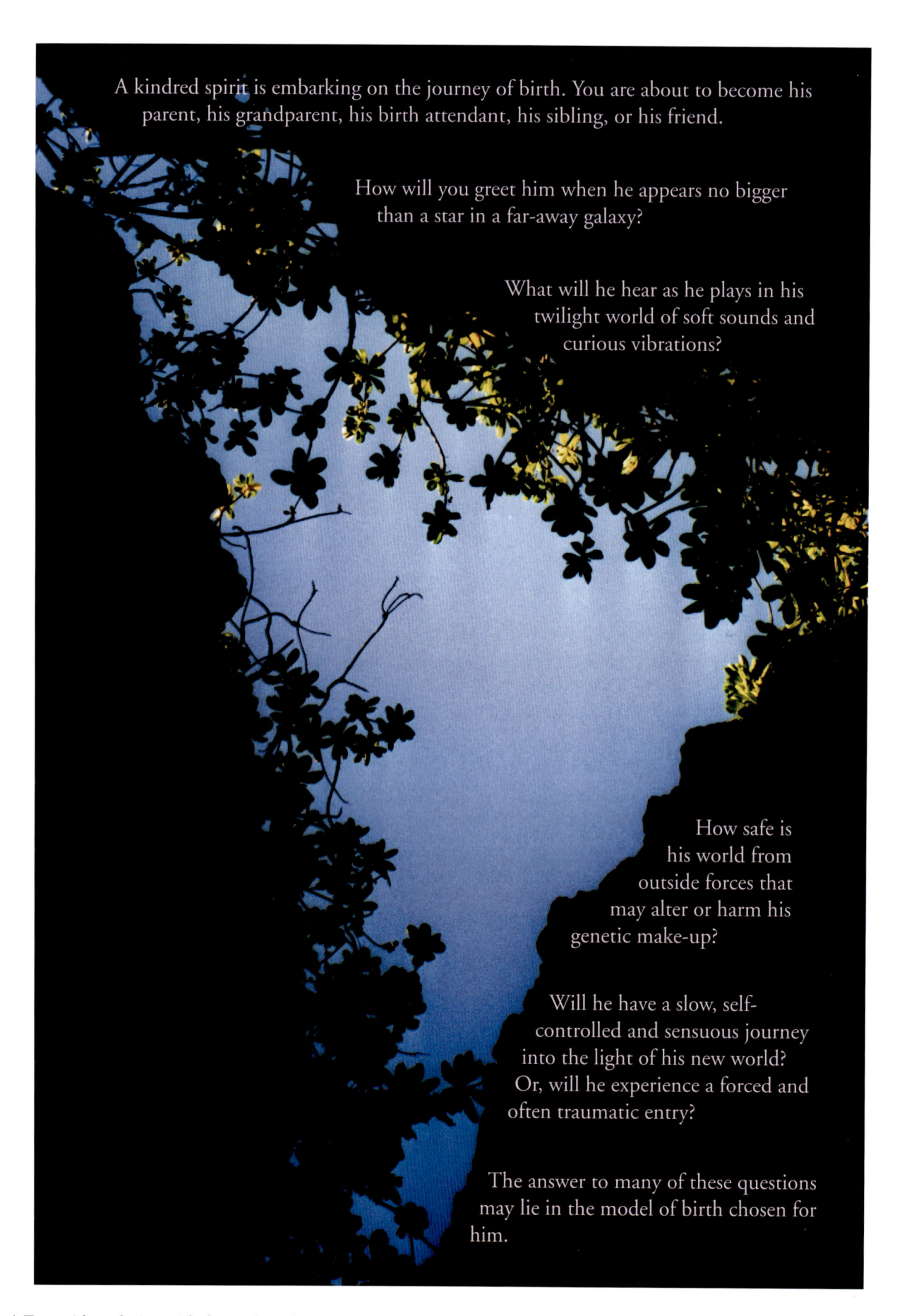

A kindred spirit is embarking on the journey of birth. You are about to become his parent, his grandparent, his birth attendant, his sibling, or his friend.

How will you greet him when he appears no bigger than a star in a far-away galaxy?

What will he hear as he plays in his twilight world of soft sounds and curious vibrations?

How safe is his world from outside forces that may alter or harm his genetic make-up?

Will he have a slow, self-controlled and sensuous journey into the light of his new world? Or, will he experience a forced and often traumatic entry?

The answer to many of these questions may lie in the model of birth chosen for him.

To avoid confusion with the mother, the masculine pronoun will generally be used when referring to the baby.

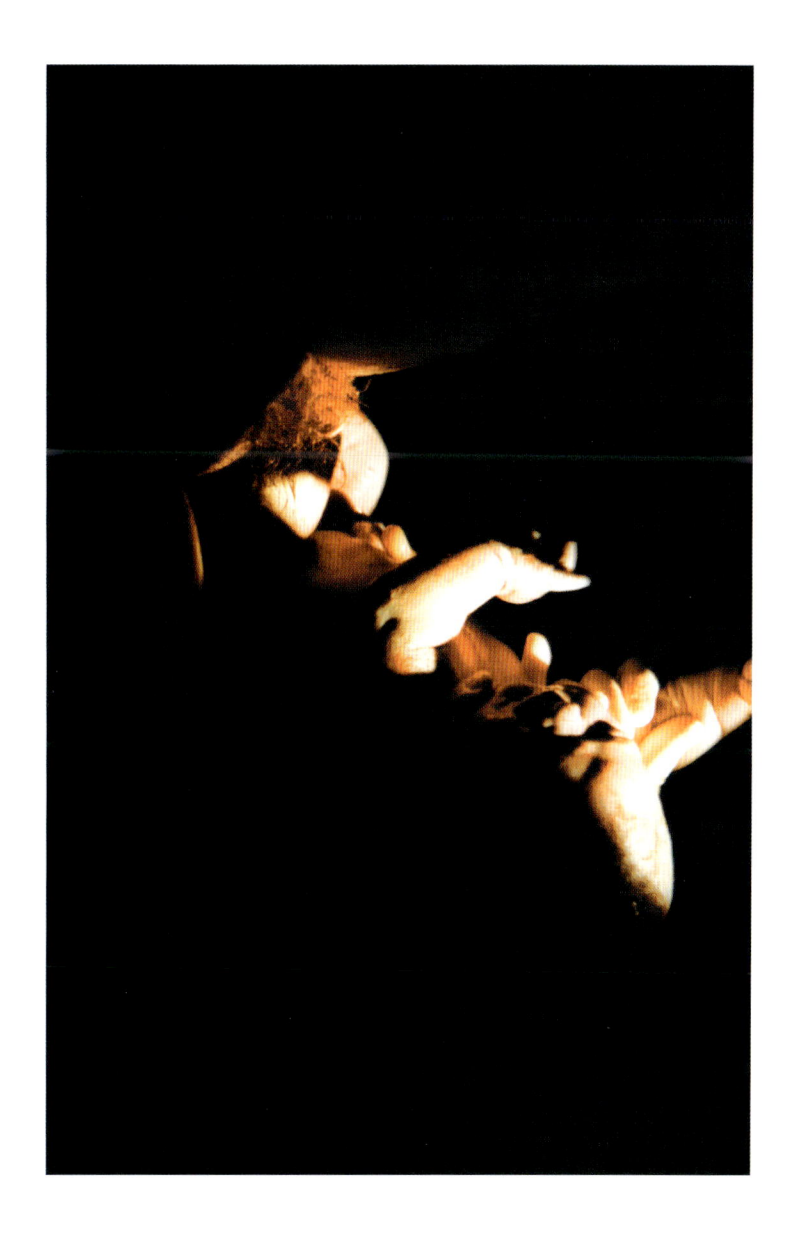

$\mathcal{B}$irth may be allowed to flow with the natural pulse of the Universal Life Force* being emitted from the Creator…

The universal life force is often referred to as Innate. Responsible for giving motion to matter, the Universal Life Force is present in all life forms and is beautifully illustrated in the intricately timed contractions of labor.

It may be managed with the use of technology created by mankind…

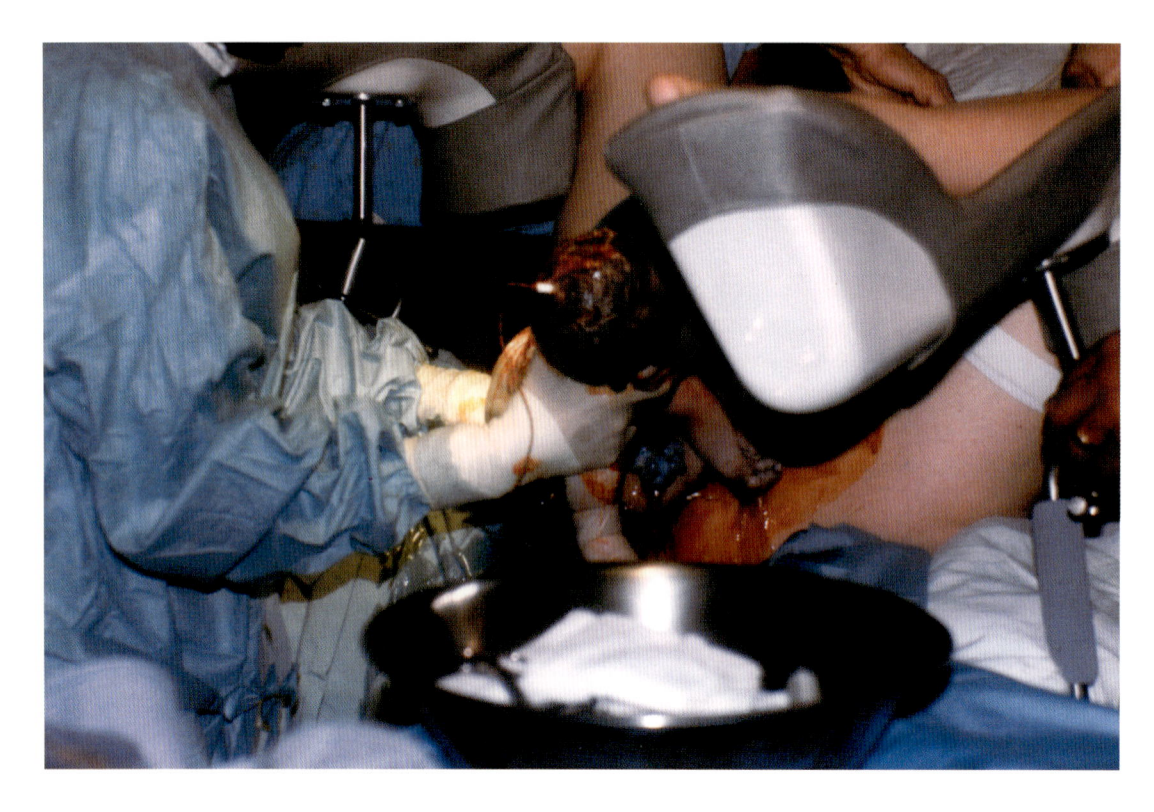

Either way, a mother and her child should be treated with love, respect and compassion for they are embarking on a miraculous journey that has an enduring impact on the future of the human race.

If we want to make a better world for our children, we must first change the way we bring children into the world.

Through the most fundamental kinds of trust—trust in the power of Mother Nature; trust in a woman's ability to give birth; and trust in the intrinsic wisdom that is acquired through personal experience—a woman can gain the confidence needed to manage her own birthing process.

Hands of Love combines the personal knowledge and wisdom of more than two dozen mothers to create a road map that will guide expectant families through nine-months of anticipation as they await the moment that will change their lives forever. This book is not an academic journey to provide parents with an understanding of the physiological process of creation; it is a spiritual journey that helps the entire family prepare for the upcoming birth by bringing to light the diversity of choices inherent in the birth experience.

Hands of Love will open your eyes to a world of possibilities. It will eliminate fear of the unknown and encourage you to take responsibility for your birth choices. This book provides a refreshing, new perspective on the birth experience and provides the reader with valuable didactic and tactile information:

- Mothers learn how to vocalize a sound that vibrates her uterus and relaxes her vaginal muscles.

- Partners learn how to perform simple maneuvers that reposition the pelvic structures and balance the uterine ligaments—maneuvers that are often successful in diminishing premature contractions, reducing back and groin pain during pregnancy and eliminating the pain of back-labor during delivery.

- Doulas learn simple techniques that help a mother during labor, such as making a tub of cold cloths to cool a mother down or visualization to help her work calmly through the intense birthing contractions.

- Family members learn how to direct loving energy from their palms into and around an unborn child—often resulting in a calm, self-controlled mother. These and many other valuable tidbits of knowledge gained from my sixteen years of experience attending more than 600 births will be at the fingertips of every reader.

The photographs in **Hands of Love** were not taken with the initial intent of sharing them with the world. Most of them were taken to record for the family the beauty inherent in a pregnant woman and the joy experienced at the birth of a child. These photographs now have the added dimension of confirming that a woman-centered birth can empower women to believe in themselves, that a family-centered birth can remove the mystery and fear often associated with the childbirth experience, and that the inclusion of a doula[1] and a chiropractor can reduce the need for excessive medical intervention.

I hope you enjoy this visual odyssey through the journey of birth and that you, too, are inspired to capture the beauty of creation and the miracle of birth.

Dr. Carol Phillips
Pre-Natal Chiropractor
Birth Photographer
Doula

1 A doula is a person who provides the family with continuous spiritual, physical, emotional, and informational support before, during, and immediately following childbirth.

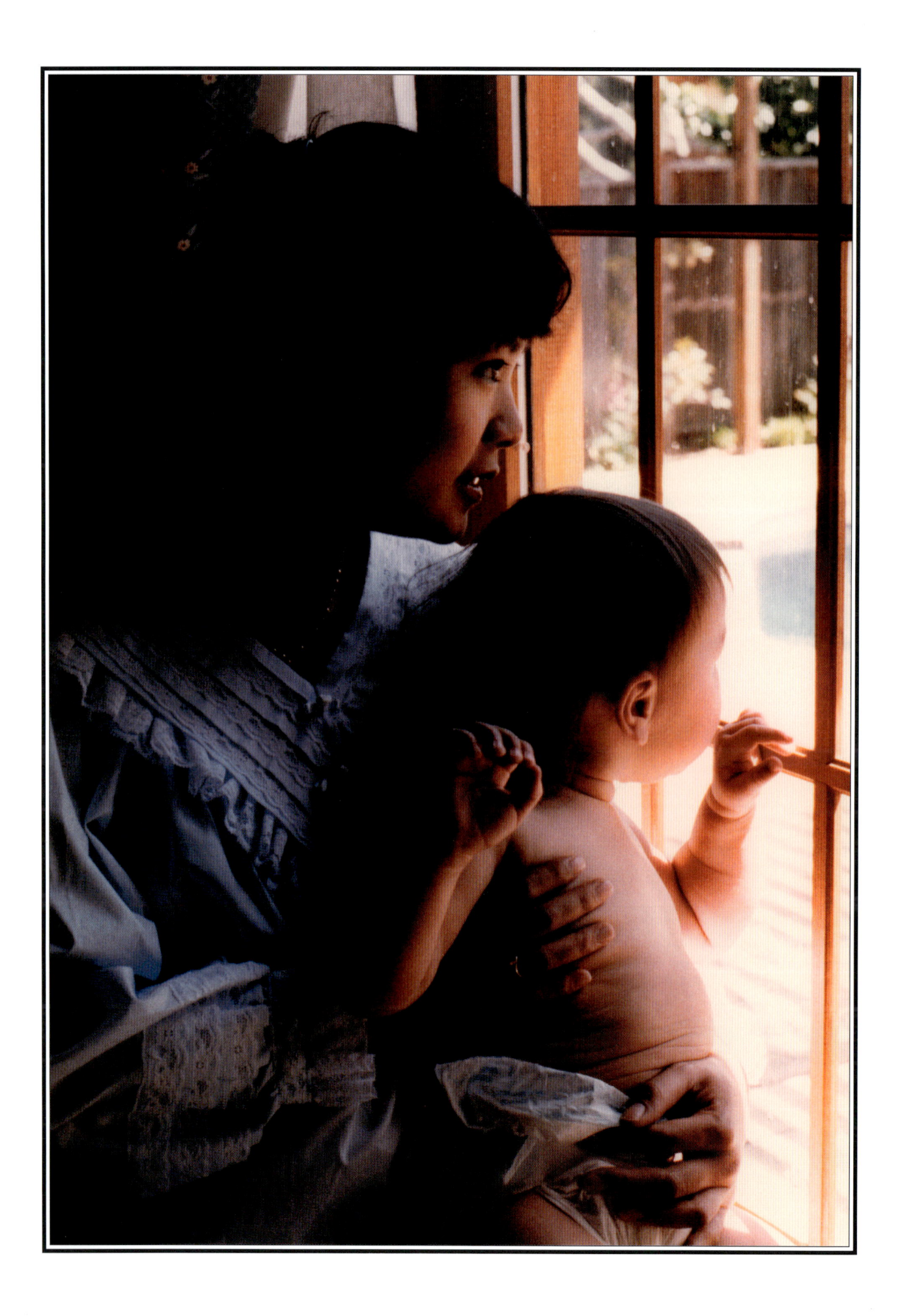

Part One

Peace of Mind

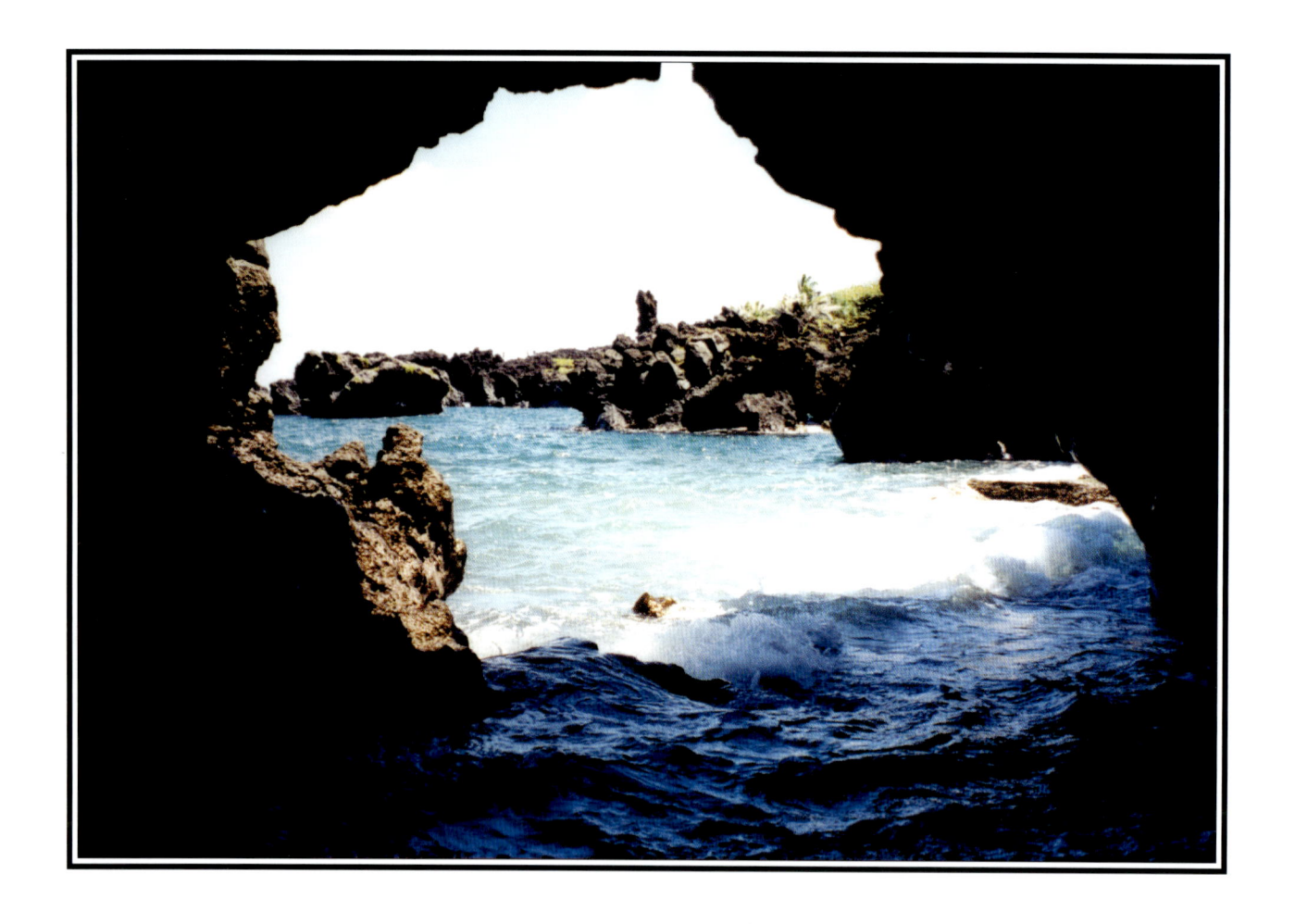

The important thing is to hold firm to your beliefs without being influenced or swayed by what others do or say. Those who live this way are strong and free of regret.

–Daisaku Ikeda

STEP 1
Decide on a Birth Model That Supports Your Belief System

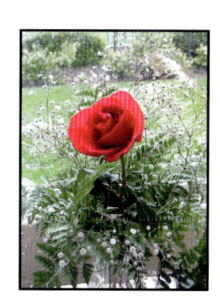

One of the first things you need to do when you become a new parent is to evaluate your belief system and investigate various birth models. Once you and your partner have a clear vision of your ultimate goal for childbirth, you will be able to adopt a model that is compatible with your beliefs and values. Making that decision doesn't guarantee that you'll have the birth you envision, but it's a start toward achieving your goal. Without clear intent, it is very difficult to maintain some kind of control over the outcome.

Women have basically two birth models to choose from. The first and most commonly adopted is the technocratic–controlled model. This is the model chosen by parents who feel their child will be best served if they leave the decision-making process to the "experts." Women at this end of the spectrum usually request epidural anesthesia and welcome the use of modern technological advances.

On the opposite end of the spectrum, for those parents who feel that birth is a natural process on the continuum of life, lies the humanistic–assisted model. This is the model most commonly adopted by parents who want more control over their child's birth experience and by parents who are willing to take full responsibility for the outcome.

The Technocratic–Controlled Model

In the technocratic paradigm, a parent accepts that the human body functions like a machine. Robbie Davis-Floyd in *Birth As An American Rite of Passage* demonstrates how this model views the female body as unpredictable and inherently defective. Consequently, it may malfunction at any time. The basic tenet of this model of birth holds that some degree of intervention is necessary in **all** births and **all** births should occur in the hospital setting. It is estimated that 90% of women in the United States embrace the technocratic model. They enter the birthing room believing that science is there to take care of them and save them from the *seemingly* unnecessary pain and anguish of childbirth.

Women often adopt the technocratic model because it's the accepted norm. They rarely question the logic of allowing others to control the process of birth and rely on medical providers to tell them what's best for them. They welcome induction, accept epidural injections, and turn to planned cesarean deliveries because it's believed to be easier and safer.

I adopted the technocratic model during the birth of my first child, Angel. I never questioned my allopathically influenced desire to turn control over to the doctors at our local military hospital. I was 20-years-old and felt I knew nothing about childbirth.

I am writing this book today, in part, because of the emotional and physical trauma my daughter and I both experienced that day. Coming to terms with my decision to relinquish control over Angel's birth has been a long journey. As a result of that decision, I have become a chiropractor and Angel has become a craniosacral therapist. We both specialize in the prevention and treatment of birth related injuries. Now, thirty years later, I realize that my decision was, in fact, part of my destiny.

January 18, 1970
Angel's Birth

I woke up suddenly with a sharp pain in my back that brought me to my feet. I clung to the dresser for support as I gasped for air. After months of premature labor contractions, I was not prepared for the intensity of the sensations that were now gripping my body. Little did I realize that in four short hours my life would change forever.

The memories of that eventful day are only flashes in my mind. I screamed "Hurry, Hurry" as we raced down the icy wooded highway, then "Slow Down, Slow Down" as I came back to this world and saw the trees flashing past us in the night. The enema and shaving are gone from my memory as the drugs that were immediately injected blurred my consciousness. Yet, nothing could blur the humiliation of being stripped of my clothing and told to pull my ankles to my chin as several medics stood at the foot of my bed to observe the process. For some reason, I vividly remember the blurred face of the doctor as he bent over me and told me what a good girl I'd been for staying home so long. I wanted to let him know that labor had just begun, but the drugs left me unable to speak. I have no memory of making a sound, but my husband said he heard my screams all the way down in the waiting room where he was forced to wait.

I have no memory of the transfer to the delivery room. Yet, I vividly remember being jerked out of my dark world when someone sat me up on the emerging head of my baby. With extreme clarity I remember screaming, "What are you doing! What are you doing!" Someone told me I was receiving a spinal block. My memory from that moment on is etched clearly in my brain and haunts me to this day. My arms were pulled out to the side where large straps pinned my wrists to the table and two rubber-appearing objects were swung up on a device at my feet. It took a minute to register that the rubber objects were my legs being strapped at the ankles to the holding device. In horror, I continued to scream out my confusion as a nurse climbed up on a stool and began applying heavy pressure to my abdomen to force the baby down. At my feet, I heard a doctor say that he was removing the baby with forceps. The next thing I remember is seeing the completely white image of my little girl, Angel, as she was carried out of the room. I was told they had to hurry because the next patient had to be brought into the delivery room. I hadn't been allowed to touch her or see what she looked like.

In recovery, I was warned not to move my head for eight hours or I'd suffer a severe headache. After that period, I would be allowed to see the baby. I lay frozen with fright and shock at what just happened to me. Suddenly, I began to shake uncontrollably. As hospital personal began to gather around the bed and cover me with heated blankets, their faces blurred as I sunk deeper and deeper into the darkness. A moment later I was floating up in the corner of the ward. I looked down and watched them working over me. I could clearly see the other women, lying in their curtained cubicles as they listened to the activity in the room. As I felt myself being pulled further and further away, I responded from deep in my soul with words that poured from my mind. "No, I have a baby girl! I have to take care of my baby girl!" Finally, a deep gentle voice simply said, "Okay." Within seconds, I was no longer looking down on the room but up into the face of a doctor as he gradually came back into focus.

It is a common belief that the widespread adoption of the technocratic–controlled model decreased infant mortality and improved the nature of childbirth in modern society. While this may be true to some degree, a look at the rate of infant mortality in the United States reveals that approximately 23 other countries have a lower infant mortality birthrate than we do. And, a glance into the Neonatal Intensive Care Units around the country reveals that many newborns may be suffering from our way of birthing.

It is not the purpose of this book to investigate, evaluate, defend or condemn medical childbirth practices. But I do want to help women regain control over their bodies and their children's births. To do that we must take a moment to review the past in order to

STEP 1: Decide on a Birth Model That Supports Your Belief System

understand what has gone wrong in the present; only then can we move forward and make decisions that will change the way we view women and birth in America and around the world.

The Evolution of Obstetrical Intervention

At the turn of the century, less than 5% of women in the United States chose to deliver within the hospital setting. Then, around 1910, women active in the feminist movement heard that an anesthetic called Twilight Sleep was being used in Europe to help birthing women have a pain-free delivery. They too wanted access to this "miracle" drug, as the fear of a painful delivery was as real for them as it is for women today. Through their efforts, the *Twilight Sleep Maternity Hospital* was established in Boston in 1915.

During the same time frame, there was an organized movement by the medical profession to bring birthing women into the hospitals and under the control of medical doctors (who had limited experience in the art of birthing). Moving childbirth into the hospitals eliminated the need for a family doctor, or midwife, to wait at a woman's home for the baby to arrive. The move gave the new medical specialty of obstetrics the ability to utilize the newest technological advances and it ensured financial stability for the emerging monopoly of medical health care.

As more and more hospitals took over the field of obstetrics, the doctors succumbed to the demands made by birthing women for a pain-free delivery. By the late 1930's, Twilight Sleep, hypodermic injections of morphine combined with scopolamine (a powerful hallucinogenic and amnesiac) and pentobarbital sodium, had become the anesthetic of choice for most doctors and women in labor. These injections were given hourly and resulted in wild uncontrolled behavior which the mother had no memory of after the birth.

By 1939, 50% of all women delivered their babies in the hospital. The American Medical Association, now having established obstetrics in their hospitals, began charging midwives with "practicing medicine without a license." The percentage of hospital births rose to 90% by mid-century. It was at that time that this country experienced a complete disappearance of the traditional ways of birthing women. (Forced underground, midwives disappeared from sight, but they did not disappear all together.)

The use of Twilight Sleep resulted in the development of restraining devices that would prevent women from harming themselves or others during labor. During 1940–1950, doctors began to discourage the use of these powerful drugs due to the potential dangers for both the mother and her child. New analgesics such as spinal blocks, pudendal blocks, and epidurals were introduced. Doctors were successful in getting women to accept the new drugs in most hospitals, but some out-of-the-way places are reported to have continued the use of Twilight Sleep up until the mid–1970's.

The standard procedures for restraining the wrists and ankles of women did not change with the introduction of new analgesics. Women, who were previously oblivious to the entrapments of delivery protocols, were now conscious during delivery, and terror often replaced the amnesia of twilight sleep.

Separated from family members, drugged, paralyzed and restrained, women had become vehicles of birth rather than the miraculous instruments of birth they were created to be, and babies suffered. From the time women began to demand a pain-free birth, babies have been denied the exhilaration of sliding out into the world to meet their parents. Drugged and manually removed from their mothers, the memory of that event is locked in the child's subconscious mind and physical body for a lifetime. Is it any wonder that fear of childbirth has become the predominant emotion for the last three generations?

A mother's body weight is the determining factor when the dosage of an anesthetic is calculated. Initially, it was believed that the placenta provided a safe barrier for the baby. We now know the placenta is an open avenue for whatever chemicals or nutrients the mother has in her blood stream. Therefore, when a mother was given twilight sleep, her baby received the same drugs at a level hundreds of times greater than the safe dosage recommended on the basis of their body weight. Imagine the shock to their systems when the drugs entered their blood stream.

In the past, few mothers failed to realize that when they received Twilight Sleep or a Spinal Block, forceps were often necessary. Women were unaware that forceps were being used because they were either unconscious or blinded by the drapes placed over their legs.

(cont.)

> Most of us between the ages of 27 – 60 years old were born in an operating room and under these circumstances. If we were in the best position for delivery, the negative effect of forceps was minimal. If we were not, the effect of our delivery ranged from obvious brain injury to symptoms that may have been insidious, slow, and obscure (i.e., learning disabilities to chronic headaches, etc.,).

When the delivery room era came to an end in the 1980's, fathers were allowed to join the mothers during labor and delivery. With this one change, love was brought back into the birthing arena. Unfortunately, technology was evolving rapidly at the same time.

In 1968, Dr. Edward Hon began the use of ultrasound technology (sonograms, electronic fetal monitoring, and dopplers), to monitor high-risk women. He was attempting to reduce the incidence of cerebral palsy by identifying and removing babies who exhibited fetal distress during a contraction.

Before Dr. Hon's theory could be thoroughly evaluated, or the technology tested for safety and accuracy, companies making the machines began marketing them to every available hospital. Electronic fetal monitoring now turned the attention of the medical staff away from the woman in labor and onto a piece of paper spilling out of the ultrasound machine. Learning to read the ultrasound tracings took practice and experience and the rate of cesarean deliveries suddenly began to rise as the incidence of "fetal distress" increased. As straps wrapped tightly around a woman's abdomen replaced the leather straps that had secured women's ankles and wrists to the delivery table, many hospitals reported a rise in their rate of cesarean deliveries from 5% to 40%.

By 1979, it was reported that 60% – 70% of women were confined to a birthing bed to be electronically monitored throughout labor and delivery, yet no research on the effectiveness or safety of the machine had been conducted. Then, in 1987, the prestigious *Lancet Medical Journal* reported that eight different studies conducted in Australia, the United States, and Europe found that "the main statistical effect of electronic fetal monitoring is to increase the rate of intervention."

Despite those findings, by 1990 the rate of women being monitored throughout labor had increased to 100%. That same year (20 years after Dr. Hon began his investigation), *The New England Journal of Medicine* published a study on the incidence of cerebral palsy. Conducted at the University of Washington, this study found that the rate of cerebral palsy was two and one half times higher in the ultrasound monitored test group compared to the unmonitored control group. This prompted an editorial in the same issue that read, "It is unfortunate that randomized controlled trials were not carried out before this form of technology became universally applied."

The incidence of frequent ultrasound sonograms and continuous electronic monitoring throughout labor began to change in 1993 after a large randomized trial involving 15,151 pregnant women found that screening ultrasonography (where you can see the baby) did not improve perinatal outcome. In other words, ultrasound technology is not an exact science and ultrasound findings are sometimes inaccurate and misleading—resulting in unnecessary, risky interventions. While research has finally resulted in the decreased frequency of ultrasound screenings, and experience has eliminated the need for continuous electronic monitoring during labor, electronic fetal monitoring (ultrasound) has become an integral part of all hospital deliveries.

We've seen many changes in the field of obstetrics since the turn of the century when more than 95% of babies in the United States were delivered at home. We've seen the rise of technology, and sadly the fall of midwifery. Moving birth into the hospital setting has resulted in advances that allow babies weighing less than 500 grams to survive. However, for every step forward there is often a step backward. Those of us specializing in pediatrics have witnessed an alarming rise in the number of babies and small children presenting for treatment with a wide variety

> The amount of amniotic fluid is greatly reduced at delivery so the ultrasonic waves may cause a baby pain as it strikes the sensitive tissue (periosteum) which covers his bones. If you were to apply the same ultrasonic waves directly to your bones you would jump away in rapid response to the burning sensation. The baby is protected somewhat by the mother's muscles and pelvis but not entirely. This could explain why babies wave during an examination—it's the startle reflex.

STEP 1: Decide on a Birth Model That Supports Your Belief System

of syndromes associated with physical and/or mental disabilities. Could it be that the same medical advances that are used to save lives are also contributing to the decline in the quality of life for many children?

The Humanistic–Assisted Model

A mother who adopts the humanistic paradigm believes she is an individual, and must be treated as such. She questions the use of routine protocols and challenges her birth attendants to make decisions based on her individual circumstances and her wishes. She believes she has the right to promote shared decision-making and accepts responsibility for all aspects of the birth process. This mother believes she is innately capable of delivering wholistically[1], while remaining open to the use of technology—if applied judiciously.

When expectant parents adopt a humanistic–assisted model, they create a birth team made up of familiar people who are willing to assist them in creating a loving and nurturing environment for the birth of their child; whether the birth occurs in their home, a birthing center, or a hospital.

Everyone in this book has adopted this model, even when the birth resulted in a surgical delivery. They all accepted the fact that in order to reduce the incidence of birth trauma in our *high-tech* society we must start taking responsibility for the outcome of birth—no matter what that is.

The families in this book will help you see that you, too, can reduce the risk of birth trauma if you begin to think of childbirth wholistically, even when entering a technocratic environment. You will learn that the power that created your baby will also help you deliver your baby, no matter where you are, if you can overcome your natural physiological response to fear and the unknown.

Here is the story of a mother who adopted the technocratic model during her first delivery. When the doctor broke her water (to speed up the final stage of labor) her baby became lodged within her pelvis; forceps and a vacuum extractor were then used to help dislodge her baby from her restricted position.

During the birth of her second child, the mother in this story was determined to achieve her goal of having a successful natural delivery. She may not have known the concept of the humanistic–assisted birth model, but that's exactly what she created for herself.

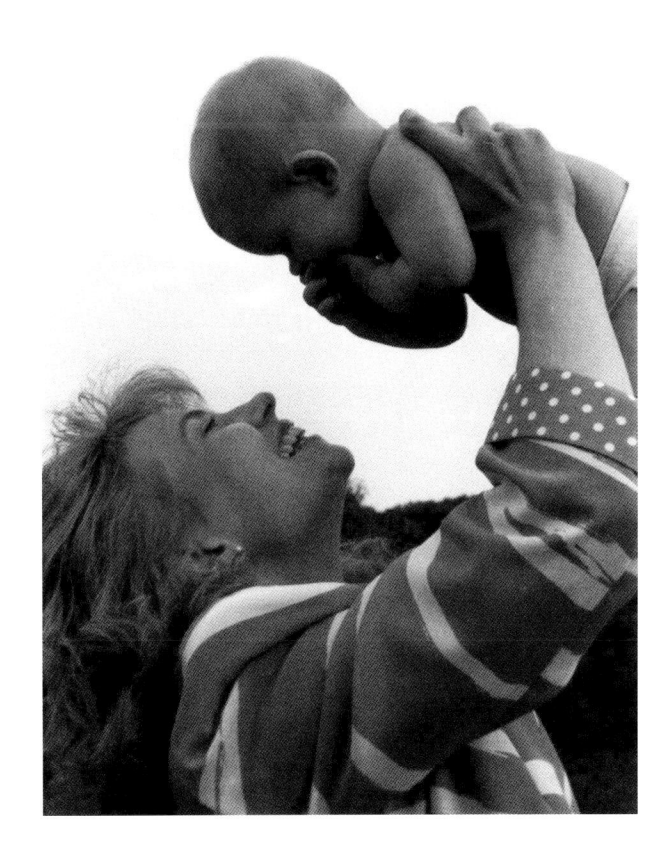

---

1 People who advocate a wholistic birth believe that the human body is a living organism with its own innate wisdom— an energy field constantly responding to all other energy fields. They believe that female physiological processes, including birth, are healthy and safe and rarely need medical intervention. Under this model, a mother's support system centers around her family rather than a medical staff. It is understood that her mental and emotional attitudes will affect her performance during birth, so every effort is made to surround her with love and security.

The Joy of Birth

Susan was at the end of her third trimester when I first met her. She wasn't aware of the benefits chiropractic care provided during pregnancy, but she had heard I provided doula support to laboring women. As much as Susan loved her husband, she had learned from her first birth, where medication, vacuum extraction, and forceps were used, that it was unrealistic to expect him to provide all of the emotional and physical support she felt she might need during the delivery.

Early one morning I received a call from Susan. She'd had three contractions, each 15 minutes apart and wondered if I would come and "check her out." I took my time getting ready and arrived 45 minutes later. Susan was in the bathroom and Jim was screaming into the phone for help. I was shocked to hear the unmistakable sounds of pushing. This was *not* what I expected.

Susan was not alone in the bathroom. Her mother, who had agreed to stay with her granddaughter while they were in the hospital, had come over as soon as Susan started having contractions. I helped Susan move into her bedroom while her mom tried to calm Jim down. Susan had progressed so rapidly that she was in no position to discuss anything. She refused to get into the car, adamantly demanded ice chips, wanted analgesic rubbed on her back, and insisted I check her cervix.

I tried to explain that I normally leave cervical checks to the birth attendant, but Susan wasn't listening. As she rocked on her hands and knees, overwhelmed by the intensity of the sensations sweeping through her body, Susan was transformed from a meek, timid woman into a fierce demanding mother taking full control of her body and her delivery. I timidly reached inside the birth canal (which was difficult to maneuver as she rocked on her hands and knees). I was shocked to feel the smooth surface of the amniotic sac just inside the opening. No wonder she was so intense and demanding. She was in the last stage of labor and the baby was coming!

I had no idea Susan would progress so rapidly and she was not prepared for a homebirth. If she had planned to have her baby at home, a midwife would have arrived with the equipment and the experience necessary to receive the baby. Now, I was left wondering if Susan would have the baby without the aide of an officially trained birth attendant. Before I could ponder any further, two emergency medical technicians came bursting into the room.

Jim had called 911 when he was unable to get Susan into the car. When the paramedics arrived they found a frightened father, a nervous grandmother trying to keep him calm, a mother unwilling to discuss the situation with them, and a doula not willing to take responsibility for the baby's delivery.[1]

Neither the older male paramedic nor the younger female paramedic had ever delivered a baby. They listened to Jim recall the terrifying circumstances he had witnessed during the first birth and decided that Susan needed to be transported to the hospital.

Susan was willing to go in the ambulance, but only under two conditions. One, she would not walk to the ambulance and two, she refused to go without me. The older male paramedic firmly explained the rules prohibiting anyone in the back of the ambulance except a patient and a paramedic. Although he was older, larger, and

---

1 The practice of obstetrics is illegal within the Chiropractic profession because we do not sever human tissue (the cord). While I would have loved to have caught the baby for her, I would have been jeopardizing my Chiropractic license if there was a complication in the delivery.

STEP 1: Decide on a Birth Model That Supports Your Belief System

spoke with authority, Susan won. She was about to deliver and she wasn't going in the ambulance without me right beside her.

The paramedic gave in, scooped Susan up in his arms, and carried her out of the bedroom. After she was strapped on the gurney and moved into the ambulance, I climbed in beside her. Jim drove separately and left ahead of us with tires screeching as he headed for the hospital.

As soon as the decision was made to go to the hospital, I helped Susan stop pushing by saying "P-A-A-A, P-A-A-A." I asked her to visualize a butterfly in front of her lips and to softly blow it away with the P-A-A-ing sound. Making this sound prevented her from bearing down. It also kept her from tightening the vaginal muscles around the baby's head.

I had to stay close to Susan's face and "P-A-A" with her to keep her focused and calm, We were heard "P-A-A-ing" all the way down the hospital corridor and into the maternity ward. We did not stop while the nursing staff explained there were no rooms available. We continued P-A-A-ing together so Susan could resist her urge to push as they transferred her from the gurney to a makeshift bed in a storeroom, while they transferred her bed out of the storeroom and into a freshly cleaned labor room, and as they transferred her onto a birthing bed.

An obstetrician, whom Susan had never met, finally entered the birthing room and sat down on the stool between her legs, which had been spread and placed into position for delivery. Susan could not see him from her position in the bed, but she sighed with relief when he finally arrived. Then we heard, "I'm going to break your water."

This nonchalant statement was interrupted when Susan immediately shouted, "Oh, no you won't! Don't you touch my water!"

The doctor shrugged his shoulders and put down the wand. He must have realized that Susan was obviously in no mood for a discussion.

Susan spent approximately two hours trying not to push her baby out and now she was finally given the go-ahead from the doctor. I looked for Jim and found him standing back in the corner of the dimly lit birthing room. Standing in the dark, he looked frightened and unsure of what to do so I asked him to come closer and rest his hand on Susan's knee. He walked right over and did as I asked.

Moments later, Susan pushed and the water sac burst, covering the doctor with the meconium-stained fluid that she had so diligently protected. The doctor said nothing. He gave me a look that seemed to say, "I'll be so glad when this day is over." One more push and the baby was out. Susan threw back her head and out of her mouth came the most beautiful laugh. Then she shouted to the world,

"I DID IT-T-T!!"

Two hours of holding back had caused the baby to have a bowel movement due to stress. He was quickly taken to the warmer and checked for swallowed meconium.[2] Luckily, his lungs were clear and he was given back to Susan within minutes. Susan was beside herself with happiness. She had succeeded in gathering the support she felt she needed. She maintained control in the midst of chaos and protected her baby from any unintentional harm. Most importantly, her baby entered the world just as she planned—through the birth canal.

---

[2] *Meconium is fecal material that looks and acts like tar. If it should get into the lungs, the baby may not be able to get enough oxygen.*

Hands Of Love

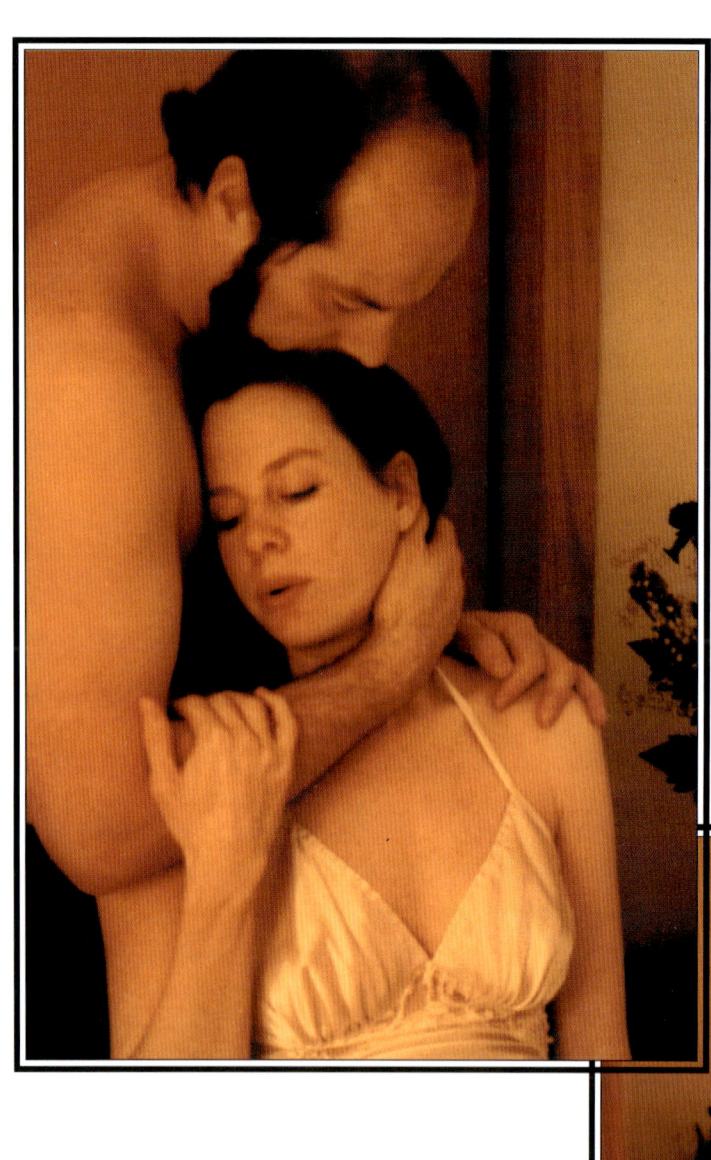

STEP 1: Decide on a Birth Model That Supports Your Belief System

The Circle of Light

The light of God surrounds them.
The love of God enfolds them.

The Power of God protects them.
And the presence of God is with them.

Wherever they are

He is.

Thank you, Father, that this is so.
(Author Unknown)

This affirmation, and the visual image of being surrounded by a white light of protection, are powerful tools for anyone who feels they are entering a situation where they need extra protection. I change the pronoun from *me* to *them* and say this in my mind as I get in my car and rush to a birth.

Hands Of Love

Here is the story of two parents, Deb and Paul, who thought they had done everything right by adopting the technocratic model for the birth of their first child. They had carefully chosen the *"perfect"* obstetrician and attended a hospital-sponsored birthing class. Then, just before the due date, they were shocked to find out their baby had moved into a breech position. Deb was immediately scheduled for a cesarean delivery. She knew nothing about chiropractic care or alternative techniques to help her baby move into a better position. Deb and Paul both felt they had no choice but to have a cesarean section. They dismissed all of their plans and turned the birth over to the medical team.

Paul will tell you briefly why that decision lead to an emotionally traumatic experience for both of them. Afterwards, both Deb and Paul will share the happy circumstances surrounding their second birth.

A Family Conquers Their Fear of Birth

PAUL: *I attended the hospital birthing classes with our first pregnancy. I went through the motions of learning how to give labor support, but I discarded everything I'd learned when the baby turned into a breech position. This was a mistake because labor started on its own the night before my daughter was scheduled for delivery. We rushed to the hospital fully expecting them to get her into surgery. But, they were busy and they couldn't fit her in for several hours.*

My wife, Deb, and I labored alone in the hospital room for many hours while we waited for the doctor to take Deb into surgery. We were so distraught. She wasn't supposed to be laboring! I didn't know what to do for her. I'd forgotten everything I'd learned at the birthing class. At one point, I went out into the hall looking for someone, anyone, to come and help us. There were so many babies being born at that time, no one was available to help.

As I stood in that hallway all I could think was, "I don't remember what to do. She's not supposed to be laboring! Someone has to come and take her into surgery. She needs help, but what can I do?" I felt totally helpless.

After the delivery, I wasn't allowed to hold my daughter, Karissa, for the first hour. Deb was so groggy from the medication that she didn't even want to see her. The trauma of that day stayed with us for years!

Several years after the birth of their daughter, Deb and Paul took steps to overcome their traumatic experience and considered having another baby. As part of their healing, they attended meetings at the local chapter of the International Cesarean Awareness Network of Minnesota. After listening to the positive VBAC (vaginal birth after cesarean) experiences of others, they slowly began to open their minds to the alternatives presented. They learned that they could and should make decisions about managing their own labor. Still, it took them three years before they were able to overcome the trauma of the first delivery and try for a second pregnancy.

During her first appointment with an obstetrician, Deb told the doctor she wanted to attempt a VBAC. She was told her attempt would be supported only under certain conditions. Deb was then informed of the many procedures that would be required as they monitored her progress and was told she would be prepped for a repeat cesarean, just in case. To Deb, all of the required precautionary procedures meant she would be allowed to try but they weren't confident she would succeed.

Deb feared that the required procedures would alter the natural flow of labor and reduce her chances for a successful vaginal birth. She knew she had to consider an alternate environment and a different birth attendant but she had no idea where to go to learn about birth options. Both she and Paul agreed that the hospital was not the right place for them to have their baby, yet they were not ready to view their home as a safe place either.

Deb and Paul needed more information about childbirth than was presented in their first hospital-sponsored birthing class, so this time, they received prenatal training in a Husband–Coached Bradley birth class. Both Deb and Paul felt the classes were extremely informative and gave them the confidence and encouragement they needed to start designing a birth support team.

STEP 1: Decide on a Birth Model That Supports Your Belief System

DEB: When I told my chiropractor that we were considering a homebirth, she referred me to her midwife, Jan Hofer. I interviewed Jan as soon as possible. After several hours of talking, I knew I wanted her to attend my birth. We were so similar in our personalities and philosophies about childbirth that I finally believed I would have the support I needed if I began my prenatal care with her. Later, I sought an obstetrician to provide back-up medical care just in case I changed my mind at the last minute. I found a doctor who agreed to provide that care, but she made one thing clear: she would help during the birth only if she were on-call that day. I hired her. What choice did I have? No other doctor would even talk to me about back-up support.

PAUL: Before we met Carol, Deb had mentioned the possibility of asking someone else to attend the birth with us. I felt very uncomfortable with that idea. I felt a doula might intimidate me and I might be pushed off into a corner, as the birth became a woman's thing. At the same time, I struggled with my concerns over what I would do in the event of an emergency or if the situation became too stressful at home. Other questions flooded my mind. Would the midwives know if she needed medical care? As the main labor support person, what would I do if I forgot everything I'd learned like I did the first time? How could I help Deb if I had to spread out my books and search for answers when a problem arose? What would I do if she didn't handle transition well? I could read and read, but would I recall everything in the heat of the moment? What if Jan was held up or had to leave quickly to get to another birth?

I wanted to help the midwife deliver the baby. How could I do that and help Deb focus and stay in control? I was still pondering over these concerns when Carol, a guest lecturer at our Bradley birth class, explained the role of a chiropractic-doula to us. I learned that a doula was a woman who helps other women in labor. As a chiropractor, Carol could also help Deb with any structural problems during labor. Suddenly, I developed a whole new level of confidence. I realized that if Carol came to the birth she would be there to support me, too. She would give me hints and refresh my memory when I went blank. She wouldn't take over my role in the birth, but would give me the freedom to tune in to Deb and the baby without fear of making a mistake.

DEB: After we heard Carol lecture, I knew she was an answer to my prayers. I was so happy when I saw Paul's excited expression and heard his insistence that we ask her to help at our birth. After Carol agreed to provide us with chiropractic-doula support, our birth team began to evolve. We hired Jan as our birth attendant and made arrangements for back-up medical support. Now we had to decide what to do with our four-year-old daughter, Karissa.

Earlier, during a prenatal visit, Jan asked what our plans were for Karissa during labor. I only knew we didn't plan to have her at the birth. Jan suggested that I not close that door just yet and gave me a book to read about the role of siblings in a homebirth. I took it home, but I didn't read it. Later, I took it back to Jan and said, "Thanks, but no thanks." To our surprise, Karissa made her own plans. We learned about them when she announced her intention to watch the delivery. We assured her that she would see the baby right after it was born. "No, I want to SEE the baby born!" Karissa made this bold statement several times before we realized that she meant it. We had to consider her feelings.

I went back to Jan and asked if we could borrow the book again. As we read about birth to Karissa, she accepted the whole process as something natural and common. She became so excited about the delivery of the baby that we slowly began to believe she could handle being there for the whole birth. We checked out several birth videos from our Bradley instructor and let her witness a birth firsthand. She was perfectly fine with all of the unusual sounds and positions. Still, there was no way we could prepare her for the intense *periods of discomfort I might go through, or an emergency situation. We finally decided we'd better include a support person just for her. My mother was the most logical person for that role on the birth team.*

My mother had four children of her own, yet she had no recall of three of those births and only slight recall of the fourth. She had her babies at a time when a mother was "put out" for the delivery. My father, of course, had no experience at all with birth. Both were skeptical about a homebirth and had no intention of being there. I asked Mom to come anyway. She loved Karissa so much that she eventually put her own fears aside and agreed. She couldn't understand why we were doing this, and felt strongly that we were taking unnecessary chances, but she loved us enough to be supportive. Dad said he absolutely would not come over. It wasn't long before Mom realized that for Karissa to watch the birth she too would have to watch. Now Mom decided she needed a support person.

Dad loves us very much, so he eventually broke down and agreed to join our birth team. Even though he stated adamantly that he would not come in the bedroom or watch the birth, we felt a need to prepare both of my parents for what they might witness. On one of their visits to town, we spent an evening watching birth videos. This was the first time either of them had seen a birth. Dad had very little to say about them. Mom began to cry. I think it was the first time she'd come to terms with the medically controlled birth of her own children. Suddenly, even Mom began to look forward to the homebirth of our second baby.

3:00 A.M.

Deb woke Paul to tell him that contractions had started. They spent the next few hours getting in touch with the rhythm of the labor, with each other, and with their baby. Deb showered and put on make-up as she prepared for this special day. The contractions were comfortable, close, and consistent. Before long, Paul began to feel somewhat anxious about being the only person on hand.

PAUL: *It was nice to have the first three to four hours alone. The initial contractions helped us to get prepared. I felt very confident. I had my stopwatch and recorded the time from the beginning of one contraction to the beginning of the next one. I felt comfortable for a couple of hours. Then, I began to get a little concerned. I didn't want to wake anyone up, but what if the support people didn't get to our home in time? I felt comfortable about my role, but I depended on all of them to do their part. Finally, at 6:00 A.M. I started calling everyone on the team. As they all started arriving, I felt my security blanket was in place and I could relax and focus on Deb and the baby.*

Deb had originally planned to walk around the house and deliver in the large comfortable bed in the guest bedroom—instead of the waterbed in their room. When we arrived, Deb surprised us by refusing to leave her bedroom and go down to the guestroom. She had chosen a spot on the floor that was about four feet wide and five feet long. With a wall on one side and her large waterbed on the other, this seemed at first to be an awkward place to have a baby. But, who were we to argue? We threw a few pillows and blankets on the floor and watched her curl up and get comfortable. Paul and I stretched out beside Deb so we could help her remain calm and focused.

DEB: *I was so happy knowing that my parents were there with Karissa and that Carol had arrived. Everyone assembled early that morning and I relaxed into my O-O-O-ing. In class, I had felt uncomfortable practicing the technique Carol taught, which would vibrate my uterus and vaginal muscles, but now I really liked it. I felt a real focus on the baby and I could actually feel my body opening up. It gave me a sense of unity with Paul and the others as they all joined me in vocalizing the O-O-tone. I felt a strong bond to everyone as they welcomed the contraction each time I said "Here we go."*

STEP 1: Decide on a Birth Model That Supports Your Belief System

I was so glad that everyone had been told what to do and that no one felt embarrassed to join in and help me stay centered. Paul surrounded me with pillows and I felt secure in my tight little space with the beautiful sound of soft music in the background.

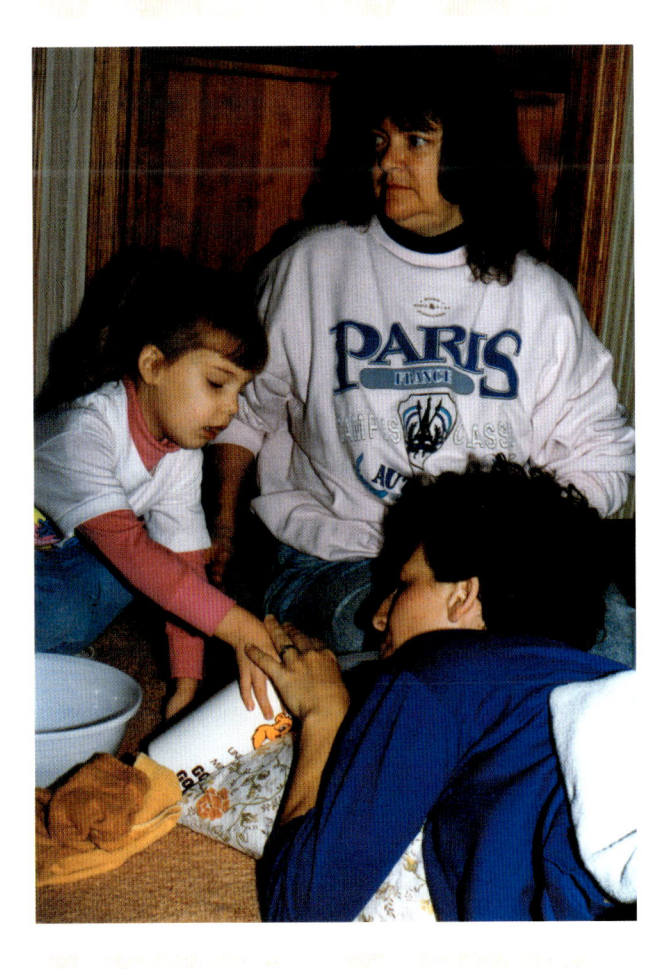

Karissa would slip quietly into the room to give me a drink, hold my hand, or just say, "O-O-O," with me. After a few minutes, she would slip off with her Grandma to make pictures for the new baby. At one point, I looked up and saw my dad standing in the door watching and my heart felt intense love for him. I don't think you could have kept him out of the room even though he had initially been so resistant. I think the strong bond he has developed with Kyla began to form as he stood in the doorway that morning.

I felt like a little mouse in the corner as I watched this family work together with love and respect. There were times when Deb doubted herself and her ability to deliver the baby vaginally. As the memories of Karissa's birth filled her mind, she would become distraught and emphatically state, " I can't. I can't." Paul would lie beside her, wrap his arms around her, and pray out loud. This calmed Deb and helped her pass through those periods of doubt and fear. I would continue laying my hands over her abdomen while I assured Deb that she was doing a great job. For some reason, the calm, gentle touch of hands over the baby helped Deb stay focused and relaxed. I hoped my actions were comforting to the baby as well, as she continued on her journey through the birth canal.

DEB: *One of my biggest struggles was with my bladder. I simply couldn't empty it because of the baby's position. The discomfort made it difficult to relax and concentrate. My midwife eventually had to use a catheter to relieve the pressure. Once that was over, I could really start concentrating on the intense contractions. They seemed so strong that I was glad my water bag was still intact. If I had been in the hospital, they probably would have broken it as it came down into the birth canal. It was comforting to know it was intact and providing a big pillow for Kyla to rest her head on while she maneuvered herself down and out. I was also glad not to be in the hospital; it would have been easy to ask for drugs when I became frightened. A C-section would have seemed like a welcome crutch when I doubted myself.*

10:30 A.M.

This had to be one of the most serene births I had ever attended. Deb's team of midwives worked so quietly they seemed invisible. Periodically, Deb's mom would slip into the room with Karissa and sit on the floor just a few feet from Deb. Karissa would wiggle herself into her Grandma's lap and together they giggled with anticipation as Deb went through the two hours of quiet pushing.

Despite his initial resistance, Deb's father maintained his position in the doorway with his arms crossed over his chest. As he witnessed the constant love, encouragement, and praise that Paul expressed to Deb, a look of absolute love and respect washed

27

over his face. During all of this, Deb appeared so serene and focused that I would never have guessed the thoughts that were going through her mind.

DEB: *The two hours of pushing were difficult. I just kept thinking, "I can't, I can't do it." I didn't believe Jan when she kept saying, "You are doing it." I thought she was just saying that so I wouldn't give up. I must admit... it did help to hear her say, "You are making progress—the baby is moving at her own pace—it is working." I went through a period of doubt. I didn't know what I was experiencing and felt I wasn't working with my body... I just didn't get it. Then all of a sudden it was okay.*

After Paul prayed with me, I realized this was not like the last birth. I could let go and stop holding the baby in. I remember realizing that I couldn't bring her back up inside of me, so I had to let her go. I also realized that no one could help me now. Only I could do this part. Then everything seemed to work efficiently.

It helped so much to have Carol's hands over the baby; her hand contact helped me know where to direct the baby and where to send my energy. When I tensed up, she would remind me to relax my face. When I did, my whole body relaxed. Suddenly everything came together and I finally felt I was doing it right. When things finally felt synchronized, Paul suggested I change to a seated position. That really kicked things into gear.

When Deb agreed to change positions I put several big pillows up against the nightstand and had Paul lean back against them as he sat on the floor behind Deb. I then put a pillow up against his chest and asked Deb to lean back against Paul. Both of them now placed their hands over Deb's pregnant belly. Deb's mom slipped in and gently supported her legs so she could relax into this new seated position. Suddenly, the water sac slipped slowly out of the birth canal. It looked like a big teardrop with crystalline fluid swooshing around inside of it. Jan placed a folded diaper under the sac to absorb the amniotic fluid when it eventually broke on its own. As the baby's head crowned, we held a mirror in position for Deb and Paul to see.

12:00 P.M.

DEB: *I felt such a sense of elation when I saw Kyla's head crown through the birth canal. It was incredible! I was doing it! Jan wasn't lying... I was making progress! Jan gave me a spoonful of honey and I suddenly felt a burst of energy and was ready to deliver the baby.*

PAUL: *I was slightly disappointed that I couldn't help with the delivery, but I was extremely happy where I was. I cradled Deb in my arms and whispered in her ear. I felt so connected and united with her as we worked together. I tried to send all of my energy and security to her. I regretted not having eye contact with her, but it still felt very good. I felt we had the emotional, physical, and spiritual connection we needed for our baby's safe delivery. I suddenly realized it might be easier if Deb squatted, so I suggested that I sit up on a chair and support Deb from behind as she rose into a squatting position. That did the trick! The squat position really opened her up. I had to strain to see Kyla delivered, but I wasn't disappointed. I knew I was right where I was supposed to be.*

Jan's hands were there to support Kyla's body as she slowly slipped out of Deb and down toward the cushioned mat. Jan then lifted the newborn up to Deb and Paul. Hands outstretched—they encircled her body and brought her up onto Deb's chest. I stood up on the bed and balanced myself as I quickly removed the chair from behind Paul so they could sit down on the floor together. I then tossed my 35mm camera to Deb's father and grabbed the video camera.

As Paul and Deb cradled their baby, Deb's mom hugged Karissa and they laughed with excitement. After absorbing all that had just happened, Karissa climbed out of her Grandmother's arms and onto the bed to get a better look. Before long, she climbed down into the tiny space beside her parents.

As they recovered from the explosion of emotions associated with the delivery, Deb and Paul turned their attention to Karissa. Paul held his newborn's head in one hand while he stroked and patted Karissa with the other. He was quick to tell her

STEP 1: Decide on a Birth Model That Supports Your Belief System

how special she was and how helpful she'd been. Karissa responded by hugging and kissing Paul before moving closer to Kyla. We all watched silently as Karissa gingerly reached out to touch her little sister.

As I continued to record this event on video, I was so thankful for another opportunity to see a baby born in a peaceful and serene atmosphere—to parents who displayed the compassion and grace she deserved. Sometimes I must watch and cringe as a birth attendant uses incredible force to pull or push on a baby's head during delivery. I often turn away when I see an attendant's wrist shake as they press down on the head to release a shoulder. As a chiropractor and craniosacral therapist, I know too well the internal trauma the baby may be experiencing. Thankfully, this little girl, Kyla, was handled with sensitivity and reverence.

Labor is not over with the birth of the baby. The third stage of labor includes the delivery of the placenta. This usually takes place within 5 – 10 minutes after the birth. Deb was an exception. The placenta failed to disengage and the midwives wouldn't pull on it for fear it would tear from the wall of the uterus.

We tried to stimulate the delivery of the placenta by having the baby nurse. Nursing triggers a release of the hormone oxytocin. This hormone will contract the uterus and expel the placenta. Deb let Kyla nurse for quite awhile. It didn't work. I've sometimes disengaged a stubborn placenta by rocking the mother's pelvis forward. Unfortunately, adjusting Deb's pelvis didn't work, either. Finally, Jan suggested that Deb curl-up with her baby and nap for awhile. Deb was too exhausted to push anymore and Jan was still not willing to pull on the cord.

For the next two hours, Jan continued to monitor vital signs as she watched Deb sleep with her newborn cradled against her chest. She finally woke Deb up and asked her to try and push the placenta out. Deb's mom held Kyla as Deb gently pushed downward. The placenta slid out easily and the birth was complete.

After examining the placenta, Jan performed a newborn exam on Kyla and helped the family get settled in. By 7:00 P.M. Jan was able to go home to her family and get some rest.

DEB: *I can't begin to tell you how nice my whole experience was with this pregnancy and delivery. Each of my many prenatal visits lasted for several hours as Jan and I sat and talked about the birth and how we wanted it to go. As the mother of twelve, she was so helpful and calm about the whole process. She and her assistant were with me from 7:00 A.M. to 7:00 P.M. on the day of the delivery and she came back many times over the next few weeks to provide postnatal care. I can't begin to count the number of hours of service she provided for her fee of $900. That is in comparison to the $5,000 that was charged for Karissa's birth. She also gave me all the love and support I felt was lacking in my first birth. And for those people who wonder—I would do another homebirth again in a minute!*

The medical model of childbirth that Deb and Paul turned away from, and the woman-centered model they turned to, had one thing in common—compassion. The difference between the hospital and the home is the degree to which that emotion can realistically be expressed.

Compassion is defined as "the deep feeling of sharing the suffering of another and the inclination to give aid or support, or to show mercy." This is an attribute that is common among all of the people who choose to work in the birthing field whether in the technocratic model or the humanistic model. The problem in the technocractic model is that we're asking people to over-stretch their ability to show compassion. If the maternity ward happens to be full at the time you arrive, you're on your own until you absolutely need their assistance. That's what happened to Deb and Paul. They relied on the hospital staff to help them cope with labor even though they were told the baby was not to be born vaginally. They felt helpless and abandoned. In the woman-centered model, there are people available who are focusing all of their attention on the birthing family.

It is difficult to share in the suffering of another without getting emotionally and physically drained. It is almost impossible to ask someone to demonstrate compassion, and share in the suffering of another, on a daily basis, and with a large number of people, without expecting those people to lose some sensitivity. This is what we expect of medical personnel. That's why I feel it is so important for us to reevaluate the adoption of the technocratic–controlled model of birth.

The natural process of birth doesn't necessarily require suffering, but it usually requires a depth of emotion and a sensation of pain that can be described by most as a form of suffering. Is the birthing mother alone in her suffering? No. We must also consider the baby and the mother's partner.

A baby feels whatever a mother feels, because the chemical reaction in a mother's body to anxiety, fear, joy, excitement, pain, etc., causes the same reaction in her baby. This is due to their shared vascular system. Whatever chemicals enter the mother's blood stream, natural or artificial, are immediately carried into the baby's blood stream in a similar concentration. If she becomes stressed, so will the baby. If she takes a drug, so does the baby. If she enjoys the experience and the exhilaration of delivery, so will the baby.

It is important that we keep the feelings of the partner in mind when we talk about demonstrating compassion. Many mothers mistakenly think the birth is going to be a romantically intimate experience for the parents and that they should be alone for the birth. This can be a big mistake for both of them. After attending a birthing class a pregnant woman may feel that her partner should be perfectly prepared to provide her with all the support she needs—physically and emotionally. Sounds good, but unless a baby makes a rapid entrance into the world (rare and not necessarily good for either of you) it's not realistic.

During active labor, a partner may suddenly feel out of control and at the mercy of nature. It's a mistake to think that anyone can suddenly become an expert in birthing, remembering everything that was said in those brief, late-night birthing classes. When the real thing happens, emotions take over and the brain may fly right out the window (I'm afraid the same thing will happen to me when it's one of my daughters giving birth).

When a woman goes into labor, her partner's hormone levels will suddenly rise, and he will instinctually feel a need to "grab the spear and protect his mate." Of course, in today's world he doesn't need to do this.

We are now asking men to ignore their hormonal instincts—to be gentle, kind, quiet, and patient, even though they are hormonally driven to endure pain and to fix any problem. During birth, a partner must sit quietly and watch the woman he loves radiate a physical strength he may never have imagined possible. This can be very difficult for some.

Men react differently during the birth of a child. Some men struggle to protect their partners from the trauma of medical interventions, while others buckle and relinquish all control to the people in charge. Some want to catch their babies, and others suffer the anguish of not wanting to witness the actual delivery. Some women are surprised to find themselves instinctively and hormonally drawn to other women when they are in labor. Their presence may make a big difference in the outcome of labor and delivery but someone needs to help a man understand this.

There will be times when a partner needs to eat, to sleep, or to go to the bathroom! He won't leave you if you're in distress, no matter how uncomfortable he becomes. He needs to know that someone will stay with you while he's gone. A compassionate doula can do this.

During a surgical delivery, men are torn between not wanting to leave their partners alone in the operating room, and wanting to be at their child's side in the nursery. Again, it helps if he knows there is someone with you who's totally devoted to you and your emotional well-being.

A lack of compassion drove Deb and Paul away from the hospital. They achieved their goal of having a spiritual and compassionate vaginal birth at home by developing explicit expectations and making decisions that reinforced their goals. They could not have made those decisions with confidence if they had not dedicated so much time and effort into the investigation of their options.

As I watched Deb and Paul cradle their newborn, I knew this family had made the right choice when they chose to have a homebirth delivery—utilizing the humanistic–assisted birth model.

In this book, I will be stressing that every parent must try to avoid making the naive mistake of putting the fate of childbirth solely in the hands of others. Learn all you can about your pregnant body. Investigate all of your options and become an educated co-decision maker.

Call the International Childbirth Education Association (ICEA) at (800) 624-4934. Their catalog will provide you with a wide variety of books, tapes, and videos that address the subject of pregnancy, birth, and parenting.

Consider attending both a hospital-sponsored birthing class and a community-based, private, birthing class. The hospital class will prepare you for the technocratic approach, and the community class (Bradley, BirthWorks, ICEA, Birth Within etc.,) will focus on the humanistic–assisted approach.

STEP 1: Decide on a Birth Model That Supports Your Belief System

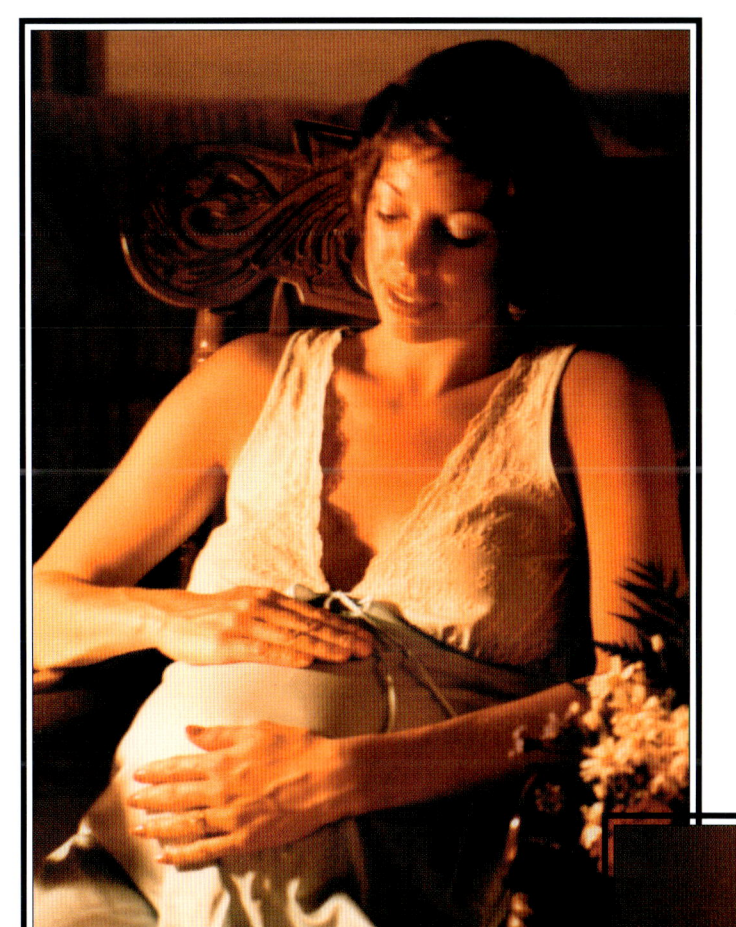

By honoring and respecting a woman's mind, body, and spirit, we will help her cultivate and nurture the potential of her unborn child.

Every pregnant woman has been entrusted with the guardianship of the next generation, and every child conceived reflects eternal hope for the future.

31

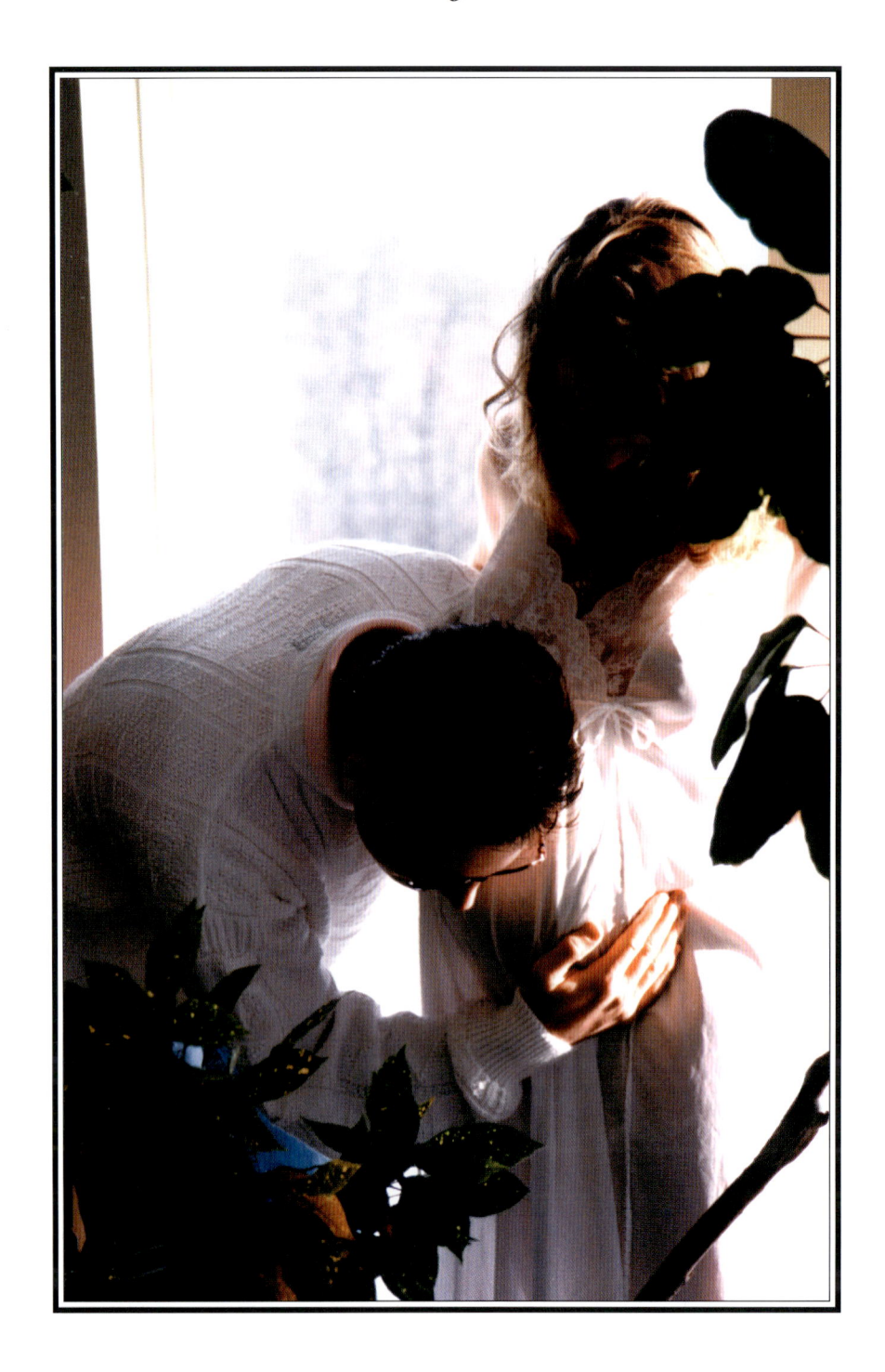

$\mathcal{T}$ake a few moments every week to go within and visualize a birth attendant who will honor creation, you and your baby—a person who will receive your newborn with the reverence he or she deserves. Choose your birth attendants wisely and trust that the person who ultimately assists with the delivery will be the one you created in your mind.

STEP 2
Choose a Birth Attendant

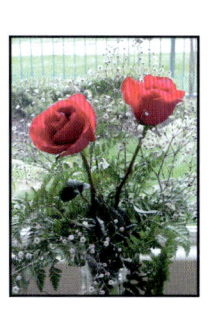

Diversity

Just as every birth is unique, so is every birth attendant. Are you aware of the many options you have in choosing a birth attendant? The person you hire may be an obstetrician (OB), a family practice physician (FP), a certified nurse-midwife (CNM), a certified professional midwife (CPM), or a direct-entry midwife. Their particular techniques for assisting in the delivery are quite different, due to each attendant's training, experiences, philosophy about birth, and the institutional policies directing their protocols.

Before choosing a birth attendant, you must decide which birth model is compatible with your personal values. If you accept the technocratic paradigm, you must choose a birth attendant who will make all of the decisions for you. If you adopt the humanistic model, you must educate yourself and hire a birth attendant who honors your knowledge and is willing to comply with your decisions. In this case, be prepared to demonstrate that you have put a great deal of thought and energy into those decisions and will accept responsibility for the outcome.

No matter which model you choose, it is wise to honor and respect your birth attendant's experience and knowledge, so you can use that to your advantage. Be willing to discuss openly any areas of conflict, but resist all forms of intimidation.

While some of you will be able to hire an attendant of your choice, most mothers are restricted by their insurance plan into utilizing an approved group practice. When using a group practice, a mother has no control over who assists in her delivery; she must trust that her wishes will be relayed to the attending physician; and she has no idea if those wishes will be honored and respected.

The uncertainty of a group practice may be distressing to some women, but there are advantages. For instance, an attendant working in a group practice can maintain a regular working schedule. As a result, the person attending the delivery should be fairly well-rested. That alone makes a big difference in how decisions are made during labor. If labor fails to progress at the expected rate, it's hard for attendants to be patient if they are exhausted, have family commitments, or just want to go home. Turning the case over to someone who has just come on duty can be a godsend to everyone involved.

Distinctions

The two most important distinctions to be aware of between various birth attendants are the amount of time they are able to spend with the mother and their ability to handle certain emergency situations.

Obstetricians (OB) attend most births in America. Therefore, their time with the patient is usually limited to the period from the time the baby's head crowns to the completion of any necessary repairs to the mother's vaginal area.

Due to their training and experience with high-risk situations, an OB will be called in to handle all emergencies, no matter who is ultimately chosen as the birth attendant. Consequently, their experience in the hospital results in a fear-based approach to childbirth. In other words, many procedures are done, *just-in-case* because complications are often common for an obstetrician.

Certified nurse-midwives and family practice physicians attend fewer births than an obstetrician and both will usually spend more time with you. However, they must also assist other women in labor, which makes it difficult for them to be with you constantly.

Direct-entry midwives, midwives who attend homebirths, are rarely under the guidance and control of a medical doctor and attend the fewest number of births. They can help you only if you deliver in your home or in an alternative birthing center. They generally work in pairs or network with other midwives so they can cover each other in case they are already attending someone else's birth when you need them. They will stay with your family from the time active labor begins until well after the delivery. Midwives are trained to judge when a woman needs emergency care and will immediately call for assistance or refer you to an obstetrician if the need arises. Luckily, this need is rare.

The legal situation with direct-entry midwives is in a constant state of flux from one state to another. Some states are passing bills to help midwives receive a license to practice and others are making it illegal. Most midwives are aware of the legal risk they take every time they attend a homebirth, but their desire to help birthing women is so great they are willing to take that risk. Finding those women will generally require diligence on your part.

As you begin your search for a birth attendant, avoid judging the skill of birth attendants by the number of babies born under their care. It is wiser to evaluate their actual hands-on experience. For instance, the average OB does not remain in the room with a patient until the baby has crowned and birth is imminent. Therefore, he or she spends approximately one hour in the labor room before the delivery. A doctor who has assisted at 1,000 births may have a wealth of knowledge concerning complications associated with childbirth, but he or she may have acquired only 1,000 hours of hands-on experience actually observing women in labor.

A certified nurse midwife who has attended the same number of births will have probably spent approximately 3,000 hours providing physical and emotional support to laboring women since they average about three hours with the patient (that average is just an observation of mine, not a fact).

Doctors and CNM's can reduce the time needed to be in attendance with a mother and her newborn because they have the assistance of nurses and pediatricians. A direct-entry midwife (or certified professional midwife) performs every task herself and averages twelve hours (generally much longer) per birth. Therefore, if she attends 1,000 homebirths, she will have spent approximately 12,000 hours observing, assisting, monitoring, and examining mothers and their newborns. Keep this in mind as you go on a search for an experienced birth attendant.

A birth attendant, chosen on the basis of their ability to support your level of knowledge and confidence, can bring you peace of mind as you successfully complete Step 2 of this pregnancy plan.

As you go through your interview process, make sure you feel comfortable discussing any issues of concern to you or your partner. If you are leery of bringing up questions about your care during prenatal visits, how will you address crucial issues that come up during labor and delivery?

Interview as many birth attendants as necessary until you find the one that gives you the confidence you need. Follow your heart and your intuition as you make your decision about a particular group or individual. Ask what protocols they are forced to follow due to hospital or licensing regulations. How flexible are their rules? Remember that there are boundaries within each profession. For example, direct-entry midwives can not accept high-risk women for a homebirth; certified-nurse midwives must follow the protocols set down for them by the obstetricians they work under; and obstetricians must follow hospital regulations, which often restrict them from assisting at homebirths.

Many of us have learned the hard way that failing to ask the right questions can result in an unsatisfactory outcome. Don't take choosing a birth attendant lightly—it may be the most important decision you make.

Twelve months and four days after Angel's birth, I delivered my second baby in the same hospital. I still had no option when it came to the choice of a birth attendant, but this time I did gain some control over my delivery. I bargained—I negotiated—I surrendered. I was allowed to labor without drugs, but the doctor insisted on rupturing my water to induce active labor; I was still forced to have my wrists and ankles strapped to the operating table, but I knew it was going to happen and didn't freak out like before. I avoided another spinal block by agreeing to a pudendal block that numbed only the vaginal area.

While I was still unable to feel the birth of my baby, I was able to help deliver her and I didn't have to be on my back in recovery for eight hours. I was so proud of myself. I believed I had achieved a natural birth and felt I had been a strong advocate for my baby and myself. I later vowed that I would someday help other women gain control over their birth experience as well.

My pride in achieving a natural birth was slightly squelched many years later when I learned that the five months of bimonthly estrogen injections I had received during my pregnancy with Wendy (I had premature contractions) may have been a contributing factor for my hysterectomy six years later, and for the removal of a large ovarian tumor fifteen years later. I learned that the amniotomy, which caused my rapid delivery (three contractions to go from 3 cm. to 10 cm.), may have contributed to her being "sunnyside up." Her birth position (occiput posterior) caused extreme swelling of her nose and face and may have contributed to her chronic rhinitis, allergy problems, and poor eyesight. I also eventually realized that being numb to the sensation of a baby sliding out of my body negated a *natural* delivery.

Despite these misconceptions, I was so pleased with the outcome of Wendy's birth, compared to my first birth experience with Angel, that I often asked God to give me the opportunity to help other women in labor. Little did I know that it would be fourteen years before I would be given the chance to help, or that in my effort to help others, I would learn much more than I would teach.

The Power of Visualization

Dr. Dick-Read wrote in *Childbirth Without Fear* that pain is whatever you perceive it to be. If you think that the sensation of a contraction building up and winding down is painful—then it is. I turned to his teachings rather than drugs during my labor with Wendy, and I decided to change my perception of labor by envisioning a similar sensation that I found pleasurable. I was living in Alaska at the time, and had the perfect visualization to use.

My husband, Bob, was allowed to be in the labor room with me, so I taught him in advance what to say. As soon as a contraction started, I would relax my hands and face, close my eyes, and listen to his voice. As he described the scene before me, I let the sensation of the contraction match his words. In my mind, I was being pulled up a rope tow on a ski slope in Alaska. At the peak of the contraction my abdomen would begin to soften and Bob would tell me to get off and ski down the mountain.

To this day, I can still remember how I imagined cold wind against my face, warm sun glistening off the snow, and tall, green, pine trees forming a path for my journey down the mountain. I was graceful and fast. It was exhilarating, and thanks to five months of premature contractions, I opened right up for Wendy.

It was too bad that my rapid dilation resulted in panic within the staff. My transition to the operating room was almost comical; couldn't have that baby coming out before everything, and everyone, was in place!

Hands Of Love

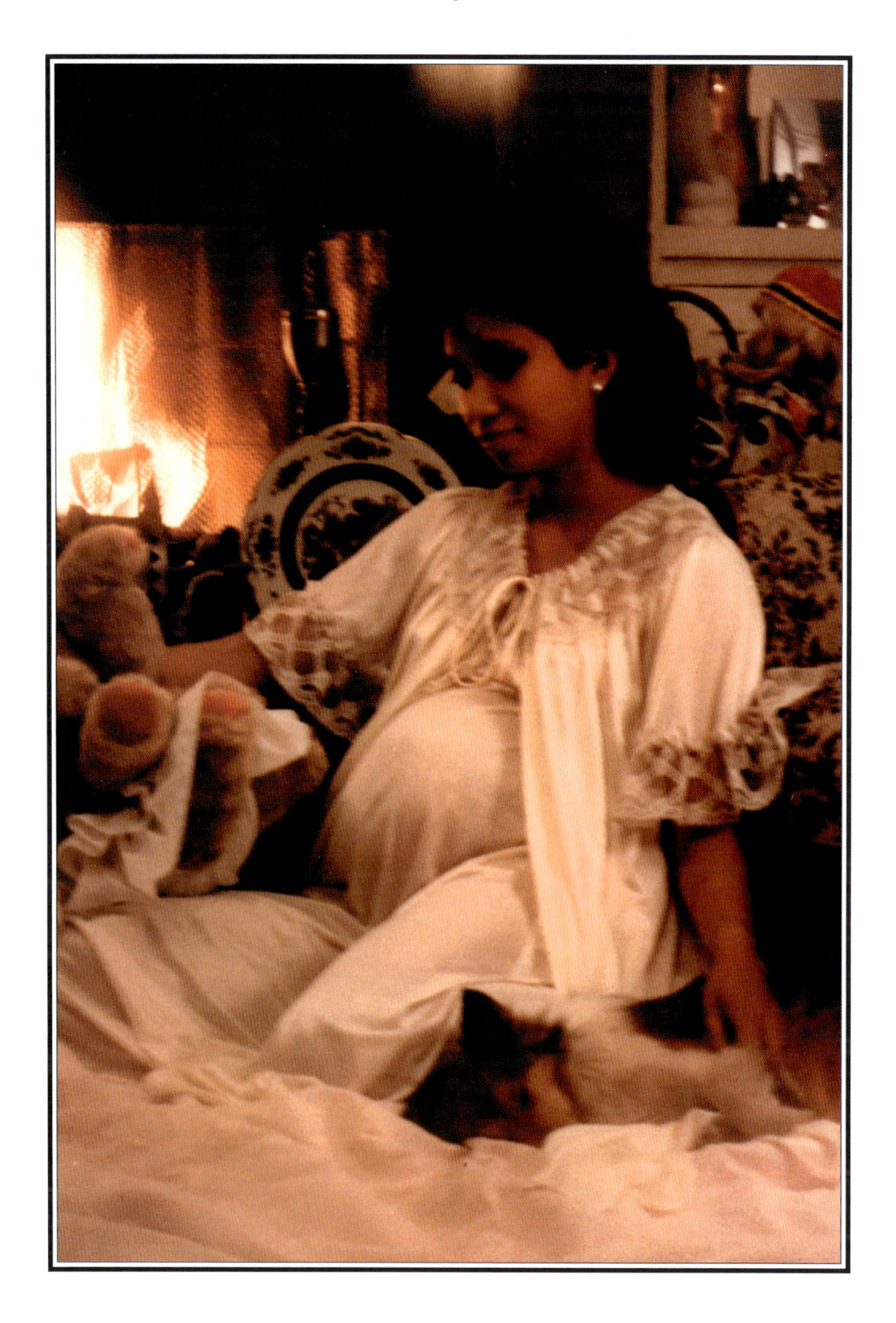

It was 1985 when, Frankie, a close friend and classmate, asked me to photograph her first delivery. Frankie didn't go into parenting as blindly as I had. She investigated her options and made decisions about prenatal care based on careful deliberation. She read many books on pregnancy and childbirth while she interviewed birth attendants. Eventually, Frankie decided it was in her best interest to adopt a humanistic birth model and deliver her baby at home, so she chose a direct-entry midwife as her birth attendant.

STEP 2: Choose a Birth Attendant

My First Birth Educator

Early one morning, Frankie woke up with a start. Without warning, her water sac had broken—soaking her bed with amniotic fluid. The baby was coming! Frankie called me right away. I grabbed my camera and left a note for my girls. My heart raced with excitement as I drove to Frankie's house. Would the baby come quickly? Would I get there in time? A baby! I was finally going to photograph a baby coming into the world!

Frankie was alarmed when her water sac broke prematurely. She had read about the risk of infection and knew that her midwife, Faith Gibson, would encourage her to go to the hospital if contractions did not start within twelve hours. Despite the fact that she now had to worry about an infection, Frankie did her best to stay relaxed while she waited for active labor to kick in.

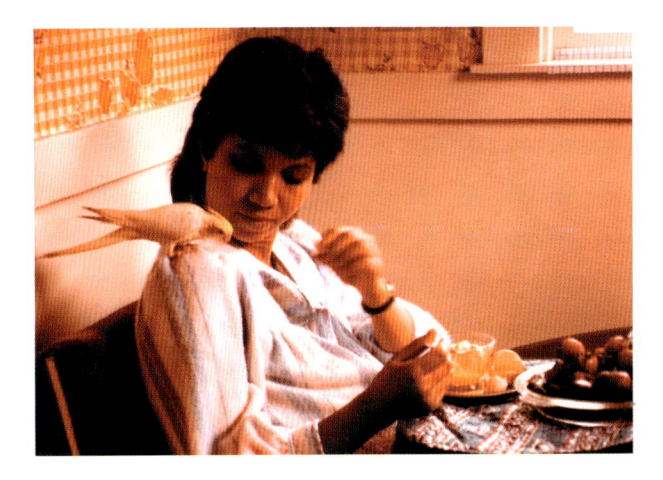

Frankie needed to provide her body with the necessary fuel to support the physical exertion of labor, so she ate a hearty breakfast of poached eggs, toast, and fruit. Naturally, we waited anxiously for the contractions to begin.

In contrast, had we gone straight to the hospital, Frankie would have been eating ice chips. If she were lucky, a lunch would have been ordered from the hospital menu. Her husband, Rafael, and I would have done without breakfast unless we left Frankie alone and went to the hospital cafeteria.

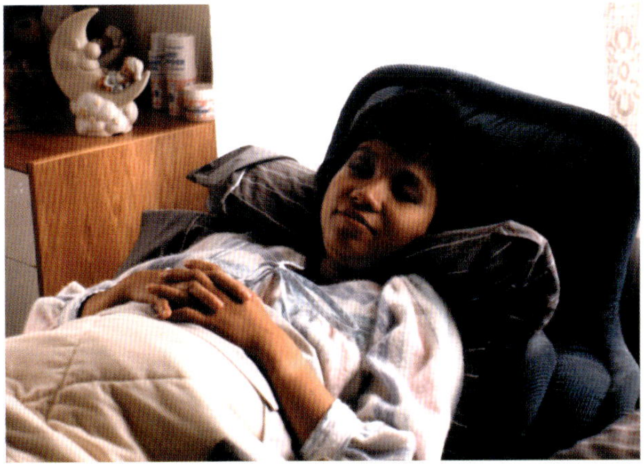

Rest is important before tackling the physical work of labor, so Frankie laid down for a nap while I prepared the living room. Rafael had already moved the couch and placed a mattress on the floor in front of the fireplace. We placed old sheets and blankets on top of plastic sheeting, and moved a large mirror into the room. Frankie wanted to watch her baby enter the world, as she planned to deliver standing. We were naive enough to believe she would be able to concentrate on watching her baby's birth.

A premature rupture of the amniotic sac may in-fact increase your risk of infection. You can reduce that risk by avoiding cervical evaluations and by remaining at home as long as possible. If you plan a hospital delivery you will need to go in for regular monitoring, whereas, a trained direct-entry midwife is fully capable of monitoring vital signs and recognizing the onset of an infection while you are at home.

The hospital environment is full of bacteria and viruses that are foreign to your normal flora. No amount of sterilization can protect you fully from the risk of infection. Therefore, if you are in the hospital you will be strongly advised to begin IV injections of an antibiotic. This often results in a "domino-effect" leading to a multitude of unexpected interventions.

And one last comment about premature ruptures. If a mother avoids cervical evaluations, remains at home, and is receiving careful monitoring of her vital signs, it may be safe for her to allow the baby five to seven days to activate labor on his own.

Hands Of Love

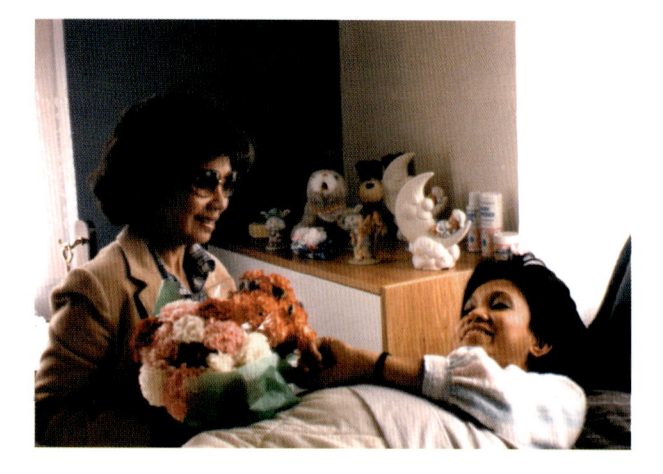

Frankie couldn't sleep. It felt like the night before Christmas and she couldn't wait to see her long awaited present! She gave up on the sleeping idea, and we decided we'd pass the time by studying. We were both preparing for finals at our chiropractic college, so we gathered our notes and started quizzing each other. While we studied, Rafael and his mother, Lordes, took advantage of this early labor period and went shopping. They bought Frankie flowers and a bottle of nonalcoholic champagne to celebrate the birth of the family's first baby. It was a touching gesture from both her husband and her mother-in-law.

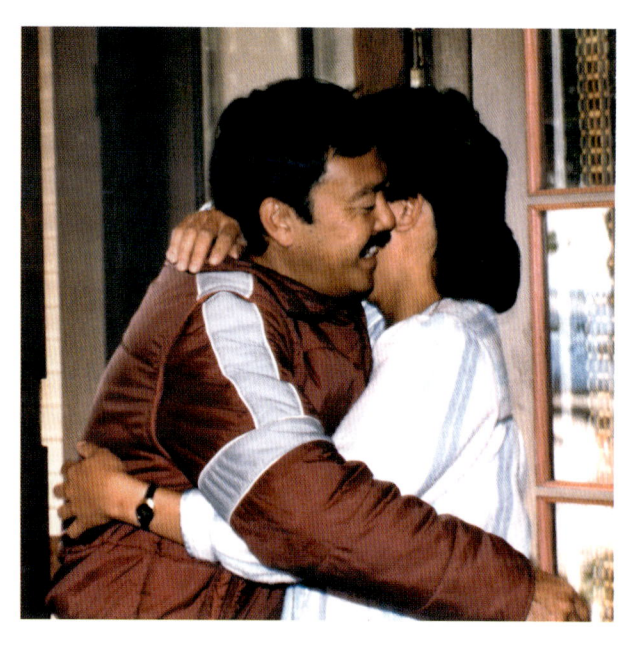

Gary, another close friend and study partner, stopped by the house to see how things were progressing. Frankie had asked Gary to help Rafael during the labor by providing additional physical support. Gary stayed long enough to see that the contractions were sporadic and weak. He decided it was safe to go on to class. He promised to check in regularly and to come back as soon as Frankie went into active labor.

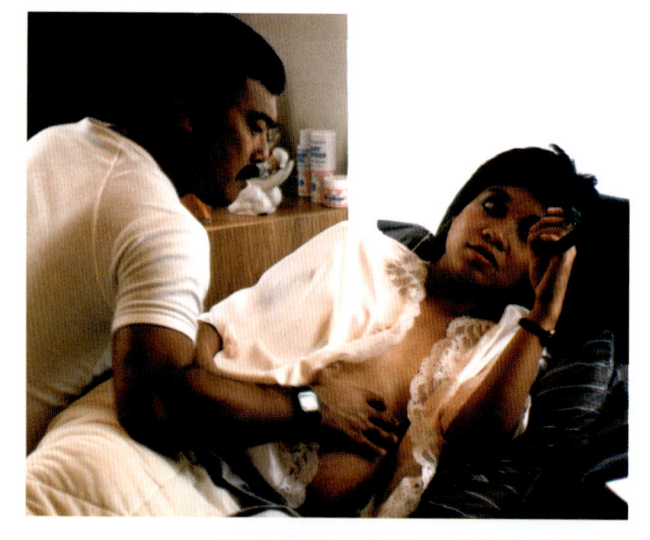

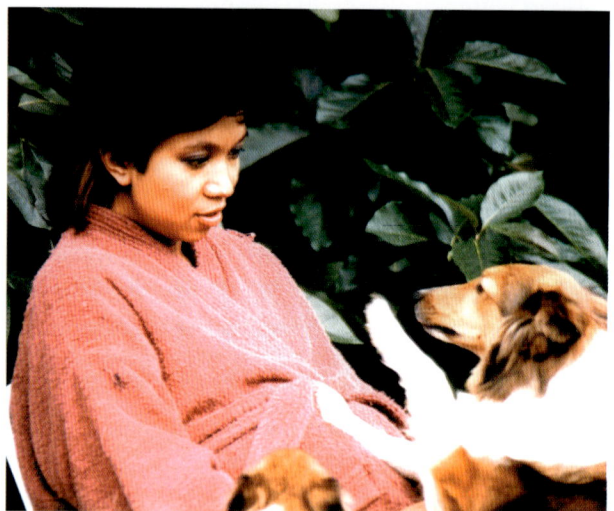

Four or five hours had passed and the contractions were still light and widely spaced. While Frankie and Rafael waited, they spent time out in the back yard with their pet Shelties. The family dogs seemed to sense something important was happening and wanted to stay close to Frankie.

Frankie decided walking might help get things going, so I grabbed my camera and we went for a walk around the block. That did it. Little baby contractions finally kicked in and we knew it wouldn't be long. How wrong we were!

Had Frankie gone to the hospital she would have exchanged her Mickey Mouse T-shirt for a hospital gown and robe. She would have been bathed in florescent lights instead of natural sunlight. We would have been limited to the corridors of the maternity ward instead of the beautiful green landscape of the neighborhood.

STEP 2: Choose a Birth Attendant

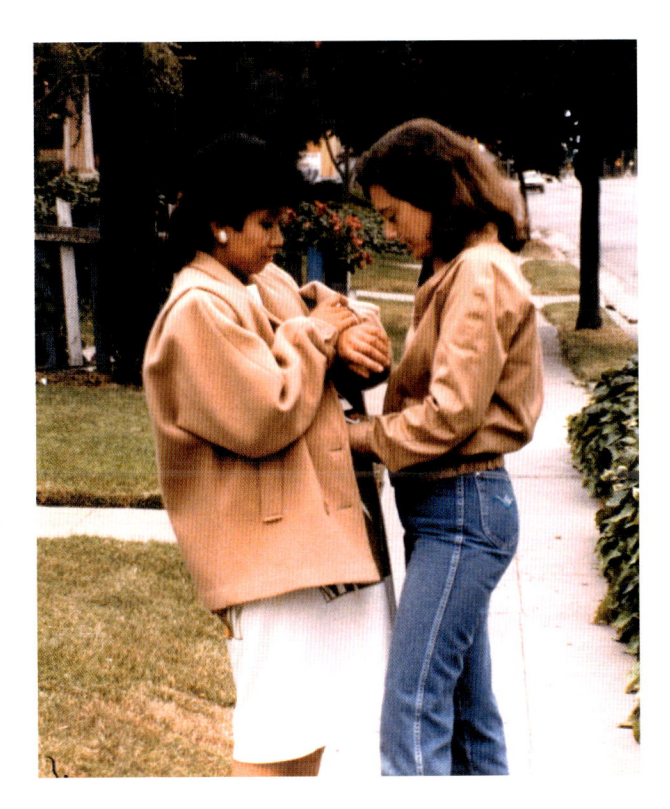

After a walk around the block, Frankie called her midwife, Faith, to let her know that labor had finally begun. She wanted to know how long the contractions were lasting; she asked us to time them from the beginning of one to the beginning of the next. Faith explained to me that Frankie was probably not able to tell exactly when the contraction started or completely ended. She told me to place my hands over the baby so I could record when the tightening sensation of a contraction would begin. Faith asked me to continue timing the contraction until I felt Frankie's abdomen return to her original state of relaxation. After monitoring several contractions, we were instructed to call her back.

Eventually, I was able to report back to Faith the exact duration and intensity of the contractions. When we told her that the contractions were not lasting more than thirty seconds, she decided she would wait for awhile before coming over. I continued monitoring contractions and soon learned how to sense them coming on and how strong or weak they were.

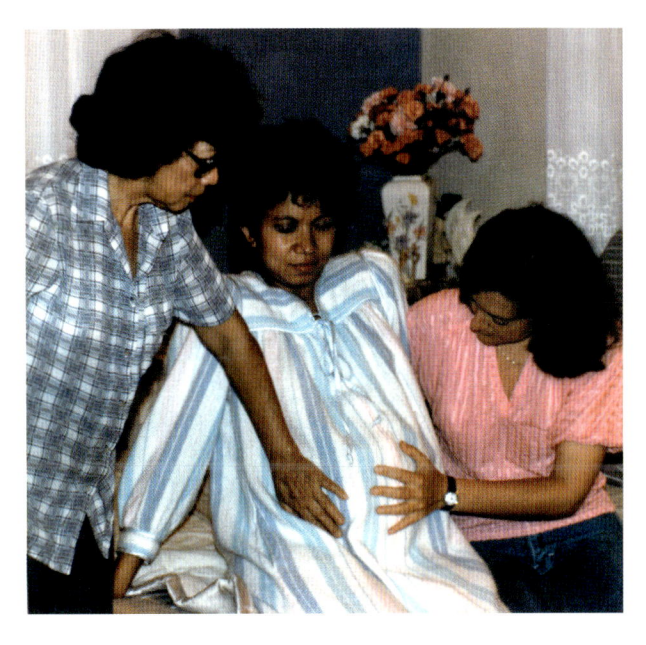

When curiosity got the best of her, I had Frankie's mother-in-law, Lordes, place her hand over the baby so she could feel the sweeping sensation of energy coming around from Frankie's back. Lordes closed her eyes and waited for the sudden change in direction. After sweeping forward, there would be another sensation of a sweeping motion coming from above-down. It would slide downward past her hand as the baby squirmed and pushed herself further into the canal. Lordes had eight children of her own back in the Philippines, but they were typical hospital births. All of this was as new for her as it was for us, and she was just as intrigued.

I helped Frankie follow all of the advice she had been given during her prenatal classes. I also used some of the visualization techniques I had learned from Grantly Dick-Read's book *Childbirth Without Fear*. As I felt the contractions, I imagined soft downy-white pillows surrounding the baby's head and warm energy passing between my hands. I was relying mostly on instinct and intuition. I'm not sure if it helped the baby, but it made Frankie more comfortable and helped us believe we were having a positive impact on the labor.

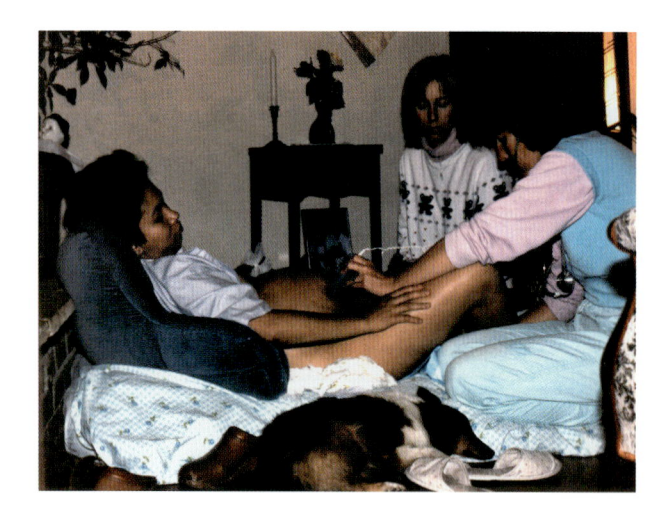

Faith and her apprentice arrived later in the day when Frankie's contractions were finally strong and consistent. They diligently monitored Frankie's vital signs as the twelve-hour mark slowly approached. Periodically, Faith would ask Frankie to lie down so she could check heart tones, blood pressure, and temperature. As soon as Frankie would lie down, Lady, her oldest Sheltie dog, would lie beside the bed. It always looked like she was trying to keep a low profile so no one would notice her. It was clear to all of us that Lady knew something was up and wanted to stay close.

When evening came with no sign of the baby, Gary picked up Angel and Wendy. They gathered up a few sleeping bags and stopped to rent several movies before coming over. The three of them set up camp in the family room as they prepared to wait, watch, help, and sleep.

In the hospital, there is rarely a comfortable place for the birth team and family members to sleep. Folding chairs, rocking chairs, and in some hospitals, a cot is available for one or two people to rest on while they wait for the delivery. Everyone else must camp out in the brightly-lit waiting room.

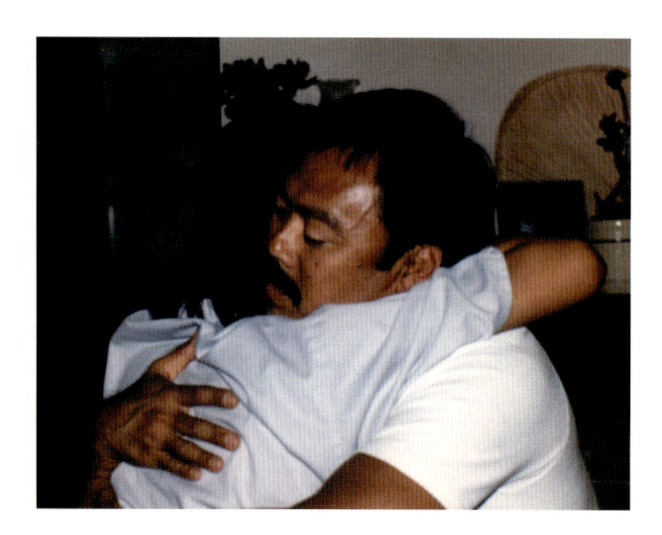

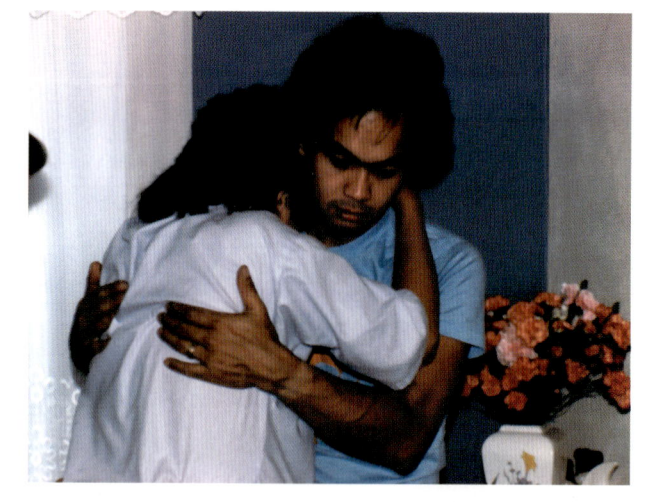

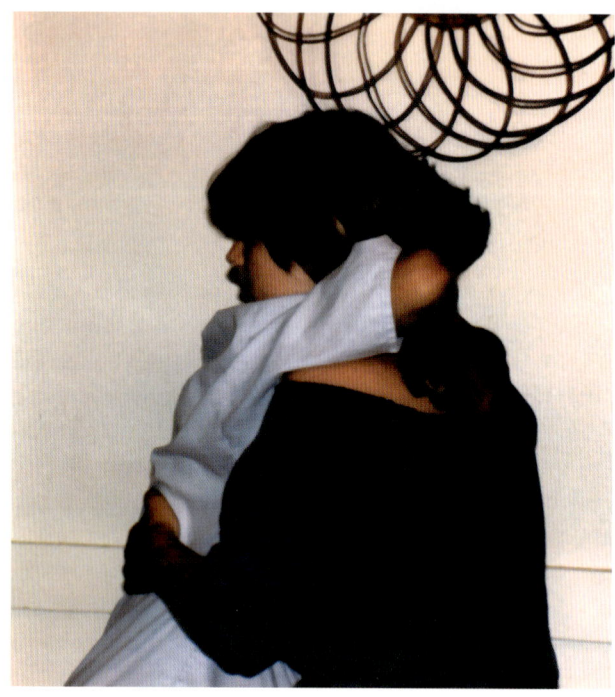

By late evening, Frankie's contractions had become so intense she insisted that standing was the only way she could endure them. Gary, Rafael, Angel and I took turns hugging Frankie as she used us for support. Lordes helped by rubbing tense shoulder muscles. As midnight approached, we were physically and emotionally exhausted. We all took turns and saw to it that someone was always there when Frankie reached out every three to four minutes for support.

Lordes had spent the day cooking. The kitchen table was constantly full of delicious Filipino dishes for anyone who got the munchies—day or night. Since it is extremely difficult for the mother and the birth team to stay hydrated and well nourished during a long labor, Lordes saved the day for all of us.

STEP 2: Choose a Birth Attendant

In the hospital, food is not an easy commodity to come by. The cafeteria is open only during peak meal times. Even when the cafeteria is open, it's difficult for the birth team to leave a birthing mother so they can eat. It's also a bad idea to bring food into the birthing room because women in active labor become highly sensitive to odors. (Make the mistake of bringing in coffee or eggs once active labor begins and you may get kicked out in a heartbeat.)

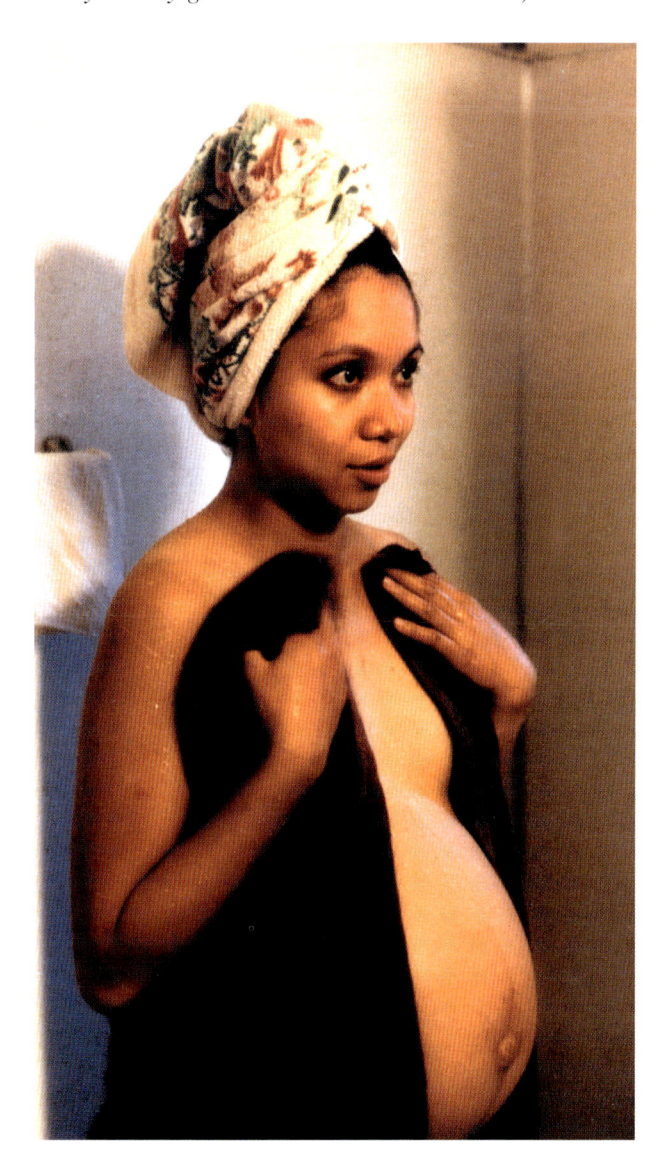

As the birth team gave in to exhaustion and began to drop like flies, Faith suggested that Frankie take a hot shower. I stayed close, in case she had a contraction or felt faint. As Frankie stepped from the shower, I took the profile shot she had always wanted. The tiny bathroom was so full of steam I could barely tell where she was. I simply pointed the camera in her direction and hoped for the best.

Twenty-four hours had passed, and still no baby. Faith continued to keep a close eye on Frankie's vital signs. She informed Frankie that ethically, she had to advise her to go to the hospital for antibiotics, because her risk of obtaining an infection was rising with each passing hour. Frankie refused, so Faith started checking her vital signs more frequently. She also checked the fetal heart tones every 10 – 15 minutes to insure that the baby was handling labor without signs of fetal distress. Everything remained stable, so Faith and her assistant sat back and continued observing Frankie's labor.

If Frankie had been in the hospital, her birthing room may have been filled with tension. Nurses, midwives and/or doctors would have been insisting that Frankie receive IV injections of antibiotics. They would have insisted on pitocin to increase the intensity and frequency of contractions, medication for pain relief, and continuous electronic fetal monitoring to observe the baby's response to the strong, pitocin induced contractions.

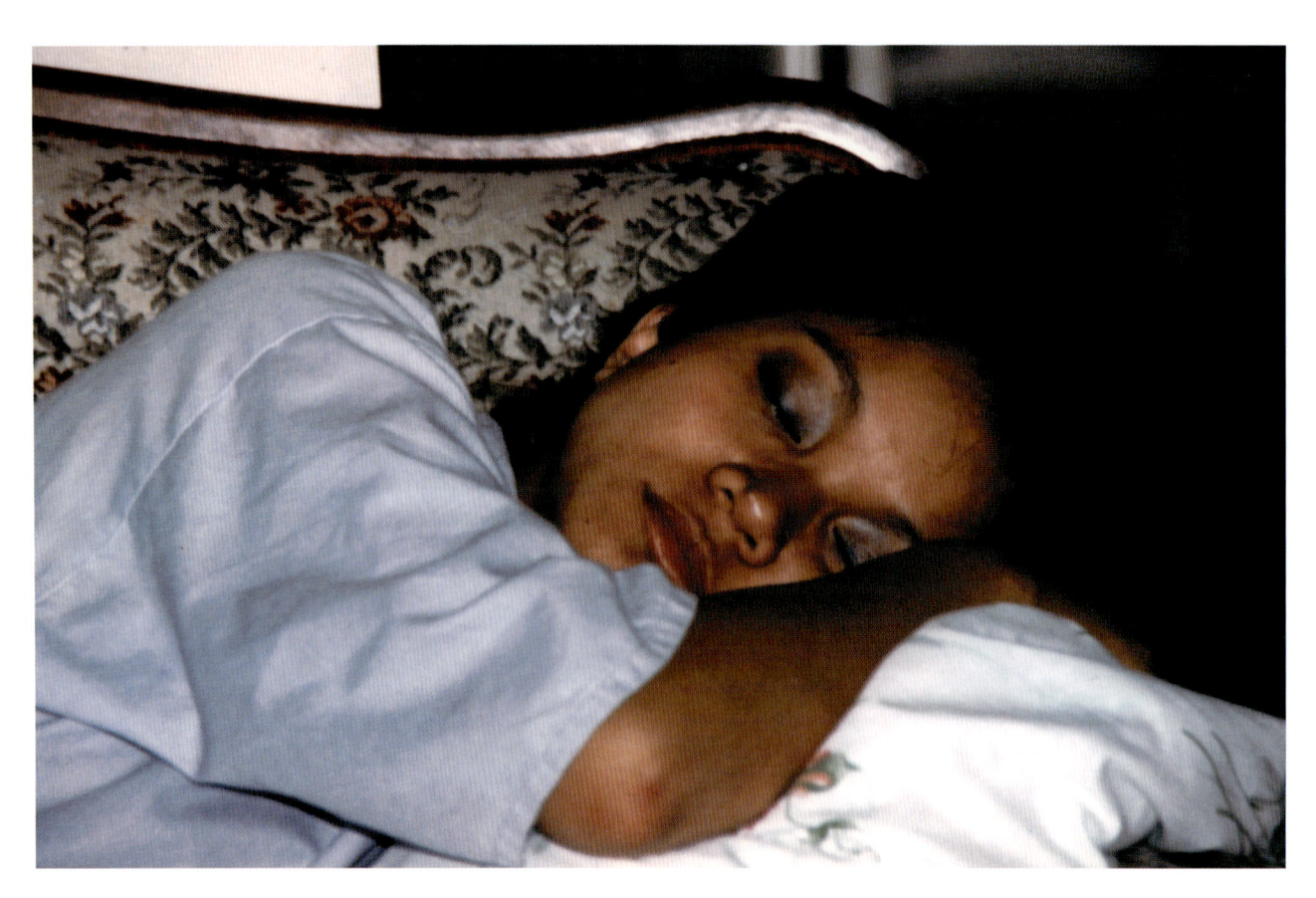

By the early morning hours, Frankie's home had become a haven for sleeping companions. Rafael needed to conserve his energy for the delivery, so he took the family bed. My girls slept on the floor, Gary took the guest bed, and the midwives slept on the mattress in the living room. Frankie and I also gave in to fatigue as we sat side by side on a love seat. She and I would doze between contractions by resting our heads on the arms of the small couch.

We had become so in-tuned with each other that when a contraction started, we stood up simultaneously, and turned to each other. Frankie would rest her head on my shoulder and we would breathe slowly through the contraction. Lady never moved from her spot at Frankie's feet, even as the blanket covering our legs fell over her body. She seemed to sense that something incredible was happening and wasn't about to leave Frankie.

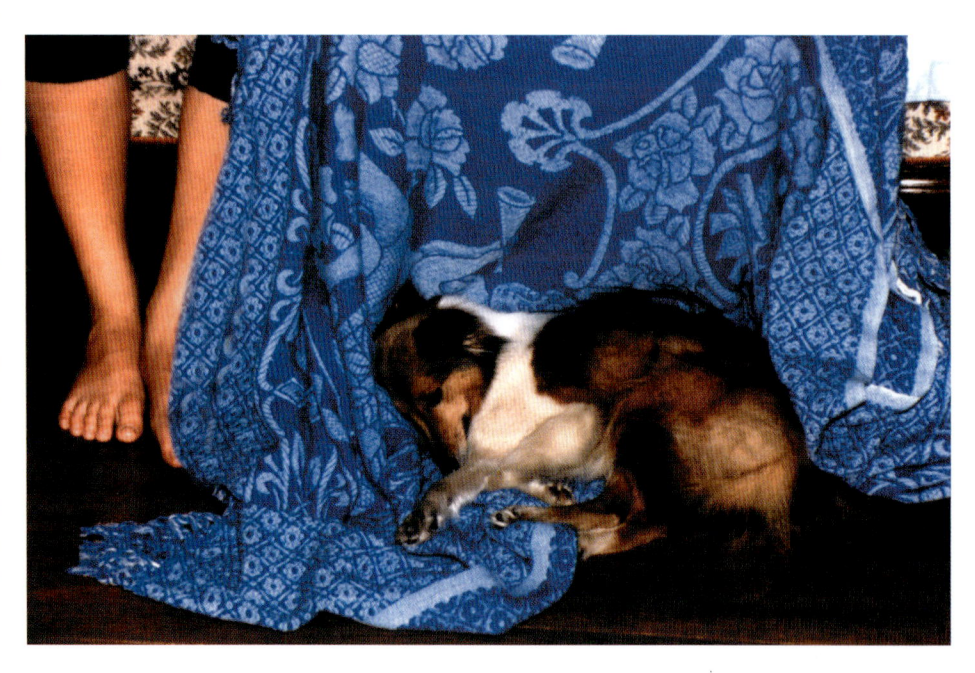

Morning came. The sun streaked through the living room and everyone slowly woke up to find that we still had no baby. Lordes started cooking again. Lady was unwillingly ushered outside when Rafael, Gary, and I took turns walking with Frankie; she was exhausted and needed to walk between two people, with her arms over their shoulders for support. We circled through the kitchen, into the living room, and back into the kitchen over and over again. We followed the same well-worn path. Frankie was losing her patience as fatigue and fear replaced excitement. She wouldn't snap at me, but when she spoke harshly to Rafael we rejoiced. (Faith had warned Rafael that women often get agitated and hypersensitive toward the end of labor.) We hoped Frankie's burst of temper meant she was finally going to transition from the first stage of labor to the second stage—delivery of her baby.

As we walked with Frankie through the kitchen and around the living room, I wondered how this was accomplished in the hospital. Pacing in the tiny hospital rooms would have been impossible. I was also thankful that we didn't have to ask her to get dressed and drive to the hospital before she could continue any further. Frankie had created a safe cocoon and had no desire to leave it.

It was now more than 30 hours since Frankie's water had broken. Faith didn't want to force her to go to the hospital, but if something didn't happen soon, she knew she would have to. She asked Frankie to lie down so her vitals could be checked. Everything was fine. This time Faith ended her exam by looking at Frankie and harshly telling her the truth of the situation. In a stern *I mean business* voice, Faith informed Frankie she could either "have her baby at home, or at the hospital," but either way—"she would have to deliver her baby."

I was shocked at the harshness of Faith's tone, but I watched in amazement as Frankie turned her fear into determination. My anger at Faith subsided as Frankie suddenly said she was feeling rectal pressure. I now realized why Faith said what she did. She seemed to know it was time to get tough with Frankie. Getting tough forced Frankie to let go of her fear. It wasn't long before she started pushing.

Frankie stood next to the mattress in the living room. Rafael and Gary provided the physical support she needed as she began to squat with each pushing contraction. To our surprise, Frankie remained calm and determined as she started pushing her baby out.

Faith showed Gary and Rafael how they could use their legs to provide support for Frankie's thighs while she was in the squatting position. In-between contractions, Frankie would stand up and give them all a rest. She was so wrapped up in the sensations of delivery that Frankie had no desire to look in the carefully placed mirror resting against the wall in front of her. It may not have helped her, but the mirror worked perfectly for Lordes and my daughter, Wendy. They were able to watch the delivery from the doorway of the family room. Angel surprised all of us by lying down on the mattress in order to look up and watch the delivery. (15-years-old and she was enthralled with the whole process.) Frankie was oblivious to everything and everyone as she focused on the sensations of her baby sliding down the birth canal.

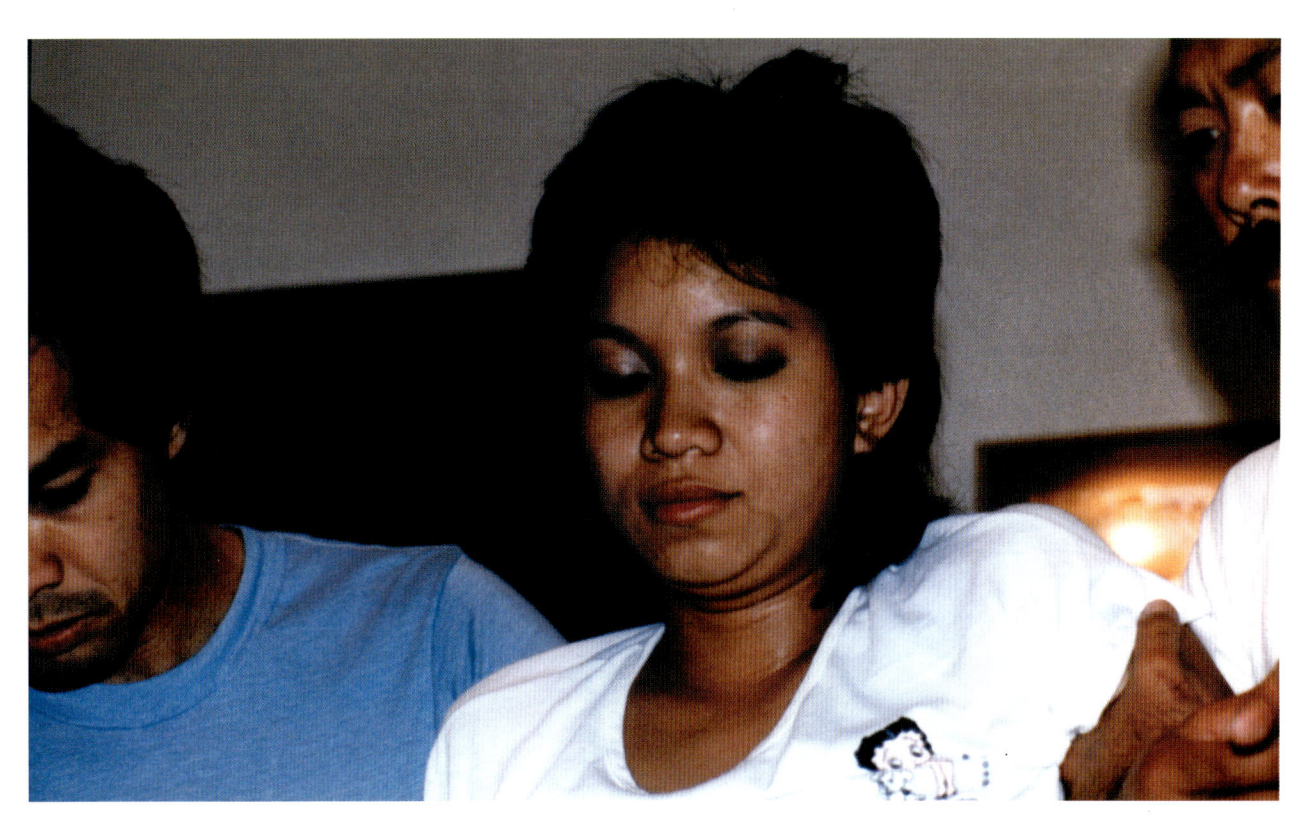

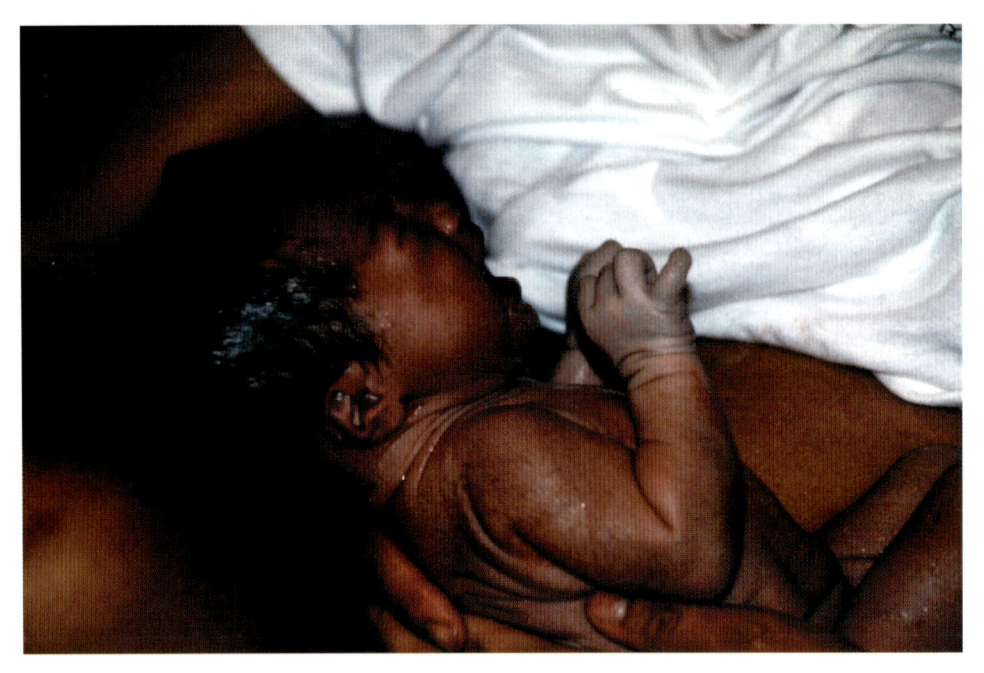

Hands Of Love

Within seconds, everyone encircled Frankie and marveled at the sight of little Ashley. We had waited for more than thirty hours to see this little girl; we had begun to wonder if she would ever come out. Faith clamped Ashley's umbilical cord after it quit pulsing and handed Rafael the scissors. He ceremoniously cut it and gave Ashley her independence.

In no time at all, the baby slid into Faith's waiting hands as she sat in front of Frankie. Afterwards, the assistant midwife eased Frankie down onto the pad we had placed on the floor. Now, with support from all around, Frankie's hands were free to take her baby.

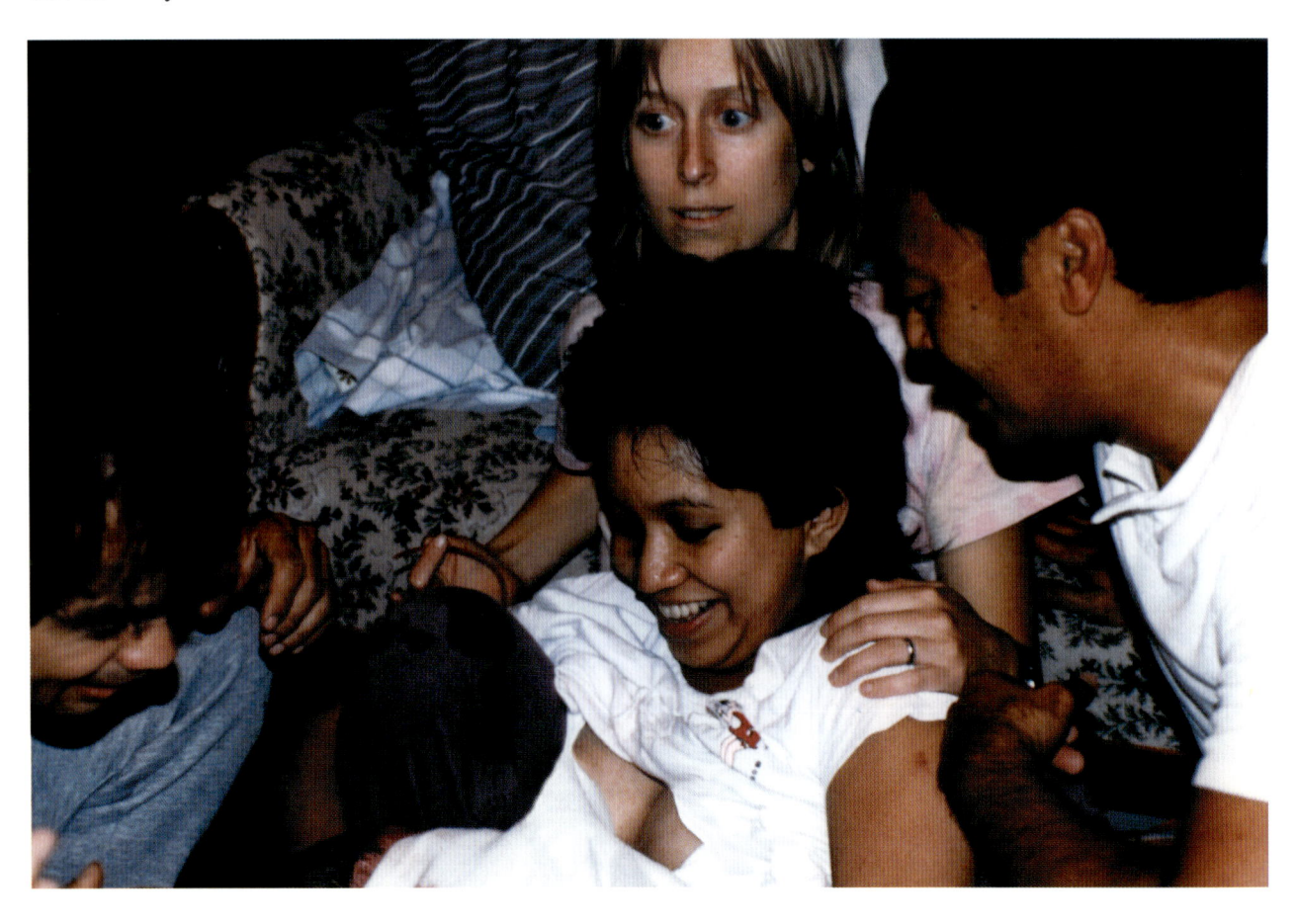

After the excitement settled down, Faith suggested that Frankie move to the mattress and finish the birth by delivering the placenta. In a flash, Rafael pulled his shirt off and took baby Ashley into his arms so Frankie could change positions. Once she'd handed the baby to Rafael, Frankie was able to move with relative ease.

STEP 2: Choose a Birth Attendant

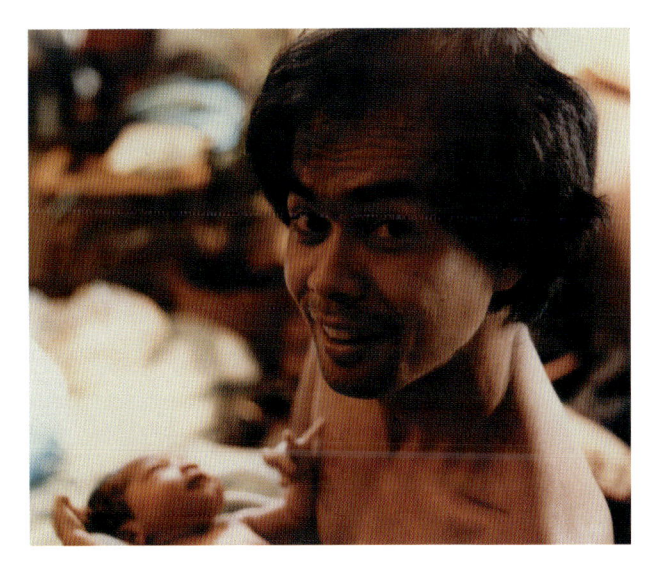

Frankie and Rafael were given plenty of time to bond with Ashley before Faith completed her role in the delivery by giving Ashley her newborn exam. I spent that time getting photographs for the family album. When Faith nestled Ashley in her lap for the exam, I marveled at how gentle and thorough she was. When she was done, Faith wrapped Ashley in a pink cloth stork-like bag and her assistant lifted her in the air for the final weigh-in.

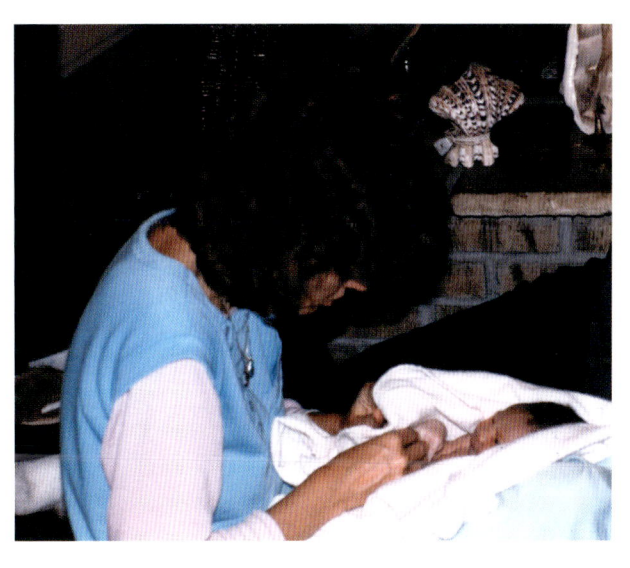

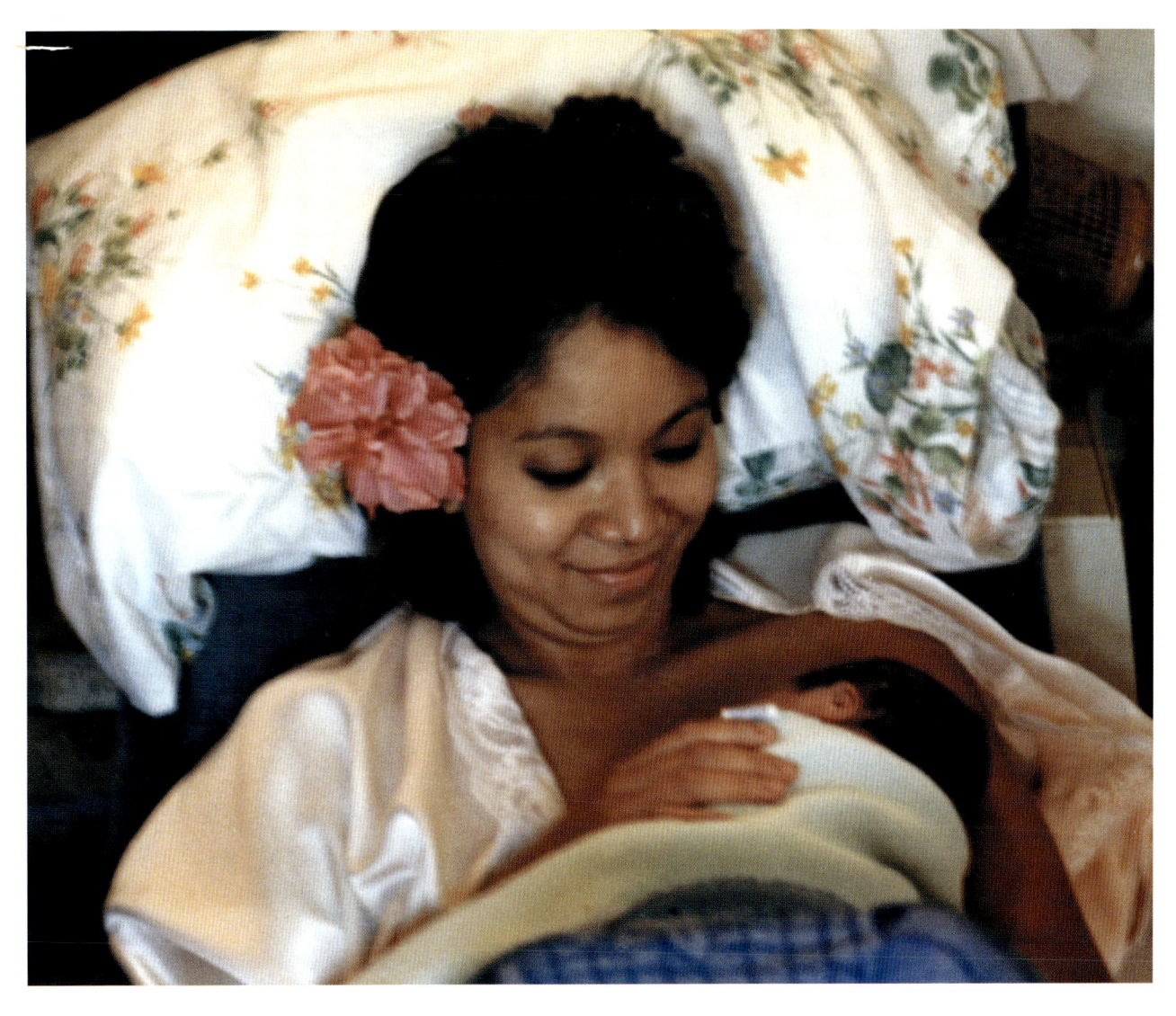

> A newborn exam in the hospital is usually rushed and abrupt. The newborn is generally moved into the nursery and weighed on a cold metallic scale, which elicits a scream and the customary startle reflex. They respond to being moved away from their mother with tears of rage and fright. They endure poking of their heel for blood, a shot of Vitamin K, and antibiotics placed over their eyes. It's a harsh and rude awakening to the world they have just worked so hard to get into.
>
> The more progressive hospitals now perform the newborn exam with the baby on the mother's chest. All routine procedures are delayed for several hours at the parent's request. (I wonder if they would ever consider the stork bag instead of the metal scale?)

While Ashley received her physical, I helped Frankie put on a silk bed jacket. The midwife assistant went into the garden, picked a beautiful flower, and put it in Frankie's hair. Lordes prepared the birthday cake with a '0' candle and poured nonalcoholic champagne into plastic glasses. It was finally time to raise our glasses in a toast to the new member of the family. We toasted to "no IV's, no medication, no pitocin, and no intervention"—just a healthy baby girl, and a happy content mother.

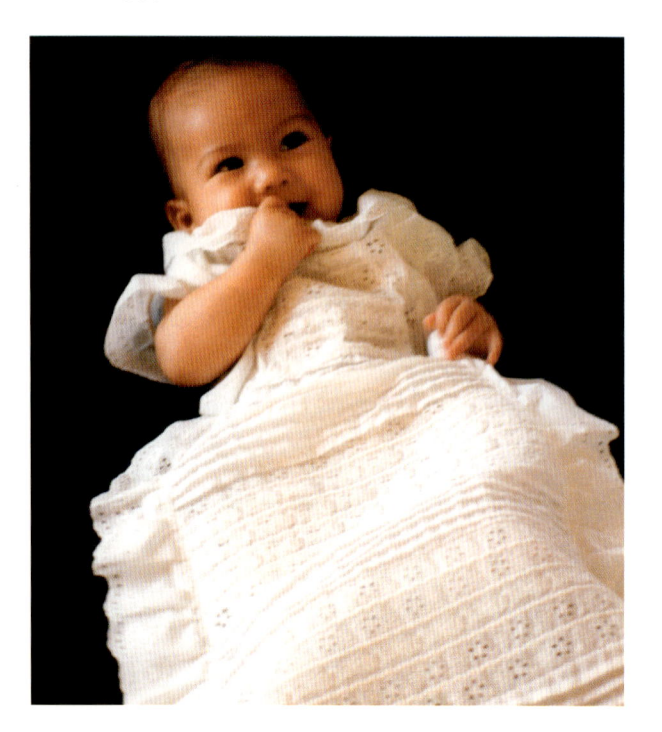

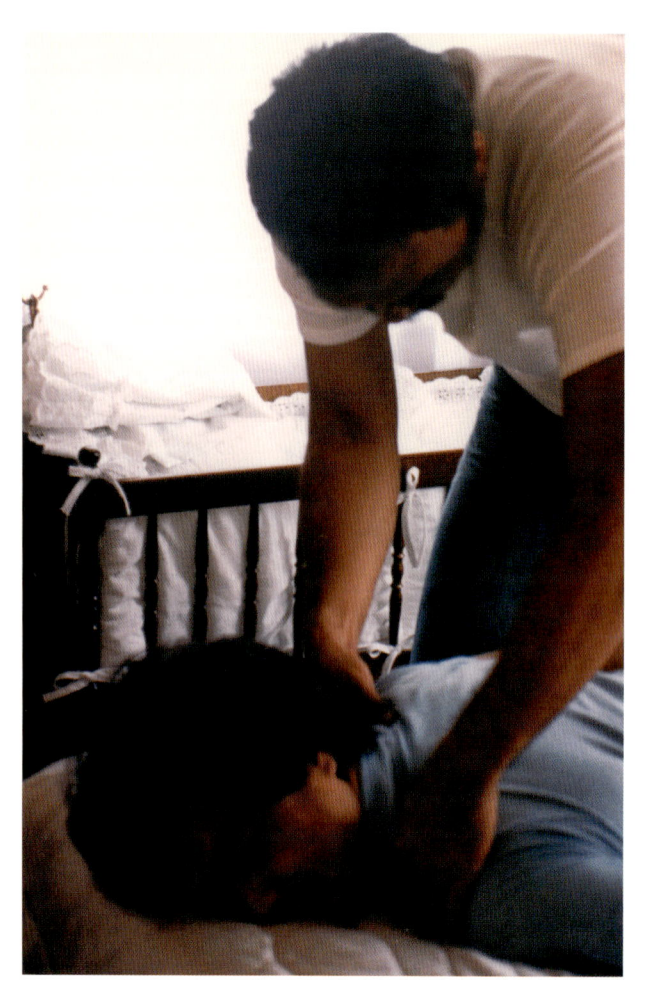

As Frankie and Ashley settled in on the makeshift bed in the living room, Rafael and I asked Gary to adjust our aching bodies. Everyone needs to see a chiropractor after providing labor support—it can be a physically challenging event for everyone involved!

After becoming a mother, Frankie decided to leave school and become a full-time mom. A few years later I joined the family for the homebirth of Farrah, who joined us within hours after labor began. I was back again within another few years to help the girls witness the gentle birth of their little brother Raffie—also at home.

Frankie may have left a career as a chiropractor behind, but she has not left the healing profession. Now that her children are teenagers, she is working as a certified massage therapist (CMT) in Cupertino, California.

STEP 2: Choose a Birth Attendant

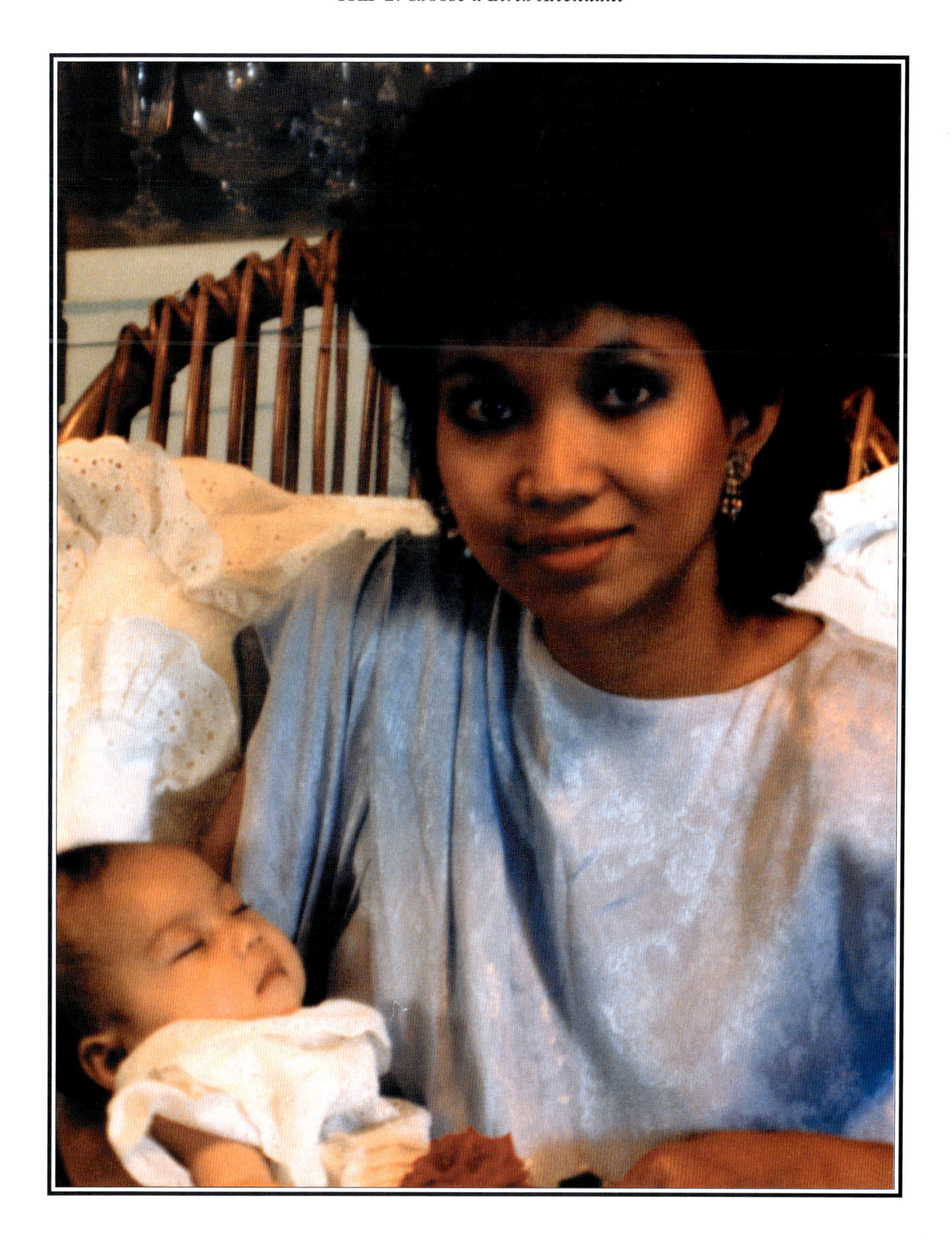

Over the next few years, I was the birth photographer and labor coach at many of the same births Faith attended. She allowed me to observe several birthing classes and taught me the natural process of labor from a midwife's point of view.

Observing Faith in action taught me how important it is to have patience during early labor. I also learned how essential it is to help a frightened mother confront her fears surrounding labor and delivery.

My intuitive respect and admiration for midwives was heightened after Frankie's birth. Faith taught me that women who embrace this profession do it out of love (they are paid relatively little in compensation for the long, unpredictable hours they spend with a family). After attending several births with Faith, I also developed a strong respect for her dedication; she knew that every time she agreed to attend a homebirth, she was risking legal action from authorities who wanted to abolish the practice of midwifery.

Several years after I met Faye, she was entrapped by the Attorney General in California and arrested for practicing medicine without a license. Faith, who was practicing midwifery primarily for members of her religious sect, was arrested and jailed after she agreed to attend the homebirth of two undercover officers posing as a pregnant married couple who were not of her faith. She went through the trauma of a lengthy and expensive trial simply because she was willing to help women give birth in a more loving and compassionate environment. She won the case after demonstrating that there was no legal statue against the practice of midwifery in California.

It is often said that midwifery competes directly with the economics of obstetrical care and is therefore in constant conflict with that profession, and with the legal system that supports the power of the medical establishment. But, there is much more to the conflict between the medical establishment and the midwifery profession than merely economics.

An obstetrician once responded to my patient's question about homebirth by saying, "Home delivery is for pizza! Why would anyone entertain the thought of moving a risky procedure such as the birth of a child, out of the hands of well-trained doctors who have access to the latest technological advances, to a person without their education and equipment?"

This comment offended the woman and resulted in her refusing any other medical care. In a way, his attitude is understandable. Most medical personnel have only witnessed birth in the hospital setting. They see trauma and crisis on a daily basis; 25 – 50% of hospital births end up in surgery and more than 90% of women under the care of an obstetrician request medication to eliminate the pain of childbirth. Doctors and nurses watch the neonatal intensive care nurseries fill up with babies on a daily basis—babies who must begin life in an incubator. These babies are attached to medical devices such as: monitors for respiration and heart rate, umbilical catheters, infusion lines for feeding, ventilators and endotracheal tubes. Of course they think childbirth is dangerous!

Doctors, CNM's and nurses acquire a fearful attitude about homebirth because they are never given the opportunity to witness birth in a home setting that is void of the melodrama typical of a hospital birth. The mistaken belief that homebirth is always dangerous is reinforced when, albeit rare, complications in a planned homebirth warrants a move to the hospital for the delivery. These rare cases may be the only opportunity for medical personnel to meet homebirth parents. So naturally, they think complications are common. The truth is that by utilizing the services of efficient, well-trained, midwives, thousands of women have babies in the peaceful setting of their home—without the need for medical intervention.

For more information about direct-entry midwifery regulations in your state, contact the Midwives Alliance of North American (MANA) by calling (888) 923-6262.

STEP 2: Choose a Birth Attendant

This next story occurred 10 years after Frankie's birth. I was teaching pediatrics at Northwestern College of Chiropractic in Minnesota, had a thriving maternal/pediatric practice and had already attended several hundred births. My role as a volunteer doula was well established in the chiropractic community and I had begun teaching postgraduate pediatric courses to chiropractors throughout the United States, Canada and Mexico. I'd come a long way on my journey to help babies come into the world in a much more humane way than Angel and Wendy had.

This next story is about a student of mine at the time who took great strides to insure her unborn child hand a humanistic-assisted birth. Barb's husband, Dean, was also determined to give their baby the best possible entrance into the world; he read every pregnancy book he could get his hands on. They investigated various models of birth, interviewed several birth attendants, and hired an obstetrician who respected their humanistic approach to birth. All of Dean's reading paid off. When the time came—he was the one to catch his little girl.

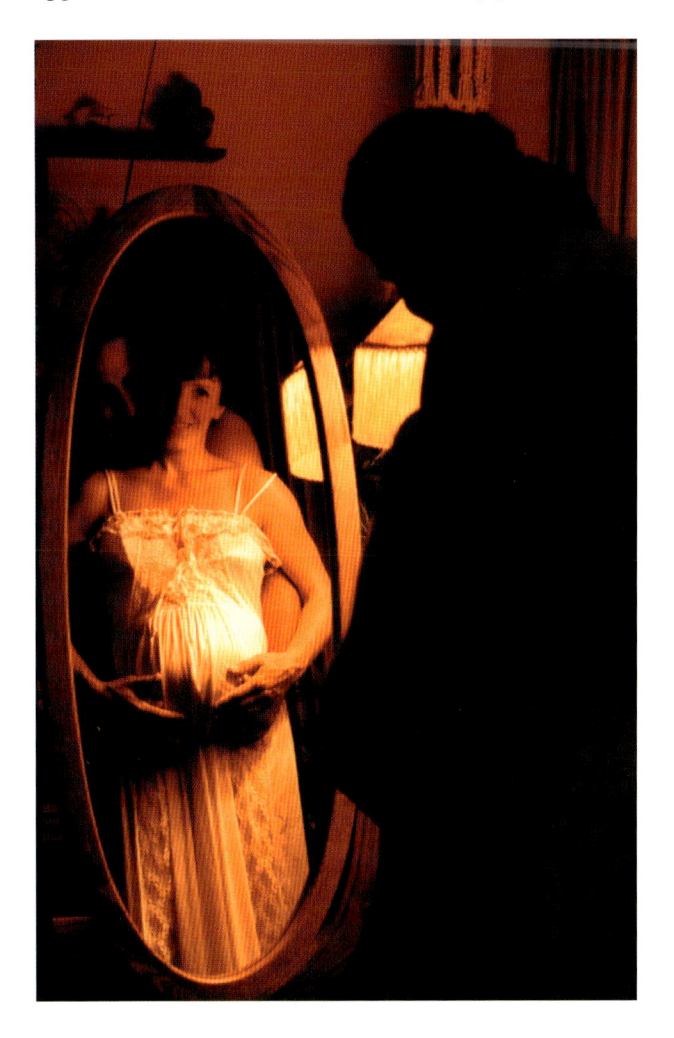

A Father Catches the Baby

BARB: *A strong contraction woke me up around 12:30 A.M. I was lying there unable to go back to sleep for about 30 minutes. By 1:00 A.M. my contractions were consistently three minutes apart, so I woke up my husband, Dean. We were surprised that labor was progressing so rapidly and wondered if we were going to be able to stay home, walk, and relax for hours as we'd originally planned. By 1:30 A.M. I knew this wasn't false labor and called my mom in Seattle. We'd heard that first babies generally take an average of 15 hours to deliver and I wanted her to see the birth of her grandchild, so I asked her to get on a plane right away.*

Mom never went back to sleep that night. She caught the first flight out the next morning and flew all the way to Minneapolis thinking she was going to watch the birth of her grandchild. Unfortunately, my baby had other ideas and Mom didn't make it in time.

The night that Barb went into labor, I had gone to their home to take a few photographs while Barb was still pregnant. By 10:00 P.M., I had gotten all the shots I wanted and we called it a night. I arrived home around 11:15 P.M. and had just fallen asleep when the phone rang. It was Dean urging me to hurry back over. Labor had suddenly begun and Barb seemed to be progressing a lot faster than expected. He wanted to gather the birth team right away.

After calling me, Dean woke up Michelle, the other member of the birth team. Michelle and Barb worked with me as chiropractic externs and Michelle was one of Barb's closest friends. Michelle, experienced and eager, had already provided labor support for another family. We both arrived at Barb and Dean's home within an hour of his excited wake-up call.

When we arrived, Barb was in the bathtub... clearly progressing rapidly. We were not greeted with the expected, "Hi, this is it!" She ignored our presence as she focused on breathing and emitting long and continuous O-O-O-ing sounds. She was unable to carry on a conversation with anyone, her face was

49

flushed and she was clearly off in another world; the sensations of labor had consumed her.

By this time in my career, I had witnessed hundreds of women during labor and there was no question in my mind that Barb had skipped the typical early stage. Her body appeared to have jumped right into the heavy-duty part of labor. I suddenly realized if we did not change their initial plan to remain at home for several hours, Barb would be having an unplanned homebirth.

I asked Dean to quickly pack the car. As we helped Barb out of the tub, we found she could not tolerate the weight of a towel due to her heightened skin sensitivity. Instead of putting on her street clothes, Barb slipped on a light maroon nightshirt and robe. Dean was hesitant to go to the hospital so soon. Barb changed his mind.

BARB: *In-between contractions, I stopped and told Dean that he'd better take me to the hospital right away or I was not going! Though we had jointly agreed to a hospital birth, deep inside I really wanted a homebirth. Dean was not emotionally prepared for that— he packed the car.*

We all arrived at the hospital around 4:00 A.M. I was happy they had chosen a hospital with a room that resembled a hotel suite. All of the medical equipment was hidden behind cabinets that complemented the room. We quickly set up soft music, dimmed the lights and prepared for the delivery. Contractions were intense and close. Consequently, Barb refused to stand up or walk around. She preferred to lie on her side, cuddle into Dean and chant the O-O-O tone that all the mothers I worked with were using. Michelle and Dean and I didn't hesitate to join her in making the now familiar sound. This helped Barb stay focused as the sensations of labor continued to consume her. She seemed far away from us and from the birthing room.

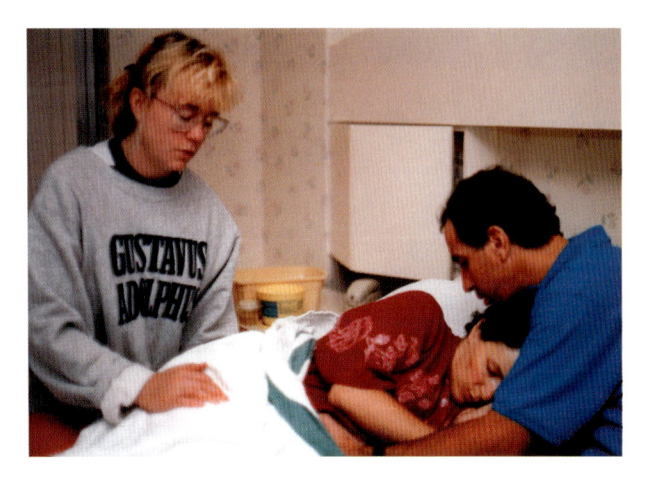

All of the nurses on duty that night were given a copy of Barb and Dean's written birth plan. Consequently, the nurses made no attempt to ask Barb to change into a gown, to bring in an ultrasound monitor, or to offer medication. Instead, they used the fetal stethoscope Barb had brought with her to check the heart tones, quietly brought in the delivery equipment table, and notified Barb's obstetrician of her progress. Standing at the foot of the bed, I videotaped the birth scene while Michelle massaged Barb's leg and vocalized the O-O-ing sounds with her. During some of the contractions, Michelle would stop, place her hands over the baby, and speak soft words of praise and encouragement to Barb.

Dr. Gretchen, looking like someone's favorite grandmother, arrived around 7:00 A.M. after completing her early morning bike ride. She assessed the scene and quickly decided to change from biking clothes to scrubs. Meanwhile, the nurses prepared the room for delivery. Since Dean planned on assisting in the delivery, they politely asked him to put on a gown and sterile gloves. I was impressed when I noticed how seriously the nurses treated Dean. You would have thought he was a very respected surgeon the way they reverently held out the gown for him to slip into and solemnly presented him with sterile gloves.

Dean's whole demeanor changed once he was in his gown and gloves. He appeared stiff and authoritative with his gloved hands suspended in the air. Yet, when he looked down to see the baby's head crowning, he suddenly melted and whispered, "Oh yes! That-a girl."

Dr. Gretchen returned and asked Barb if she wanted an episiotomy. Barb was so caught up in the turmoil within her body that she just muttered, "Oh, I don't know." We all knew Barb did not want an episiotomy unless it was medically necessary, so I suggested that Dean do perineal massage. He immediately turned and grabbed the oil from their backpack. During the last few months of pregnancy, Barb and Dean had been faithful with their nightly perineal-stretching exercises. Therefore, Dean felt confident about stretching the perineal area to help the baby come through without tearing Barb's tissue. With the serious nature of a doctor, Dean bent down and began to oil and stretch Barb's vaginal tissue around their baby's crowning head.

Barb was so quiet it was hard to tell she was pushing until she stopped and gasped for air. Her hands

STEP 2: Choose a Birth Attendant

rested lightly on her abdomen as she used her mind, body, and spirit to ease the baby out as smoothly as possible. All of a sudden, Dr. Gretchen broke her silence with words of encouragement. "Keep it coming babe... come on sugar... down past the burning... push it away... now stop... pant!" Barb suddenly realized someone was speaking to her. She seemed puzzled with the sudden command to stop pushing. Suddenly Dean was holding the baby's head as he urgently demanded, "Pant, honey, pant!" Then, just as quickly, he started shouting, "Oh cutie—she's here, she's here!"

Dr. Gretchen placed her hands under the baby's head and told Dean, "You're going to have to scoot around here real quick if you're going to do this, sir. Place your hands like this under the body." Dean scampered around to the other side of the bed so he was better able to support the baby's body. As soon as he had the baby's head back in his hands, Dr. Gretchen turned to Barb and said, "Now, give us a little push Barb." As I sat at the head of the bed holding Barb in my arms, I whispered, "Let her slide, Barb, just let her slide." Michelle picked up a camera and quickly started getting photographs of the birth. Dr. Gretchen suddenly shouted, "Barb, open your eyes! We have a baby type!"

Barb quickly pulled her nightshirt up to her chin so she could cradle her beautiful baby girl against her chest. Barb had not torn or bled, so Lauren was pink and shiny against Barb's bare skin. As Barb looked down and caressed Lauren, she smiled and said, "Hi, baby. Hi, little one. Welcome to the world."

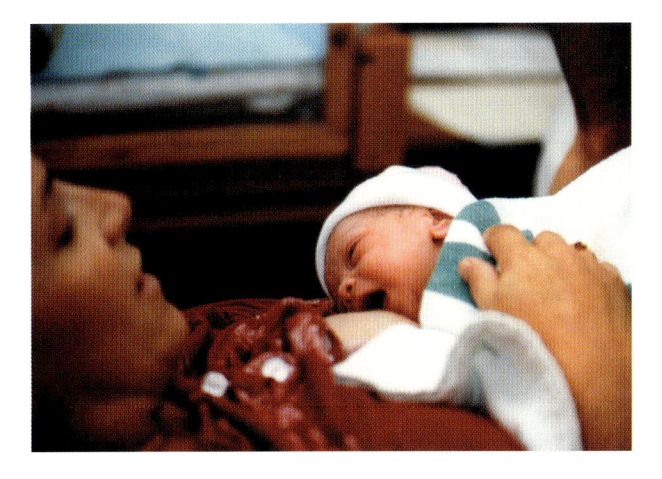

Lauren was never taken off of Barb's chest. The warmer sat unused. The nurses came to Barb's bed to measure, monitor and place bracelets on each of them. Dean performed the "cutting of the cord" as Barb looked on. She was patient with everyone up to that point, but as soon as Dean was finished, she demanded that he remove the gown and gloves as quickly as possible. Dean removed everything except his jeans and climbed into the twin bed with Barb and his daughter, Lauren. Barb needed to concentrate on delivering the placenta, so she handed Lauren to Dean. Lauren was upset momentarily, but quickly quieted as she buried her face in her father's hairy chest.

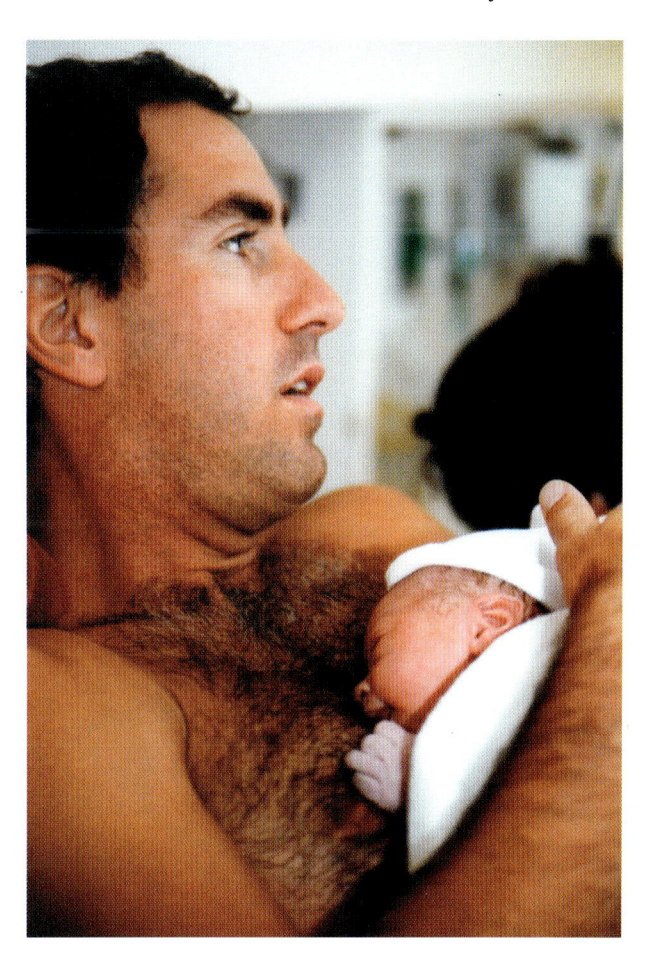

As Lauren settled in, she allowed Dean's heartbeat to soothe her. I then made the mistake of interfering with her serenity. I wanted to get one good photograph of her face before I left, so I asked Dean if he would turn Lauren around.

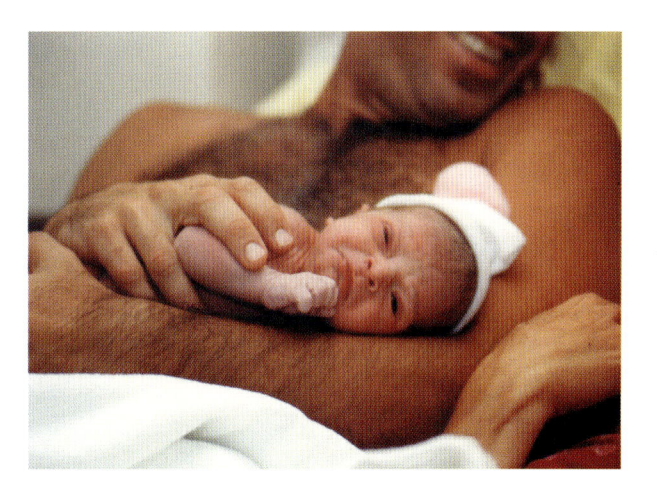

Hands Of Love

I left at 7:30 A.M. because I had to teach an 8:00 A.M. pediatric class before going on to treat my clinic patients. Staying up all-night and then going to work was really becoming a hardship. However, the thrill of witnessing a new spirit entering the world through hands of love made it all worthwhile.

Several weeks later, I returned to Barb and Dean's home. We set up the living room as it was on the night of Lauren's birth and took new pictures for the family album.

Dr. Barb, Lauren, and Dean now live in Seattle, Washington, and Lauren has remained a healthy, bright, and happy child since her peaceful entry into the world.

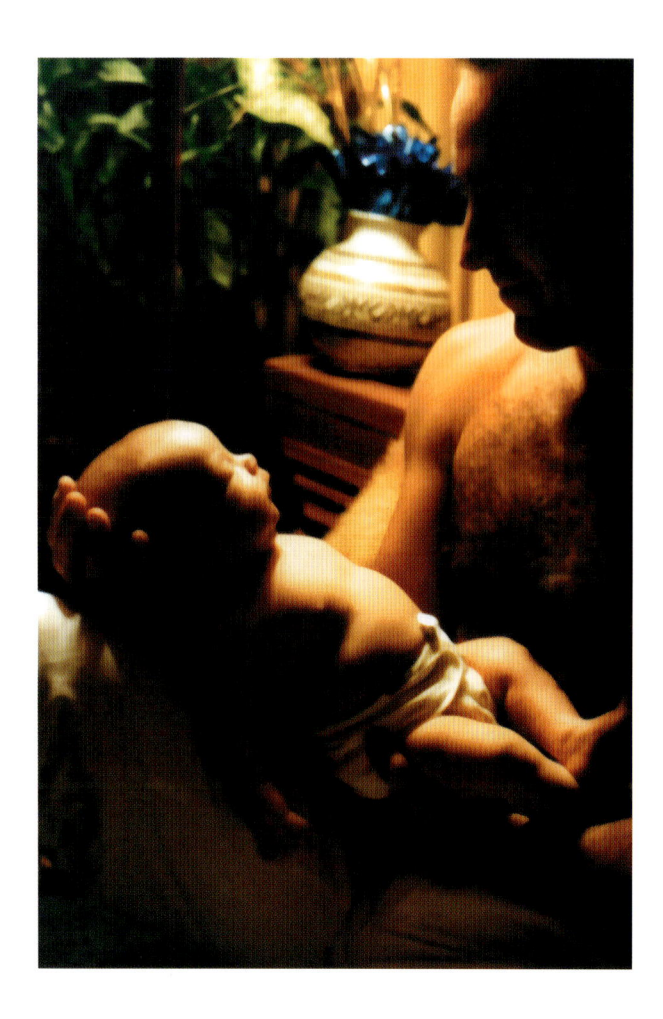

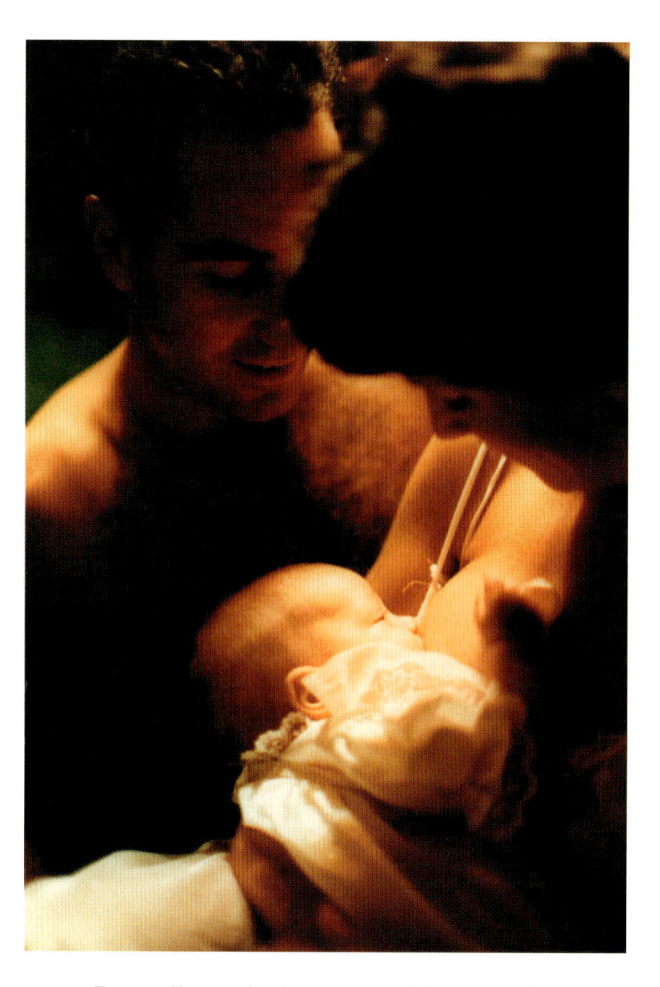

Regardless of whom you ultimately choose as your birth attendant, you should feel confident about your decision. If you choose homebirth with a midwife, remember to hire a physician who can provide hospital care if you need it. Tell them you're planning a homebirth and need their back-up support. If they refuse to give you additional prenatal care, hire someone else who will respect your patient rights. Later, if you decide to go to the hospital, you'll have someone you trust waiting for you.

If you choose a certified-nurse midwife, or a family practitioner, and find you need additional medical care, they will already be working intimately with an obstetrician.

Cover all your bases and be prepared for any possible scenario. When everyone involved with the birth works together as a team, everyone wins—especially the newborn.

STEP 2: Choose a Birth Attendant

A Parent's Prayer For the Birth Attendants

To Our Creator
We ask that all those who enter this sacred space do so with hands that are gentle, kind, and loving.

We pray that you will help them show reverence for the birth process while acknowledging their limited role in assisting with the birth.

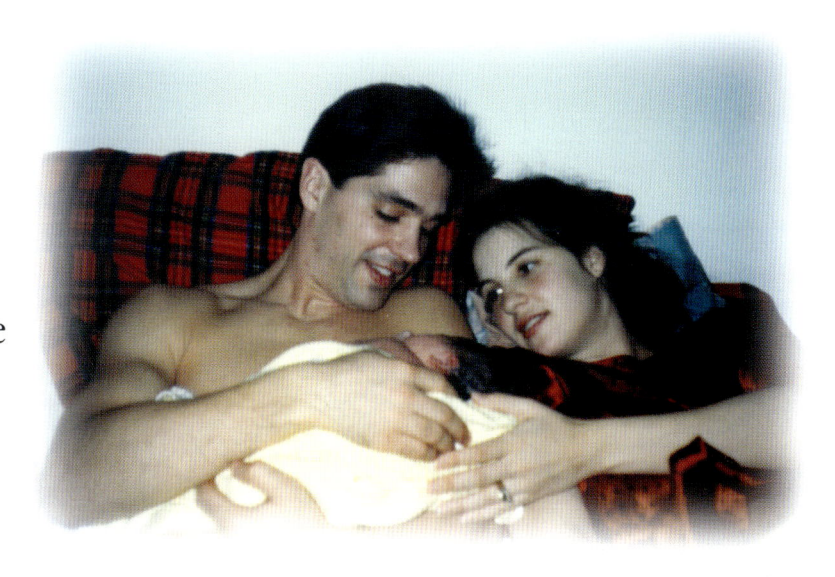

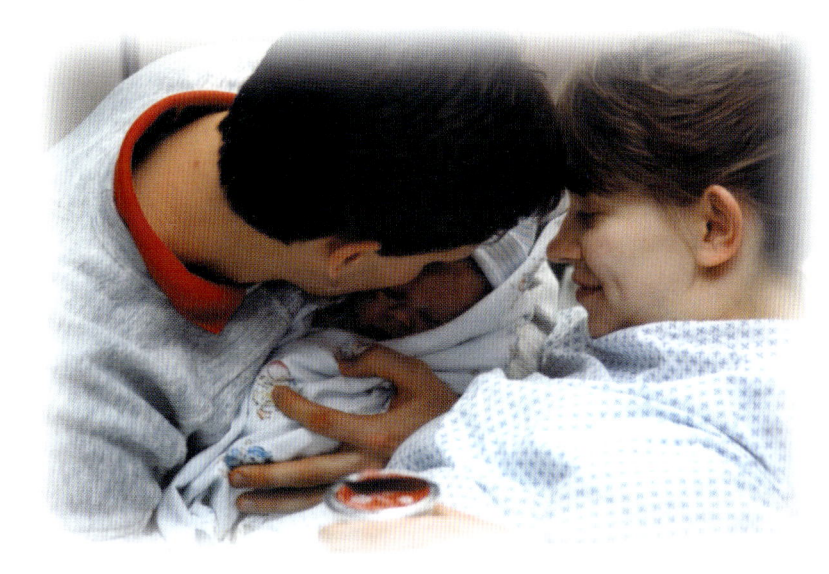

Please help them trust our judgment, respect our wishes, and protect us from harm. Please help them as they guide this newborn up, and into, our waiting arms.

Thank you for being here on this special day. Thank you for hearing what our hearts have to say.

Hands Of Love

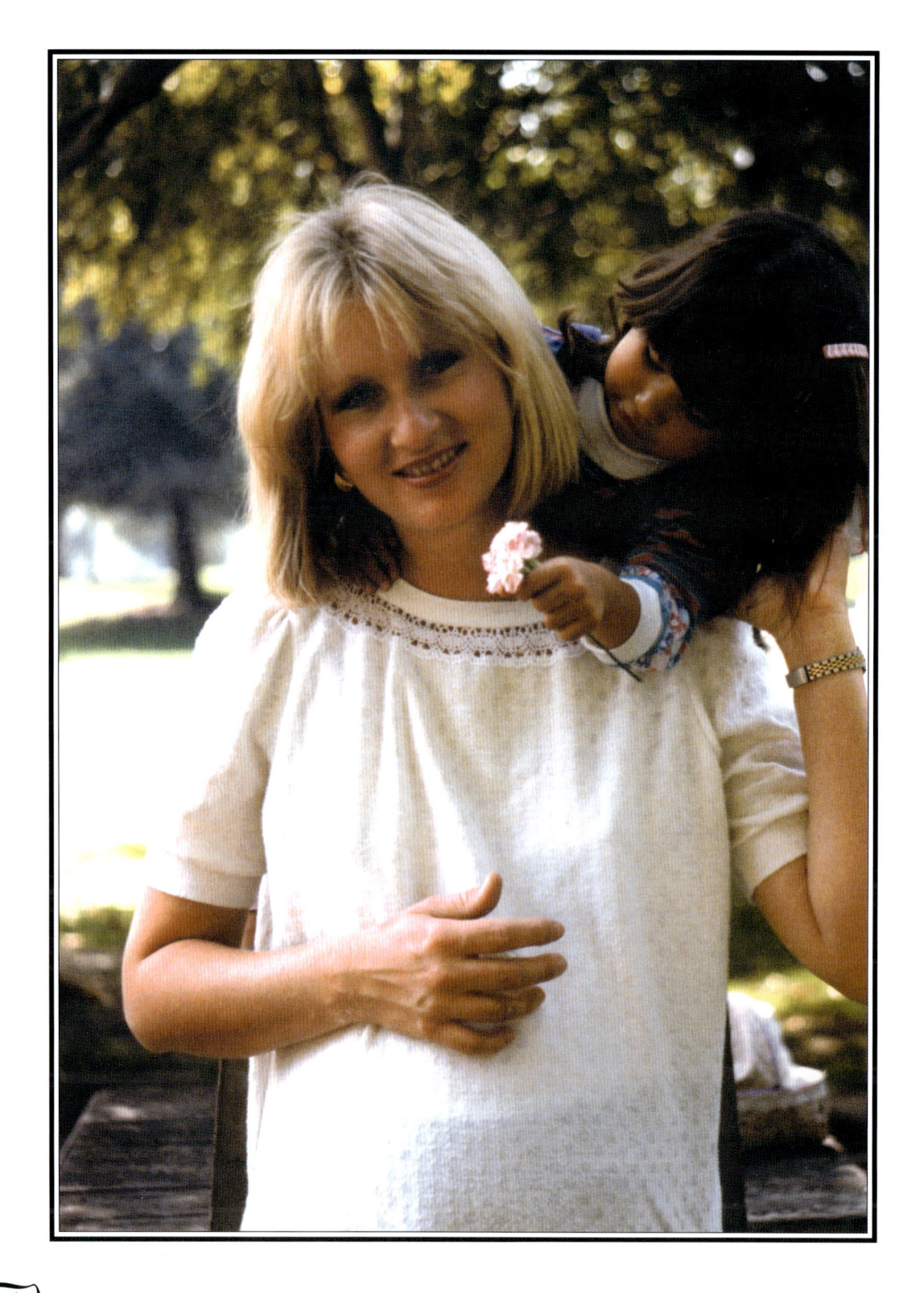

𝒫lan on surrounding yourself with people who will express the love they hold in their hearts for you and your baby. Seek out a doula who will help your birth team engage the miracle of childbirth with confidence, peace, and trust in the intelligence of nature.

> **STEP 3: Create a Birth Team**

STEP 3
Create a Birth Team

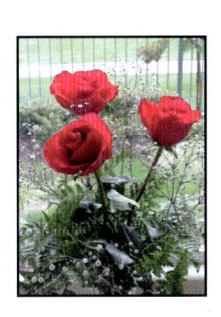

Now that you have chosen your birth attendant, it is time to create a birth team that will help you achieve your goals. There are several reasons why you might consider surrounding yourself with a team of carefully chosen people.

The first reason is that you have no way of knowing if your labor will be swift and uncomplicated, or long and exhausting. Your partner may need time to go to the bathroom, eat, or take a power nap. During those times, you need continued support by someone who can focus solely on you and your needs.

A second reason for creating a birth team is that your partner needs the support of someone who has labor and delivery experience. He needs to know that someone else will be there to help him cool you down if you overheat, to apply ginger packs if your muscles are in spasm, or to suggest alternate positions that will help the baby descend down the birth canal.

And, thirdly, you need to surround yourself with people who will intuitively enfold you with love radiating from their heart to yours.

If you are a first time mom, you are probably worried that other people may somehow "replace" your husband. He, too, is probably worried about that. Trust me. That will rarely happen. No one can give the form of emotional support he gives because no one is as intimately involved with you as he is.

Men react very differently when they attend the birth of their child. Some men get so excited, and so charged by the flood of testosterone hormones that are swarming into their cells, they can hardly contain their need to do something physical. I have arrived at some homes to find the father vacuuming the entire house, grating enough ginger for ten births, and on one occasion, disassembling the entire stereo system to take to the hospital. They can't help it. They are as hormonally driven as a woman is with her flood of oxytocin hormones.

I once attended a birth the eve of Easter Sunday when a father allowed his natural flood of hormones to give him the courage to stand outside the door of the birthing room and stop the doctor from speeding up his wife's labor with pitocin. The doctor wanted to get the birth over with so he could be home with his family. The father was not going to allow it, nor would he allow anyone into the room who would give any indication that his wife was not "performing quickly enough." We were totally unaware of the situation outside the door; we just knew that Dan was helping in his own way. (It's unusual in a first birth for a man to have the courage and strength to voice what he feels in his heart is right for his wife and child.)

I remained with his wife, Jean, as she quietly and lovingly labored through the night. She delivered her baby in the early morning hours—on her mother's birthday. You can see a picture of Jean on page 178 with a picture of her deceased mother in the background. That picture sat on a table in her hospital room with a large Easter lily. Emily was destined to be born on Easter Sunday, her grandma's birthday—not before. Dan allowed that to happen.

Members of a birth team know when to help, and when to back off. In my experience, they intuitively know how and when to give emotional or physical support to both parents. With their help, the father is free to give as much as he can, or to pull away when he needs to.

If this is your first birth, you might be asking yourself, "What about the nurses, the midwife, or my doctor?" Yes, you will have the services of your birth attendants, but they can rarely give you undivided attention from the onset of labor until well after the delivery. Here are several reasons why you need your own birth team. 1) If you decide to deliver in a hospital setting, you will spend most of the early stages of labor at home—alone. Once admitted to the hospital, you will have nurses available to take your vital signs but they have other patients to attend to. 2) Even if you decide to remain at home for the delivery, your midwife will usually wait until you are in active labor to arrive. And, should another patient go into labor, she might have to leave soon after the birth.

Your birth team will assemble as soon as you call for them. They will devote their time and energy anticipating and fulfilling your needs. They will be intimately and emotionally connected with you, your partner, and your baby. The birth may be an exciting new adventure for them and their excitement will help you through the long weary hours if you begin to wonder why it is taking so long.

Here are a few recommendations for creating a birth team and several stories that will allow you to see for yourself the joy, fun, and incredible support a birth team can provide.

Recommendation #1: Include a trained doula.

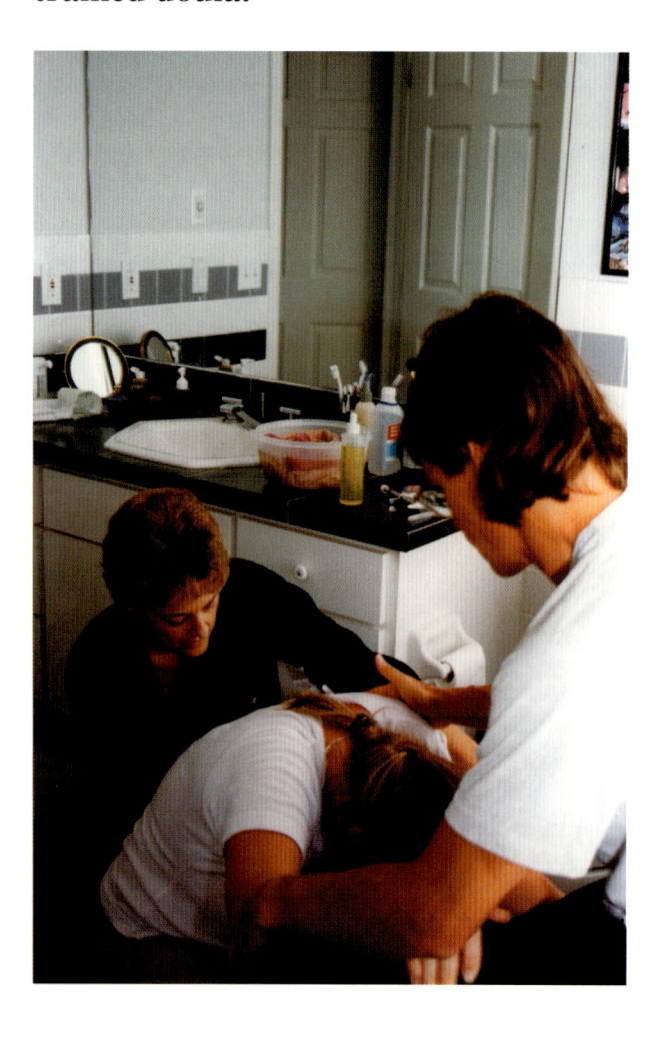

A doula is a traditional term for a woman who functions as a surrogate mother for birthing women. Historically, mothers and aunts fulfilled the role of a doula. They were able to do this because knowledge of birth practices was handed down from generation to generation. This changed when birth was moved out of the home and into a hospital setting. With the advent of the maternity ward, mothers were no longer allowed to be with their daughters. Thus, modern mothers do not have the firsthand experience of our historical mothers. We must now train women to provide the emotional support that once came so naturally.

A doula differs from the medical caregivers in that she will provide continuity of care. Her shift will not end at a certain time and she will rarely leave to care for another birthing mother. She will not take the place of your partner; she will only assist your partner by providing the emotional and physical support you both need.

A trained doula will train other members of the birth team. She will serve as an advocate who can help make educated decisions about recommended interventions. She should not make those decisions, nor should she communicate decisions to the medical staff. Her role is simply to help you and your partner discuss all options and answer any questions she is qualified to answer. I strongly advise you to interview several doulas prior to hiring the one that feels like the best fit. As one doula instructor, Amy Gilliland, would say, "Choosing a doula is an 'inner' thing not a 'values' thing."

Many doulas will bring into the birth arena their own skills in areas such as Massage Therapy, Chiropractic, Craniosacral Therapy, Acupuncture, Aromatherapy, or Homeopathy. Thanks to the research of Dr.'s Klaus, Kennell, and Klaus, the benefits of doula support are no longer a well-kept secret. Since the publication of their book *Mothering the Mother*, doula-training workshops have sprung up all across the nation. Insurance companies have conducted their own research into the benefits of doula support. Their studies confirmed that the presence of a doula reduces the need for intervention, as the mother is more relaxed and confident in her ability to deliver her baby. Thus, some insurance companies are now paying for their services and some hospitals are starting to provide doula support for birthing mothers.

STEP 3: Create a Birth Team

Here are a few key principles to keep in mind when choosing a doula:

1) A doula should honor the role of the partner and make every attempt to help him/her remain comfortable with his/her role in the birth. Try to avoid a situation where he/she feels pushed out of the birth scene.
2) A doula's goal is to decrease the need for medical intervention, but not to interfere with the care provided by the birth attendants who have been hired by the parents.
3) It is the responsibility of a doula to introduce herself to the birth attendant and birth team members, to explain that her role will be to nurture the mother and assist in any way she can, and to assure them that she will not interfere with the care given by the primary care providers hired by the family.
4) A doula helps the parents by providing additional information about recommended procedures, but limits involvement in the discussion to topics in which they have received special training in.
5) A doula should support any decision the parents make during the labor—regardless of her own personal beliefs.

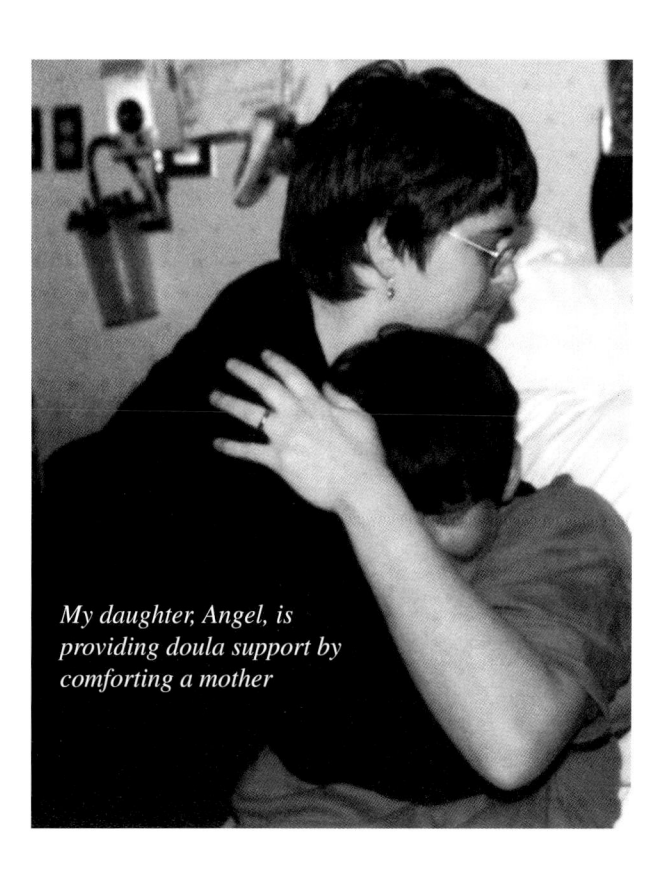

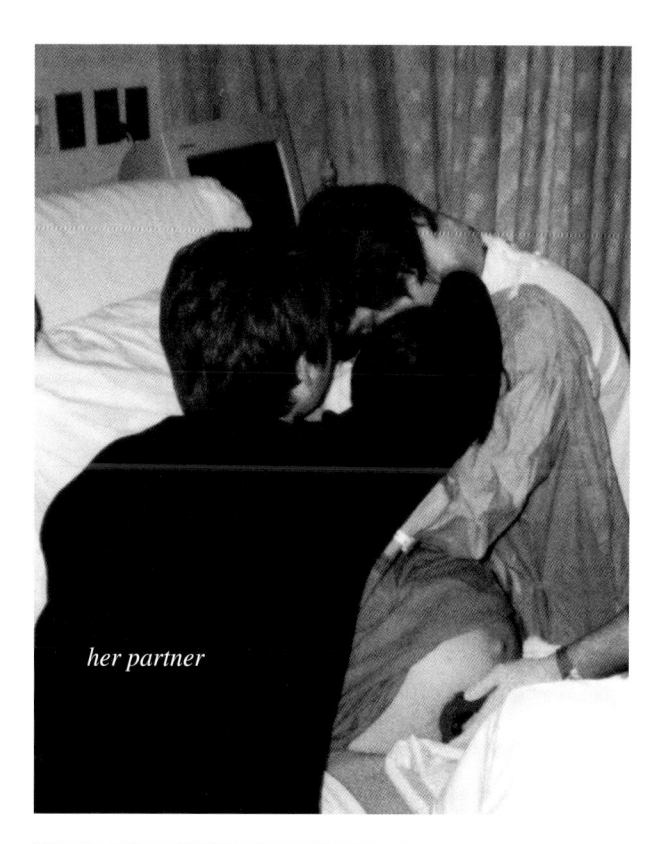

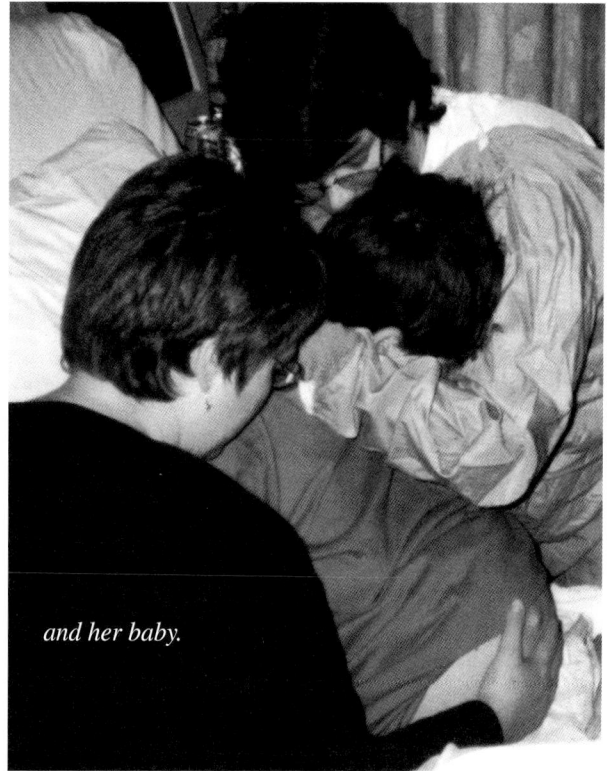

her partner

and her baby.

My daughter, Angel, is providing doula support by comforting a mother

Recommendation #2: Consider the possibility that your parents may want to be present for the birth of their grandchild.

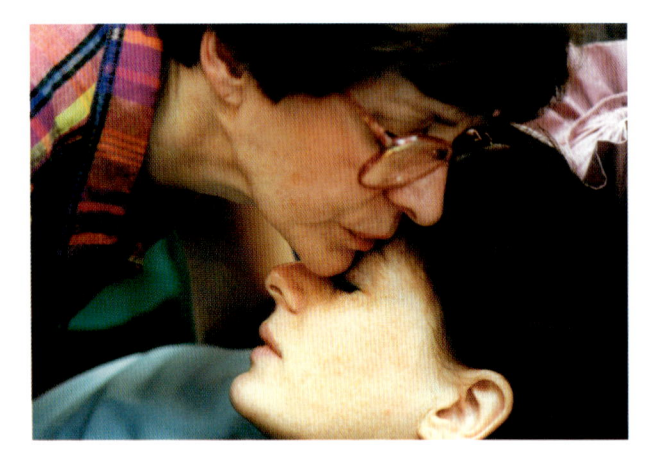

On many occasions, I have witnessed the positive influence of parents who arrived unexpectedly after the onset of labor. When encouraged to share their love and skill at nurturing, they proved to me the power of parental love as their presence alone improved the outcome of the birth.

A Mother's Intuition

Heidi, Steve, and I had just returned from the hospital. After examining Heidi, a doctor advised us to return home. In spite of Heidi's extreme back pain, he felt she was in the early stage of labor and it was too early for admission. Heidi's mother, Peggy, surprised all of us when she appeared in Heidi's bathroom where she and I were kneeling on the floor. Heidi was rocking on her hands and knees while she cried softly from the pain in her back. The pain was severe enough to cause constant nausea. I did not know at that time in my career how to help the baby turn into the proper position. I could only rub her back and rock with her.

Peggy whispered that she had an intuitive feeling about coming to the house right away. She looked at me and asked if she could hug her daughter. "Of course," I replied quickly. Peggy knelt down and wrapped her arms around Heidi. When she felt her mother's embrace, Heidi collapsed tearfully into her arms and the baby moved. The pain subsided enough to stop the nausea, so Heidi moved into the bedroom.

As nightfall took over, Heidi and Steve lay curled together on their bed in the dark bedroom. I sat at the foot of the bed and quietly observed the sleeping couple. Peggy rested in a chair next to Heidi's head. Whenever she stirred to warn us that another contraction was beginning, everyone would spring into action. Peggy would stand up beside the bed, and Steve would rise up on his knees.

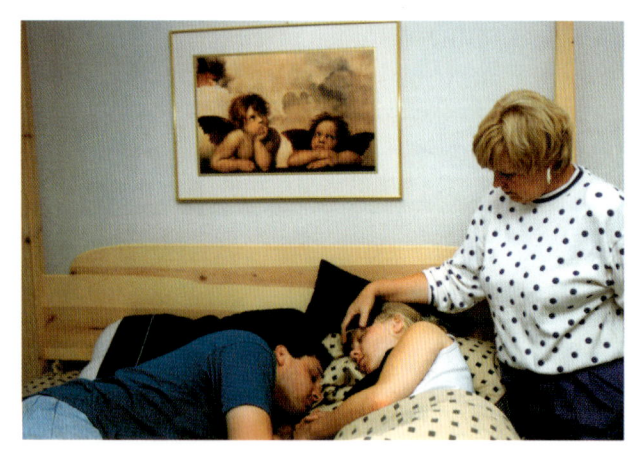

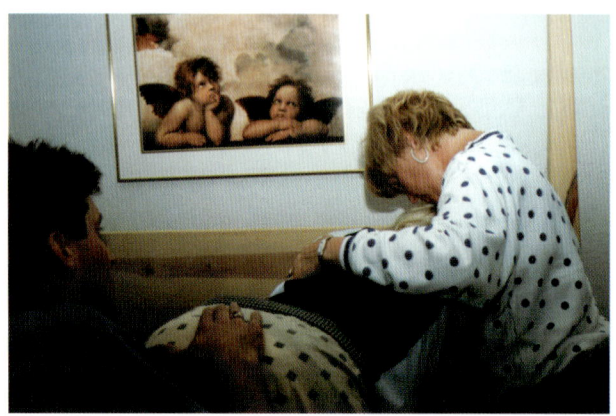

Unable to bear the pain in her back while reclined, Heidi would quickly roll over and come up on her hands and knees. In the twilight of the room, her instinct was to lunge forward and place her head on her mother's chest. Peggy was always there as Heidi lunged for that comfortable secure place where she could breathe through each intense contraction. Steve, a chiropractor, was quick to get behind Heidi and traction her sacrum to ease the pain in her back.

I watched (and listened with amazement) as Peggy, rocking Heidi in her arms, softly sang a lullaby that she had sung to Heidi when she was a child. After the contraction subsided, Heidi and Steve would lie back down next to each other and wait for the next contraction. Peggy was suffering from back pain and scoliosis, but she maintained her position at the side of the bed for what seemed like hours. I knew the bending over and rocking must have been agonizingly painful for her, and I was deeply moved by her love and devotion. She demonstrated that a mother's intuition about the needs of her child remain strong and true—even when the child becomes a parent.

STEP 3: Create a Birth Team

During one contraction, the flash of my camera gave me a glimpse of a large painting of Angels hanging on the wall over the bed. The Angels appeared to be watching over Heidi, Steve, and Peggy as they rocked through each contraction. I knew without a doubt that God had sent Peggy. She brought comfort and security into the birth that no one else could have provided at that time.

At one point, I relieved Peggy so she could run to the restroom. When Heidi stirred, I stepped up to the bed. She lunged forward, fully expecting to nestle into her mother. Instead, her head rested against my less-endowed chest. Not the same thing! She never let on, but, as I rocked her through the contraction, I'm sure I wasn't able to provide the comfort and security Peggy gave so instinctively. I did the best I could, but I could not sing her the lullaby, or generate the same degree of love. Needless to say, I was so thankful when Peggy returned to assume her role!

Later, when we decided it was time to return to the hospital, Peggy felt her role was complete so she returned home. (We were praying they wouldn't send us back home!)

At the hospital, Heidi requested medication to help reduce the back pain that hindered her ability to help the baby move down. Heidi chose a medication (intrathecal morphine) that would also give her baby relief from the unrelenting pressure of the contractions that were unsuccessful in moving him past his lodged position in the birth canal. A few hours later, Heidi gave birth to their son, Taylor.

Below, Heidi and Steve show the range and intensity of emotions that often accompany the birth of a baby; a woman can go from anguish to euphoria in just a few moments.

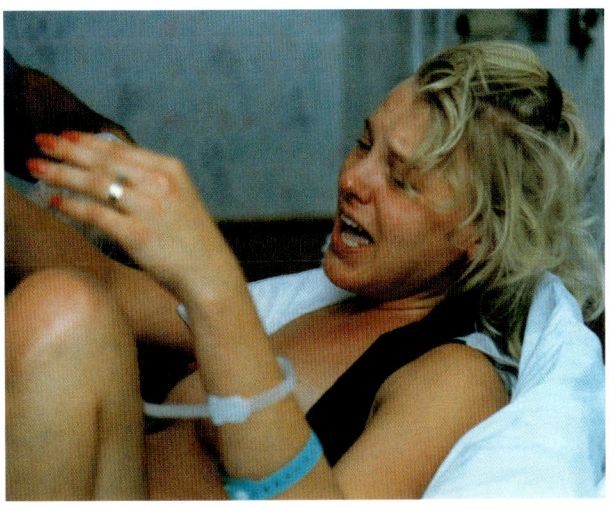

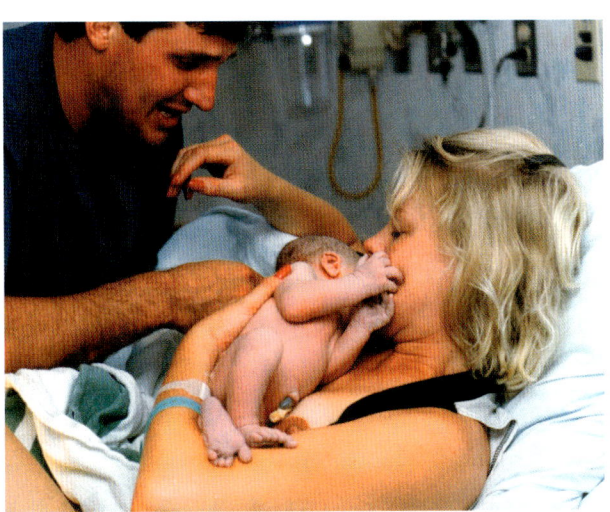

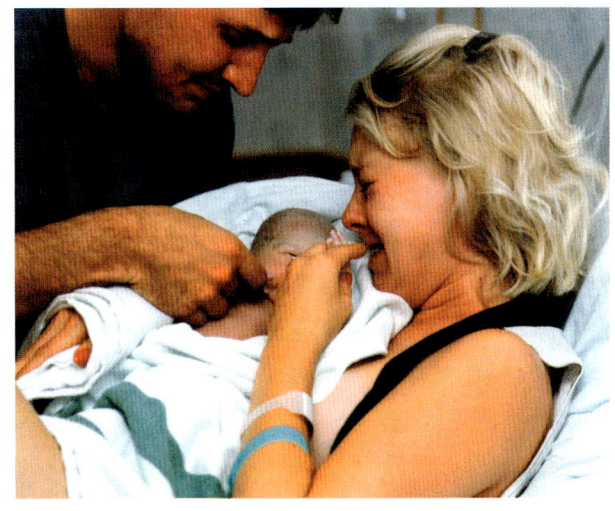

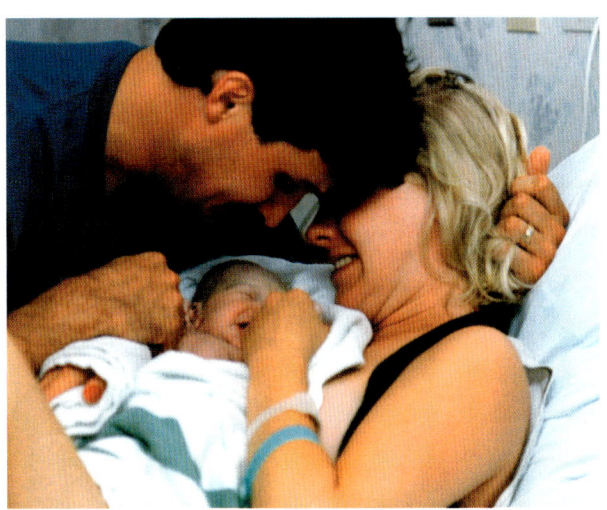

During one birth I attended, two parents showed up at the hospital to wish their daughter good-luck. The woman's father had not attended the birth of his own children and had no intention of witnessing the birth of his first grandchild. But, sometimes God has a plan, and in this story, the plan incorporated both the woman's mother and her father.

During this birth, Christie's father, Bill, taught me one of the most valuable tools I use as a doula. His training as an Olympic-boxing trainer came in handy as he watched me struggle to keep his daughter cooled off during the heat of labor. His suggestion on how to prepare a tub of ice water and cold cloths is one of the first things I do when a woman transitions into active labor. Let me tell you about that birth.

A Father Knows Best

Christie was still in the early stage of labor when I showed up to adjust her and help her get prepared for active labor. After the treatment, Christie's intuition nagged at her. She felt strongly that we needed to go in early and get settled into the hospital. Her apprehension was more than just first time jitters, so we went ahead and drove the five minutes to the hospital. We supported her decision in hopes that she would relax once we got her settled into her room.

Todd set up his sound system and turned on their ocean tape. The bright, sun-filled room was suddenly filled with the soothing sound of ocean waves that were rushing onto the beach, retreating, and rushing back again. Within ten minutes, Christie was lying in bed with the ultrasound monitor strapped to her abdomen and was told she would have to stay in that position. This was the very thing she had hoped to avoid, but the nurse felt there was something not quite right about the baby's heart rate in any other position.

Todd and I did everything we could to keep Christie relaxed and comfortable in her restricted position in the hospital bed. Christie, herself, worked hard to keep her spirits up, and despite her discomfort, she managed to keep her fear under control.

About an hour later, Christie's mom and dad surprised us with a visit. They had come as soon as they heard we had arrived at the hospital. Loretta wanted to wish her daughter good luck with the delivery; she had no intention of staying. Christie's dad, Bill, was uncomfortable being in the room and sat on a stool behind a curtain. Bill sat with his arms folded across his chest in a protective manner. From his position, he was only able to get a tiny glimpse of the birth scene.

I didn't realize Christie's parents weren't invited to the birth. Therefore, I immediately started teaching Loretta how she could help by placing her hands over the baby. Christie's dad continued to sit behind the curtain and wait for Loretta; it wasn't long before curiosity got the best of him and Bill started peeking into the room.

After learning there might be a complication with the baby's heart rate, Loretta made no move to leave and continued to do whatever she could to help her daughter stay calm and focused. From his post behind the curtain, Christie's dad waited and watched.

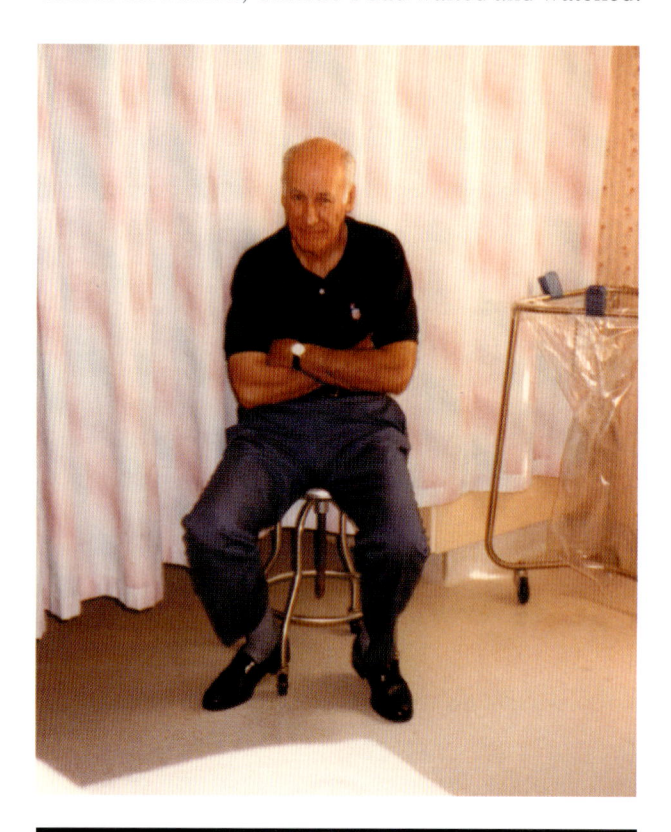

As women transition in labor they often get extremely hot. One of the most helpful things a doula can do is to wipe her forehead with a cool cloth and to place one around the nape of her neck. The cloths will not remain cold very long so it's important to keep applying fresh ones. Up until this birth, I would make many trips back and forth to the sink to run the washcloth under cold water.

STEP 3: Create a Birth Team

After watching me make several trips to the sink, Bill hesitantly spoke up and suggested a different procedure. He told me to fill the square tub on the night stand with approximately three inches of crushed ice, add just enough water to cover the ice, place a washcloth over the ice, then place three washcloths into the small amount of ice water resting above the cloth-covered chips.

What a brilliant idea! I now had a small tub of ice water right beside the bed and I could keep Christie cool with my constant supply of fresh cold cloths. The crushed ice didn't stick to the cloths because of the one I had spread out on top of the ice. And, I didn't have to make trips back and forth to the sink! After getting it all set up, I asked Bill to take on the job of cooling her off. He jumped off the stool, came out from behind the curtain, and stepped in just like a trainer working on an athlete. (Though I doubt he looked at his Olympic athletes with the same adoring expression I was witnessing.)

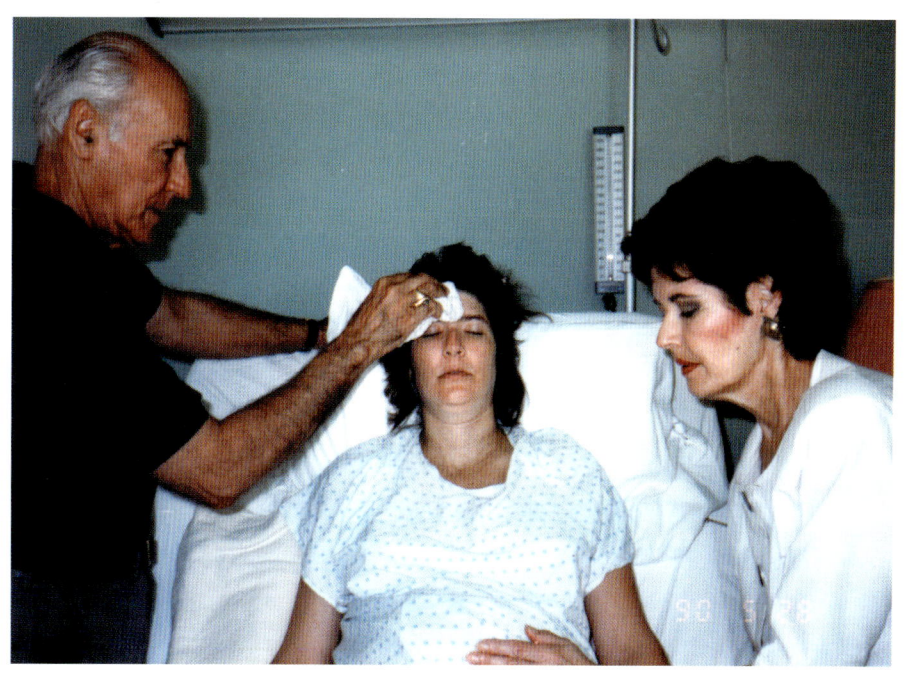

As the hours clicked by, Loretta kept soothing Christie by directing energy from her hands into the baby. Todd held Christie's hand and talked softly to her during each contraction, while her dad continued to apply cold cloths to her face and neck. When Christie complained of leg cramps, her dad would start rubbing her legs to ease the pain.

I kept turning the ocean tape over to keep the soothing sound of waves constant in the room. As Christie closed her eyes she could truly imagine she was standing on the beach with her baby watching the ocean swell and recede over and over again. The crashing waves helped diminish the screams coming from the room next door to ours. (I wanted so badly to go next door and help—if anyone needed a doula, that mother did.) Thankfully, everything was under control in this room and my role now seemed to be limited to being the family photographer.

With all this love, Christie was handling labor beautifully. Nurses kept checking on the baby's heart rate by watching the monitor out at their desk. Periodically, one of them would come in offering pain medication, but Christie adamantly and repeatedly refused it. If her baby was suffering from fetal distress, she didn't want to do anything that would compromise his ability to handle the delivery. Besides, she wasn't experiencing enough pain to consider robbing herself of the experience of childbirth.

Another complication cropped up when the nurses started checking Christie's cervical dilation. Different nurses kept showing up to check her. We found out later that the nurses couldn't agree on whether Christie was dilated to 1 centimeter or 10. They finally called in her family practice doctor to see what she thought. She couldn't be sure either, which made the nurses feel better, but perplexed everyone. Her doctor then called in an obstetrician.

The obstetrician felt the suture lines on the baby's head and felt that the water sac should be broken. She kept trying to break the water with a wand, but it wouldn't give. She finally decided to wait until Christie had a contraction to break the sac. She sat there patiently waiting, but as soon as the contraction started she surprised everyone by pulling her hand out of the canal and ordering the medical staff out into the hall, immediately.

No one had realized at that time that Christie's uterus had inverted and the baby's head was being pushed into the wall of the uterus instead of the cervix. This was discovered only after the specialist felt the real sac slip around from behind the spot she thought was the cervix. She suddenly realized that the amniotic sac she was attempting to break was in fact the uterine wall.

When the specialist suddenly realized the gravity of the situation, she demanded that the entire medical team meet out in the hall immediately. Todd left Christie's side to join them. The doctor stopped him and demanded that he remain in the room as they discussed the situation, but he refused. If any decisions were going to be made, he wanted to be in on it. He listened as the doctor told everyone to start setting up for an emergency cesarean. If the wall had been ruptured they would have to operate immediately.

Thankfully, Loretta and Bill remained calm as they joined me in assuring Christie that her job was to stay present with the baby and help him continue his journey down the canal. Together, we helped Christie remain calm and focused. The cesarean was unnecessary and called off when it was discovered the doctor had not ruptured the wall of the uterus as she had feared. When we changed Christie's position and sat her upright, the uterus corrected itself and her baby began a rapid descent.

Everyone scrambled to get the room ready for the delivery. Another specialist who had come in from another hospital took a seat at the foot of the delivery bed. There were so many medical people there I couldn't even begin to tell you who they were. Christie's family doctor stood at the side of the specialist. Her role in the delivery had been passed over when she called in an obstetrician. Suddenly, the baby's heart rate dropped dangerously low and the obstetrician announced, "I'm taking this baby out!"

I looked up, and with a shocked tone in my voice, I asked him what he intended to do. He simply put his hand in the air and said, "Give me the vacuum."

Christie opened her eyes and looked at him with fear written all over her face. When she saw the vacuum being handed to the doctor, she took a deep breath, closed her eyes, and pushed with all of her might. Suddenly, Todd, her parents, and I saw her determination to get her baby out before the doctor could attach the vacuum. We started shouting. "Go, Christie! You can do it! You can do it!" We were not at all quiet or subtle with our cheering. This was not like all the other births I'd attended where we had wanted the baby to be greeted with quiet, gentle voices. No, this baby was coming in with a cheering squad!

We weren't the only supporters to recognize Christie's wish to spare her baby the trauma of being vacuum extracted. Her family practitioner, a tiny Asian woman, stepped in front of the specialist to prevent him from getting to the baby. She put her hands out and helped the baby ease his way out of the canal all by himself. As he came out everyone saw the cord wrapped tightly around his neck and body. I heard several people say, "Oh, thank goodness she kept refusing pain medication."

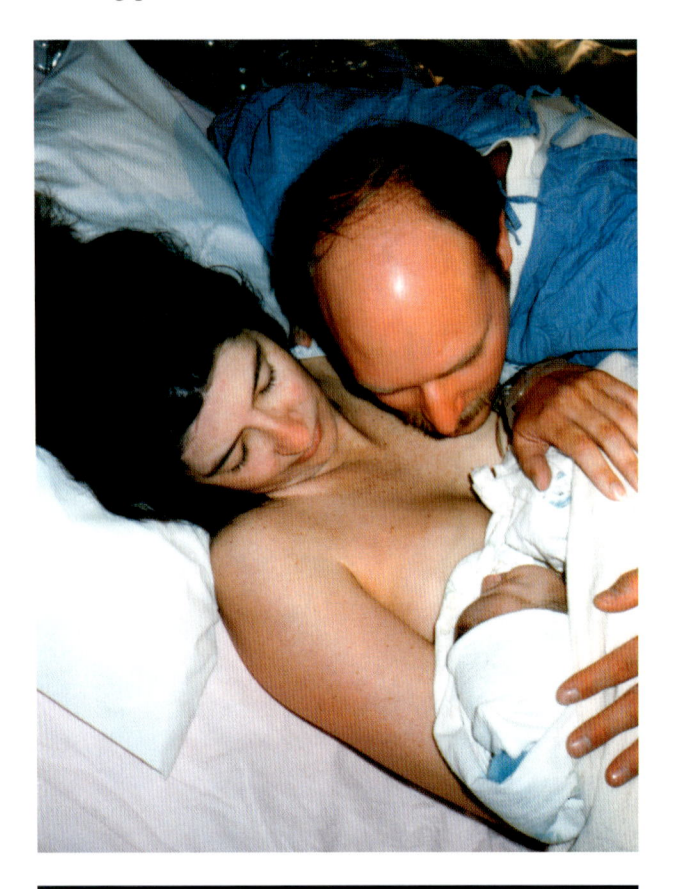

Pain medication will generally lower a baby's heart rate. That's why the nurse's will monitor a mother and her baby so carefully once they inject it. Generally, the lower heart rate is not significant enough to worry about. But if a compressed cord already compromises the baby, it could become life threatening. Christie's intuition to go in early kept her from compromising his life.

Christie's instinct to protect her baby from the vacuum was also accurate. Even under normal circumstances, the vacuum can be harmful to the baby's cranial system. If the baby doesn't slide right out with a slight tug of the vacuum, the doctor will pull harder. This has the potential to overstretch the dura mater that protects the blood vessels. The wall of the blood vessels can tear and cause a leak into the cranium. The vacuum can slip off easily

STEP 3: Create a Birth Team

> and may have to be reapplied several times before the baby is successfully extracted. This will result in rapid changes in cranial pressure that will negatively affect the entire craniosacral system.
>
> You will know a baby has suffered this type of injury if he develops a hematoma (a blood clot that applies pressure to the brain) somewhere on the head. If the body is not able to seal off the tear, it will continue to leak, which can eventually lead to brain damage.
>
> The cord was wrapped tightly around the baby's body. If the doctor had pulled hard to remove the baby quickly, he could have also pulled the placenta off the wall of the uterus. By allowing the baby to control how he maneuvered through the opening, there were no complications. The baby was just fine.

A bond was formed that day between this child, his parents, and his grandparents; nothing can compare with being present and helping at the most crucial moment in a child's life.

When things calmed down, I asked Christie's dad what he thought about witnessing the birth. He shook his head and said, "I have a whole new appreciation for my wife Loretta, but once is enough. I'll stay home and baby-sit for the next birth." And, much to Christi's dismay—he did.

Recommendation #3: Give siblings the opportunity to join the birth team.

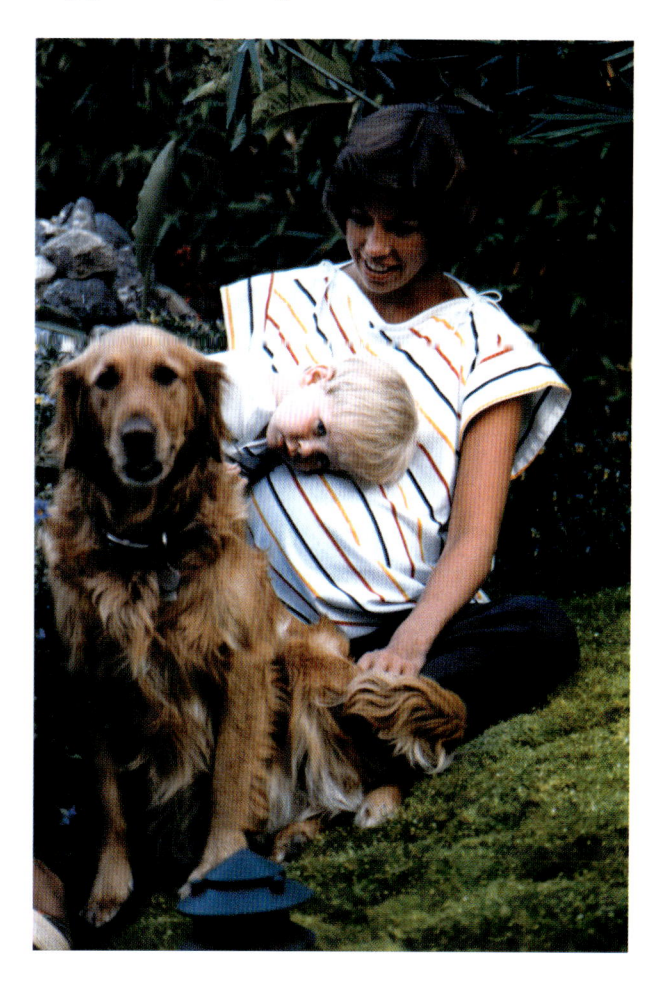

When a child witnesses the birth of their sibling, they have the opportunity to develop a strong bond that can't be broken. I have worked with many families who allowed their children to be present for the birth of their sibling. They report that the older child is protective toward the new baby and rarely demonstrates typical, developmental regression.

Hands Of Love

> It's common for an older toddler to lose ground in their potty training efforts, to want a bottle again, and to revert back to baby talk after the birth of another child. This doesn't seem to happen when they are involved in the birth and when the mother remains at home after the birth. Having a mother gone for several days, and then returning home with a newborn, can be traumatic for a small child who has not been away from his mother for any length of time. Anger expressed toward the baby may simply be a way of showing his mother how he feels about her leaving him for so long.

her eyes to look at her, Ashley lifted Frankie's blouse and announced, "There won't be much blood, Mommy." She dropped her mom's blouse back down and went on about her business.

A few minutes later, I suggested that Frankie move from the rocker to the bedroom. Ashley watched intently as her mother walked quickly over to the foot of the bed. As soon as she stepped onto the thick bedding we had set on the floor, Frankie's second baby came sliding out unexpectedly.

Ashley squealed with delight as I grabbed for the slippery body of baby Farrah. As I handed Farrah up to her mother, I realized that Ashley was right; there was no blood.

A stream of relatives came and went throughout the day after Farrah's birth, and each person wanted to hold the new baby. When I returned later in the day, I found Ashley sitting next to one of the guests as they held Farrah. Ashley had diligently sat with every visitor throughout the day with her hand resting protectively over her sister's chest. No one could convince Ashley that the baby was safe and she could go play.

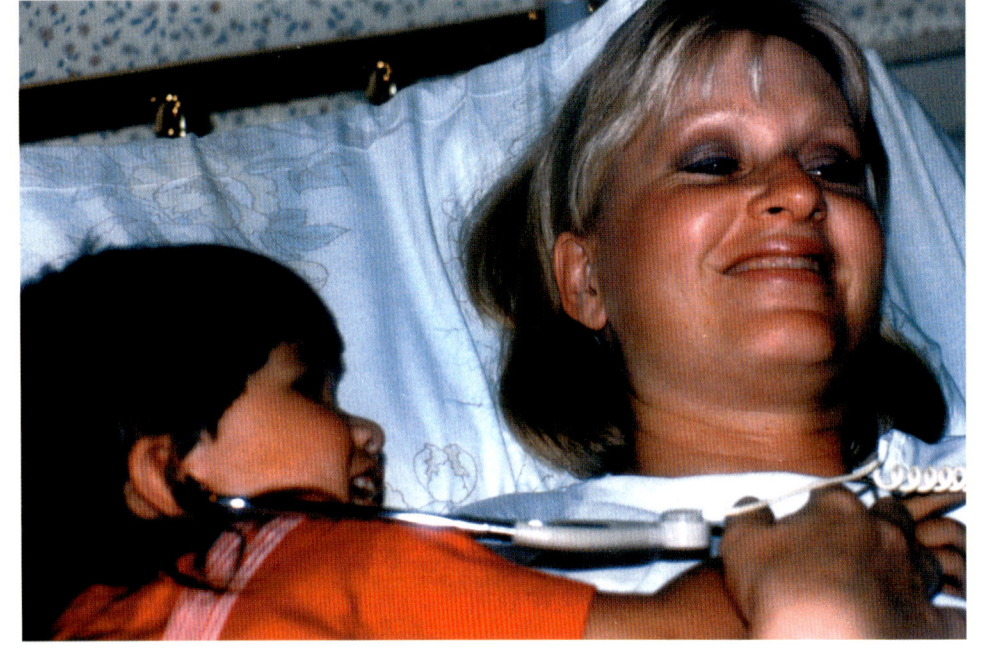

Many mothers do not consider the possibility of siblings attending the birth because they worry that the child will want attention and will not allow her to concentrate on laboring. It has been my experience that even young siblings recognize something special is happening when a mother is in labor. Rather than demand their mother's attention, siblings observe the action of others, and often mimic them by vocalizing with a mother or softly touching her belly during the contraction.

For example, remember the birth story of Frankie and her daughter, Ashley? During Frankie's second labor Ashley, who was just a few years old at the time, walked up to Frankie and stood there waiting for the contraction to subside. When Frankie opened

My friend, Vicky, and her daughter shared in the excitement of child birth by listening to the baby's heartbeat together. When a child is allowed to participate in this exciting event, sibling rivalry can be greatly reduced.

STEP 3: Create a Birth Team

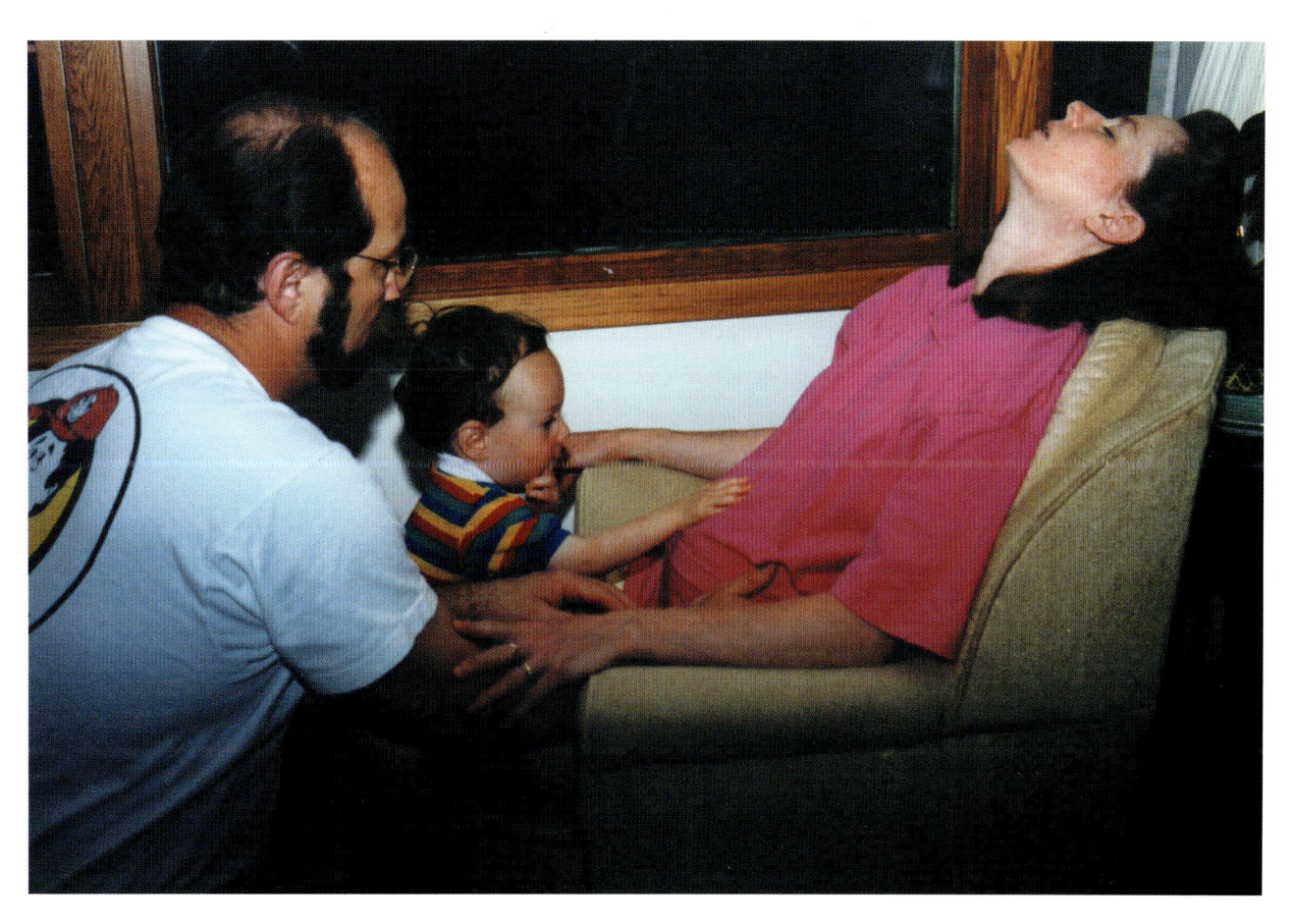

When I arrived at the home of Dr.'s Anne and Larry Spicer their son, Weston, was helping Anne get through an intense contraction. Anne's parents had arrived a few hours after the onset of active labor to give Weston a little labor support. Free to come and go, he would slip over from time to time to give his dad and mom a helping hand.

Interestingly, Anne had assumed the same position while she was in labor with Weston; during the wee hours of the morning, Anne had leaned back on the couch and listened, while Larry played a soft melody for her on the piano. I believe that somewhere, deep within Weston's subconscious, he remembered that night; he intuitively placed his hand over his brother and vocalized the O-O-O tone. Without any instruction, Weston was welcoming Brandon into the world just as we had welcomed him.

Hands Of Love

Here is the story of a family who allowed their toddler to view a birth at home, and to actively participate in providing a nurturing environment for his mother.

Luke

Written by Carol Rettman

Around midnight, I had been lying down with my husband Leon and my two-year-old son, Luke, when suddenly I felt a strange sensation. My water had broken and had begun leaking. Gosh! This was not what we expected! I told Leon I thought the water had broken and Luke sat right up in our bed. With excitement he asked, "Is the baby coming?" Somehow he knew the water breaking was significant. He then held our hands and walked downstairs with us to call our midwife, Brigette.

Brigette encouraged us to get some rest before the contractions started. We all went back to the waterbed and tried to sleep, but Luke was silly, giggling, and kissing me a lot. I finally asked him if he was excited and he exclaimed, "Yes!" After he calmed down and fell asleep, we moved him to a futon bed. Leon and I continued to sleep/rest as the night went on and we worked through contractions as they came. By 4:00 A.M. the pain was increasing and we decided to get the birthing tub prepared.

Around 7:00 A.M. we ate breakfast and went for a walk. It was a beautiful day with sunny skies and very little snow. We enjoyed the fresh air and green trees all around us. After walking for an hour or more, we returned home and the two midwives, Jan and Jeannie had arrived. They checked me and found I had dilated to seven centimeters. We decided to rest a bit more; Leon went to the futon and I went to the waterbed. My birth team had assembled and joined me in the bedroom. We all enjoyed the silent anticipation of transitioning to the next stage of labor.

Later, I walked through the house and worked through more contractions. I was expecting to have a difficult transition as I did with my previous pregnancies, but that never happened. (Carol's second baby is not in this story because she died during delivery from cord compression.)

We wanted to get the baby to engage more, so the midwives suggested we go into the shower and let the water hit the top of my tummy. It worked! Soon afterwards, I left the shower and Leon and I entered the birthing tub.

I remember being irritated by what seemed to be "idle talk" in the room. Luke seemed to be the only one who was totally focused on my comfort at that moment. I guess that was the point of transition.

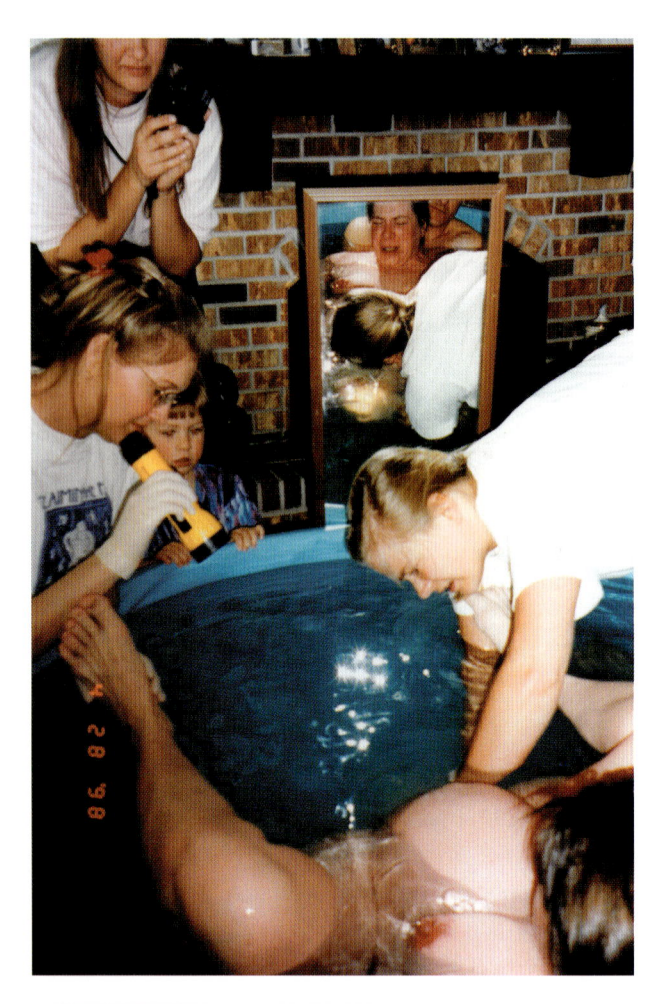

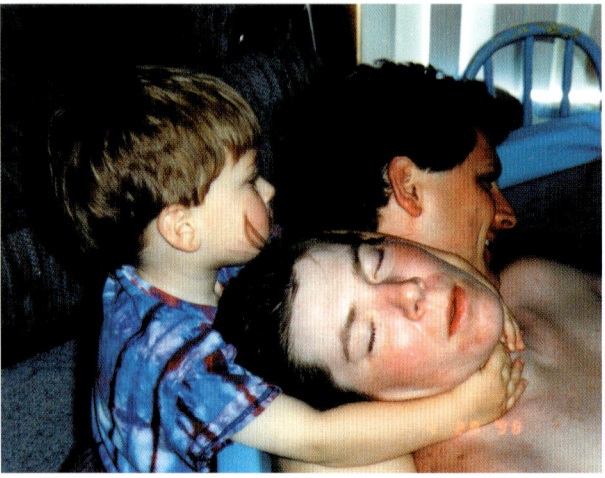

My goal was to be patient when the baby crowned, and with encouragement from the midwives, Kerry and Brigette, I put my hand on the baby's head. It was a gentle distraction for me and it allowed the baby to ease himself out. Luke climbed up on top of the couch to get a better view of the delivery and at 1:49 P.M. our beautiful baby boy, John, was born.

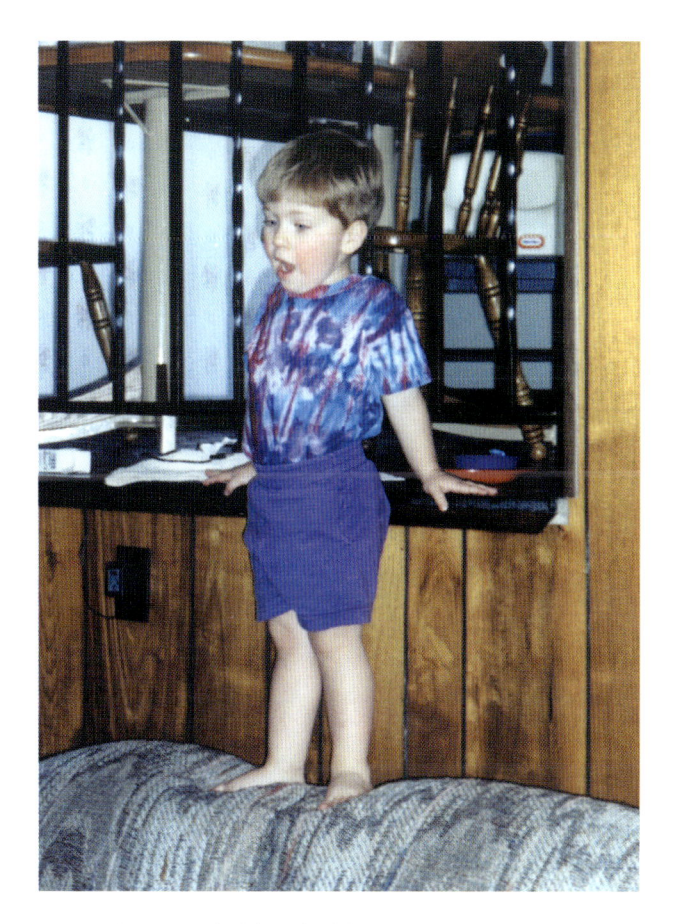

STEP 3: Create a Birth Team

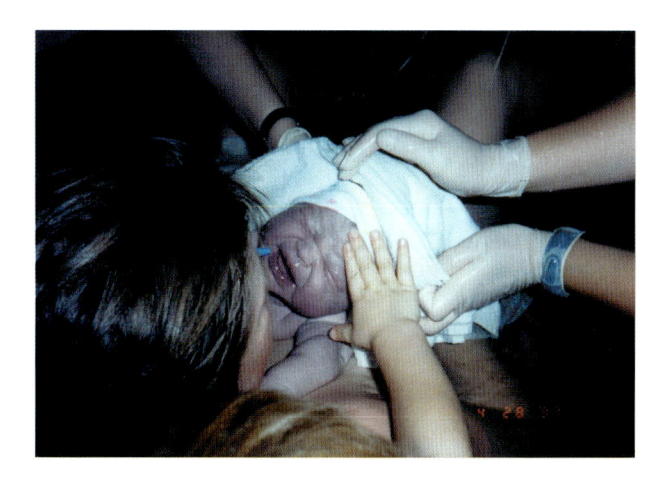

By early evening we transferred upstairs to our big futon bed. Luke joined us and fell asleep next to his new baby brother. It was a day we'll always remember and treasure!

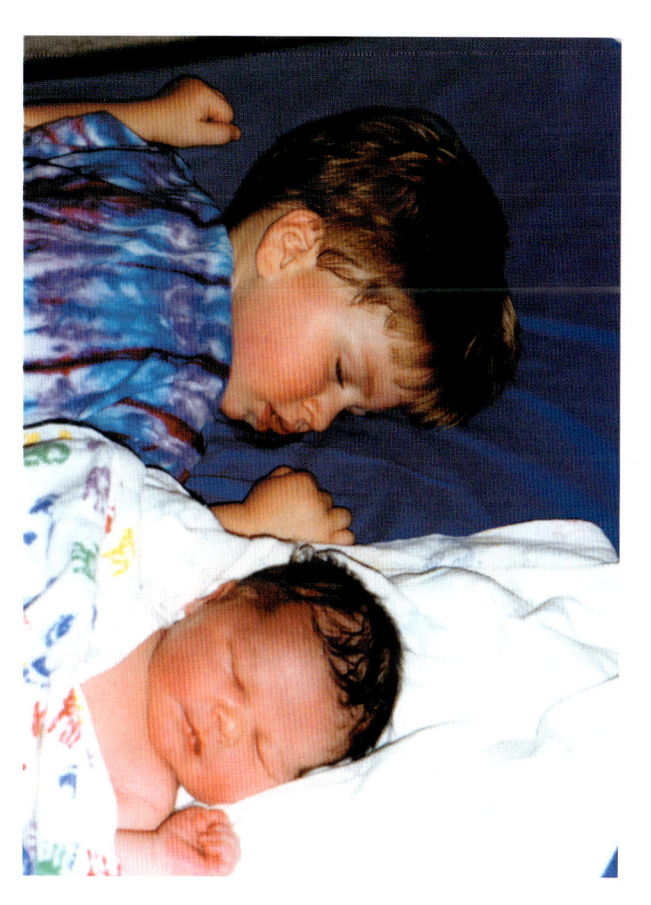

As Leon held us in his arms, Luke came to the side of the pool so he could reach out and touch John as if to say, "It's okay, baby." Shortly afterwards, Leon, John, and I stepped out of the tub. After I'd had a chance to size him up, I bundled John in blankets. He was 22 inches long and weighted 11 pounds and 6 ounces. A new record and a beautiful gift from God! Oh, he was so precious.

Many siblings regress in development after the birth of another child. Luke not only failed to go through that typical sibling regression period, he potty trained himself right afterwards. John is now seven months old and Luke is still an extremely protective and loving brother. John has never suffered from any form of illness since his birth, though he did have some cranial molding problems that required craniosacral therapy (his extremely large head had to do some shifting as he worked his way down the canal). Otherwise, thanks to a gentle loving entry into the world he has been a healthy, happy infant.

67

Hands Of Love

Parents who are thinking about including their older children at the birth usually quiz me by asking questions such as: 1) "Will my older child resent or reject the baby if he thinks the baby is causing my pain?" 2) "If complications arise that require fast action on the part of the medical team, should my daughter remain in the room?" 3) "Isn't childbirth too private to be shared with a child?"

These are valid concerns, but based on my clinical experience, I'd have to answer no to every question. My experience has been that siblings who have their own support person enjoy the event and will turn to their personal companion for guidance and assurance if they need attention or have questions. Their support person knows when to take them out of the room and when to stay. As far as the privacy goes, that is an individual decision that only the mother can make. My personal feeling is that we, as parents, should be the ones to prepare our children for life-changing events such as birth and death. Most boys and girls will experience childbirth sometime in their adult life. If we remove the mystery and fear of childbirth, our children will have the opportunity to enter the arena of birth with personal knowledge and confidence.

A colleague of mine welcomed her young son to the birth of his sibling. Afterwards, she sent me the following letter and pictures so I could share them with you. Here is how she felt about including an older child on the birth team.

Kevin

Written by Dr. Meg Simans

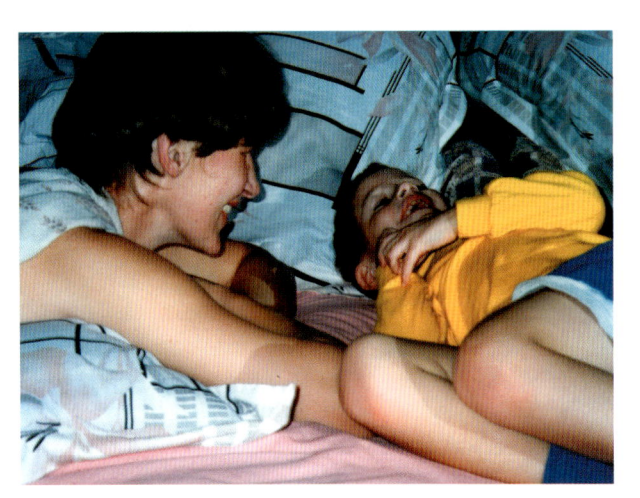

Dear Carol,

*My son's name is Kevin. His age at the time of my second birth was three years and seven months. The picture of he and I on the bed was taken during transition. Kevin came running up to the bedroom to see how I was doing. He patted my belly and said, "The baby is still in there!" Then he ran back downstairs to be with Grandpa, his "labor support person." Kevin kept telling us to be sure and call him when the baby was coming out. He **definitely** wanted to be present.*

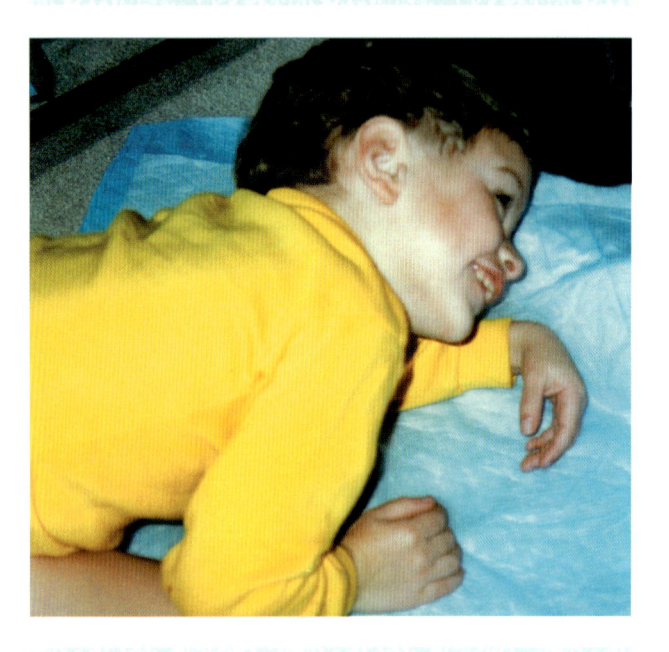

When the baby's head crowned, Kevin came sprinting up to the bedroom and got right down on the floor with the midwife, watching his baby brother, Corey, be born. Kevin saw the gush of amniotic fluid, blood, Mommy in pain, etc., all with smiling dimples and laughter, and a huge overwhelming sense of excitement beaming from his body.

I feel so fortunate to have experienced birth at home. It's the best! We are not having more children. However, giving birth so naturally, so comfortably, and so beautifully makes this a bittersweet decision. I can honestly say that giving birth at home was FUN!

With love, Meg

STEP 3: Create a Birth Team

Sarah

I once attended a birth where a five-year-old adopted daughter came with her own labor support person. With the help of her labor companion, this little girl, Sarah, visited the gift shop and brought back a basket of flowers. She spent time looking at the babies in the nursery in-between her visits to check on her mom. She watched TV in the waiting room and roamed the hospital floors.

When she entered the birthing room, she was quiet, observant, and only spoke when her mother, Alison, acknowledged her presence. Alison would always greet her daughter with warmth and admiration for how patient she was during the long hours of waiting. During one brief visit, Sarah whispered to me, "Can I help?" I said, "Sure." Before I could say anymore, Sarah was down on her knees rubbing her mother's exposed foot. After her mother voiced her appreciation for the wonderful foot rub, Sarah smiled and tiptoed out of the room.

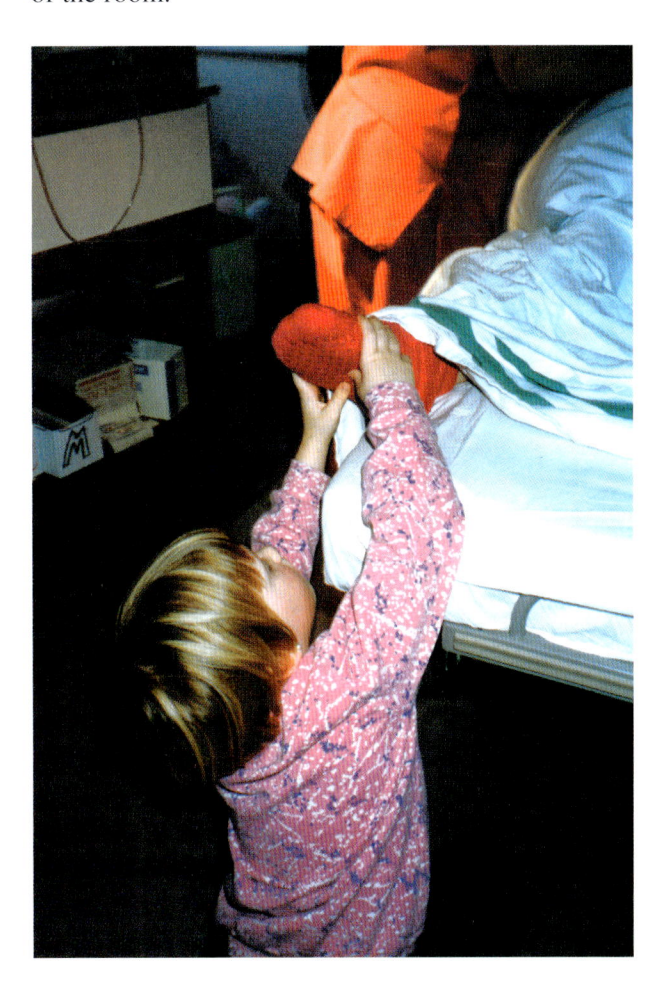

Alison had tested positive for a bacteria that can be fatal to a newborn—beta-hemolytic strep. Sarah sat quietly up on the nightstand watching her mother struggle to overcome the nausea, weakness, and exhaustion caused by an adverse reaction to the intravenously administered antibiotics.

Somewhere deep in Sarah's mind, I'm sure she was recording how a mother works through a difficult childbirth. Her mother never cried out. She never screamed. On the contrary, she was always loving and supportive of Sarah's presence in the room.

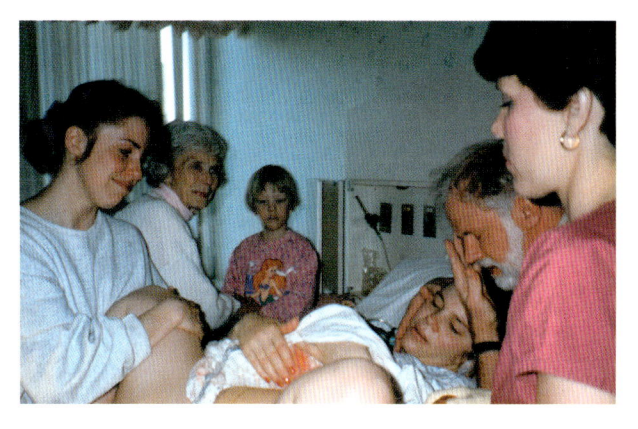

In the end, Sarah shared with her parents a very important time in their life. She saw the agony and the bliss. She saw her parents working together in a loving manner, and she saw her new baby sister come into the world. As an active participant rather than an absent outsider, she was spared the trauma and uncertainty that may have come into her life if she had been excluded from the life-changing miracle of her sister Zoie's birth.

Hands Of Love

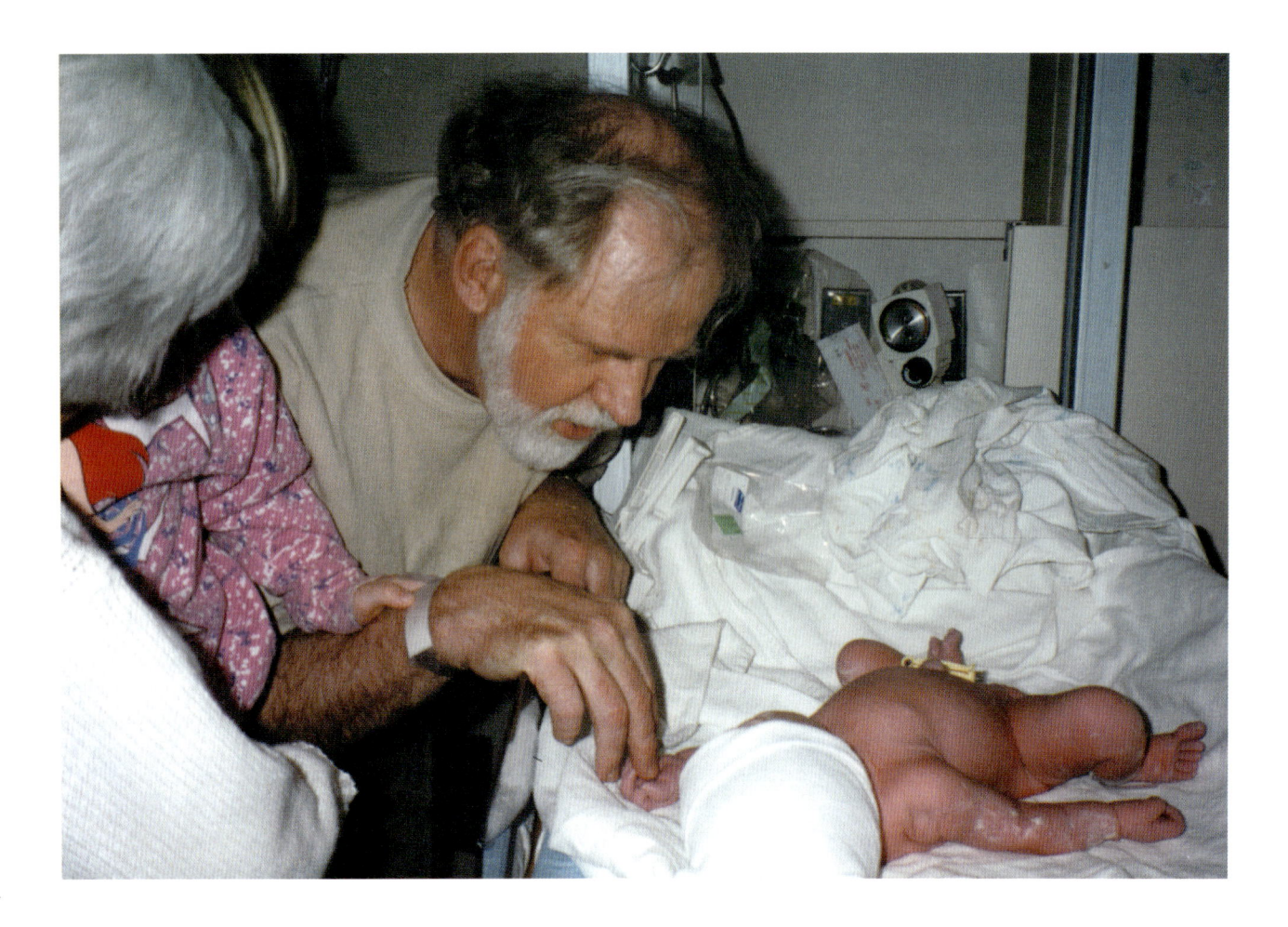

Sarah is held by her labor companion as she watches her dad welcome his new baby girl into the world.

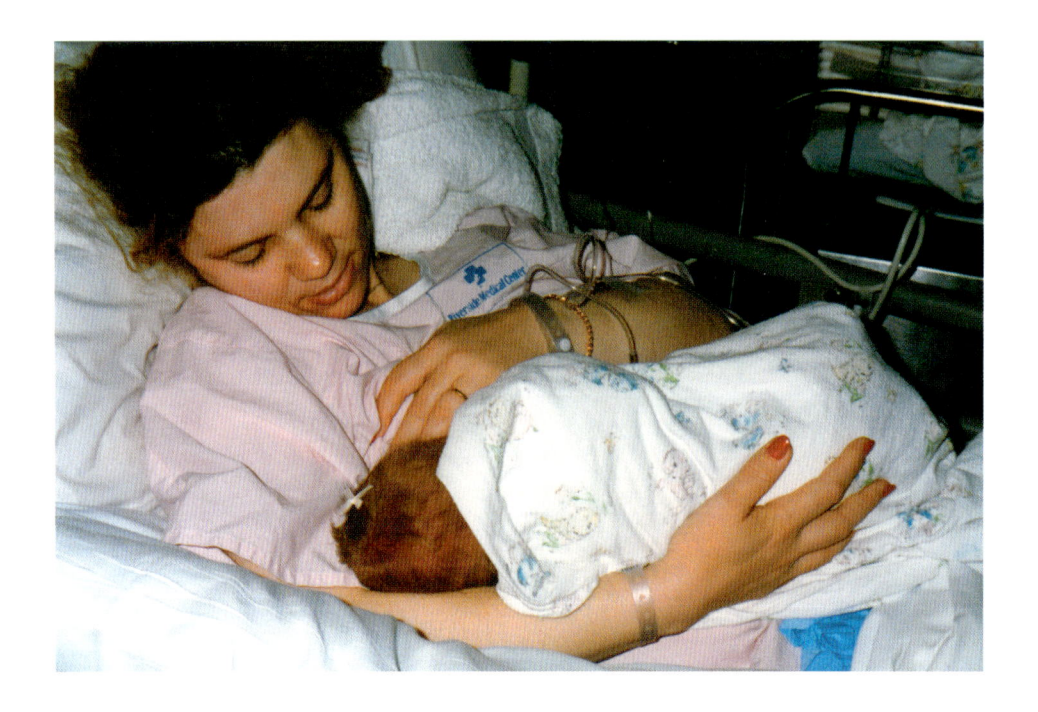

Sarah looks on as her sister, Zoie, nurses for the first time.

STEP 3: Create a Birth Team

Gretta and Luke

On another occasion, I was called over to help a patient who was having trouble maintaining active labor. She had gone to the hospital earlier that day, but was sent home for "failure to progress." I went to her home, adjusted her spine, and relaxed her pelvic floor muscles by doing Craniosacral Therapy. Afterwards, Jeanne's labor kicked in so quickly there was hardly enough time to get her back to the hospital. As we were leaving, I encouraged Jeanne to bring her two older children with us. I knew the baby could come at any minute and felt they would benefit from watching the birth. Jeannie agreed. Luke and Gretta grabbed their coats; we all giggled with excitement as we scrambled into the car. Approximately ten minutes after arriving at the hospital, Gretta and Luke witnessed the rapid birth of their little brother.

The baby's palate had molded incorrectly from his position in utero. After delivery, he continued to cry until I placed him on a pillow on my lap and encouraged him to suck on my finger. The bones at the roof of his mouth slowly moved into their proper position and his suck normalized. After about ten minutes of working with him Gretta took him from me and was able to hold him for a few minutes before he started crying again. This time, Jeannie took him and encouraged him to suck on her finger. Before long, he gave up her finger for he was now able to take her breast and nurse peacefully.

A few weeks after the birth, I received a picture and two letters from Luke and Gretta. Here is what they wrote.

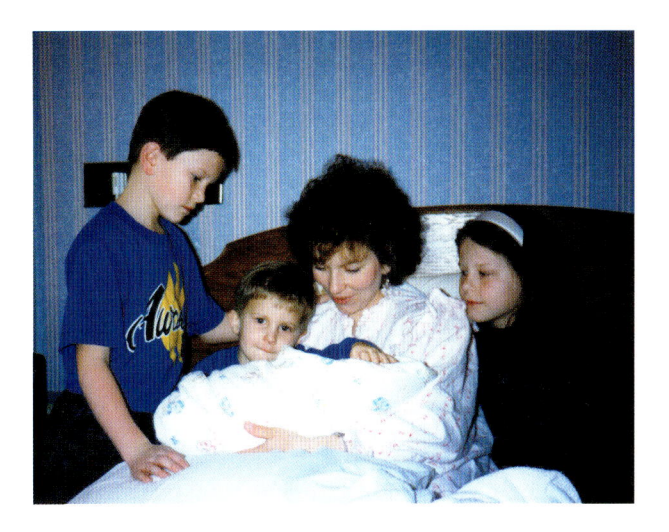

> Dear Dr. Phillips,
> Thank-you so much for letting me come to the birth. You really made being there special. Being there will be a great memory! It sure comforted my mom and me when we knew you were going to be there. Thanks for everything.
> Sincerely
> Luke

> Dear Dr. Phillips,
> Thank-you for making it posabul for us to see the birth! It made my mom and me feel more better when we new you wer coming. Thanks for helping my mom too. I like having michelle take care of us. I cannot wate until we see you agen.
> Love from
> Gretta

A few years later, Gretta and I worked together to provide labor support for her mom and dad at the birth of their fifth child. This time Gretta wasn't there just to observe the delivery; she was an active participant on the birth team and did an incredible job of assisting her parents in creating a birth environment that was full of love and compassion. When the baby decided to come, the medical staff stood off to the side as Gretta helped her father lift their new baby up into Jeanne's arms. There wasn't much for the rest of us to do but stand back and watch. It was an experience I will never forget.

Here is the story of a family who allowed their eight-year-old to videotape the birth of his sibling, Izabella. It may have been a struggle for his mom, but he was as cool as... a big brother.

Alex

Written by: Jody Peterson Lodge

People thought I was crazy when they heard of my plans to have my son attend the birth of his sibling—seven years his junior. But I felt strongly that if this, *up until now, only child* was going to welcome a new baby into his home, he would have to witness this little person's arrival. After all, not only was a new life about to be born, but his, mine, and ours was about to change dramatically.

My husband, Chuck, and I had been taking Bradley classes, but I felt they were too graphic and intimidating to share with our son, Alexander. No matter how "beautiful" the whole thing was portrayed, I didn't want to scare him. Therefore, we arranged to take a birthing class for siblings at the hospital. They used dolls and a watcher-friendly film of a woman giving birth. Alexander got the idea, without all of the intimate details.

Chuck and I agreed that when we arrived at the hospital, the baby should give her big brother a "birth day" gift—something to entertain and distract him. We also hoped a gift would help Alex realize he would always be special, even if he was no longer our only child. We also arranged for my mother, who had photographed his birth in excruciating detail, to be there with him. Together, they would videotape the arrival of this new baby.

I had asked Carol to become my prenatal chiropractor and delivery doula soon after our initial meeting in the summer of 1995. I had initially selected her based on her skill and unique qualifications. After six months in her care, I felt I would also benefit from her intelligence and optimistic belief system. She soon convinced me that childbirth didn't have to be as painful as my first delivery.

During the last few weeks of pregnancy, I experienced many episodes of false labor. I grew increasingly frustrated every time the contractions stopped until Carol explained that this was the ideal way for the baby to make his way down the birth canal; soft and slow was ultimately good for everyone.

I was four days overdue when I had my last prenatal visit with Carol. I was playing the waiting game and was just plain miserable. By then, I had done my research and informed Carol that I was going to use herbal stimulants to get active labor started. I wanted to get the show on the road. I was ready. Carol adjusted my aching body, balanced my cranial system and soothed away my anxiety. She encouraged me not to take the herbs and told me that the baby would come when it was ready.

By 9:00 P.M. that night, I finally went into labor. I called Carol right away when I saw that I had passed my mucus plug. Next, I called my mom. I told them to hurry. They each had a long drive to our home and there was a typical Minnesota snowstorm waiting in the wings.

A soft snow was falling and a fire was ablaze in the fireplace. Tony Bennett was crooning Christmas ballads on the stereo. Outside, the crystalline ice glistened in the dark (Alexander had strung little white lights on anything faintly resembling a pine needle). Inside, a gigantic Christmas tree made the living room look cozy and inviting.

After packing and showering, I dressed for the photo session in which I would soon be *co-starring*. Nearly complete, I held off on one important detail. When Carol arrived a few moments later I asked her to do the honors of painting my toe nails fire engine red. A first for even her!

When my mom arrived at the house a short time later, my contractions had finally fallen into a regular pattern. They were regular but not strong enough to keep our little birthing party from indulging in huge bowls of chocolate, chocolate chip ice cream (which had become a basic food group during my last trimester). When the contractions hit their peak, I simply stood up and started O-O-O-ing. Without so much as a thought, everyone would stand up and "O-O-O" with me until the contraction was over. Then the talking, laughing, and eating continued without skipping a beat. Alexander enjoyed this part of the party!

Around 11:00 P.M. Carol said we were having too much fun and decided it was going to be quite awhile before the big event. She insisted that we get some rest. Oddly, it seemed as if everyone was a lot more tired than I was. Chuck and Alexander said their goodnights and went to catch a few winks in Alex's room. My mother and I headed for the loft, while Carol curled up on the sofa below.

I couldn't sleep. The contractions were getting more intense. It was hard to get serious though, because my silly mother was spooned against me whispering how brave I was. She kept saying things that were sure to keep me laughing. Carol listened from the sofa below. She mixed laughter with threats as she told us to get some sleep.

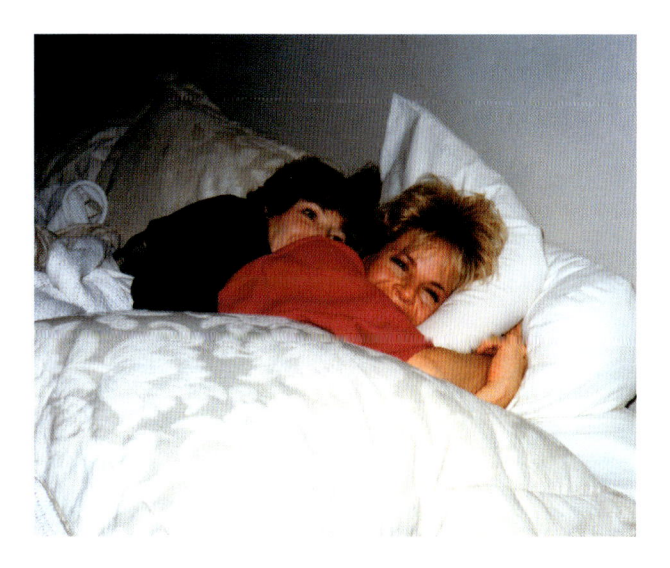

After close to an hour of unsuccessful rest, Carol crept up the stairs with the video camera. Mom and I felt like two schoolgirls getting caught with our hands in a cookie jar.

Minutes after Carol came upstairs, the pain of labor became really intense. As in my first labor, my lower back was tremendously painful. I could not fathom lying down. I got up with every contraction and wrapped my arms around either my mom's neck or Carol's. I would hang from them, which elongated my torso while I chanted my O-O-O-ing sounds. With all of the commotion, Chuck and Alexander were soon up. I stopped joking around! A look of worry now crept over Alexander's face.

It was just past midnight and I wanted to get to the hospital. Fearing we might have hours of labor ahead of us, Carol encouraged me to stay home awhile longer. I tried to remain good-natured, but I was firm. It was time to go. By 1:00 A.M. we were ready and had everything loaded in the car.

Driving in separate cars, we found ourselves caravaning on the icy highway for the forty-minute drive to the hospital. There was silence as Chuck, Alexander, and I rode alone in our car. I was no longer in a mood to talk. In fact, I could barely remain seated. I twisted and moaned the whole way there, honestly believing I was dying. I was unable to say anything, fearing that I would psychologically damage Alex forever. Oh, the things I wanted to shout and didn't.

We piled out of the car at the hospital. Realizing that I was no longer able to walk, I was rolled into admissions by wheel chair. Although we had pre-signed everything, it seemed there was another maze of paperwork to plow through before they would *let me* have the baby.

My mother (the queen of positive thinking) continued to whisper to me how brave I was. It was a wonderful distraction, although the only thing I kept thinking was, *as if I have a choice*. I knew whatever Alex witnessed would remain in his memory banks—connected to this baby—forever. I had no choice but to be brave.

Finally, we were in the birthing room that we had selected weeks earlier. A big room. Big enough for everyone on the birth team to walk around and sprawl out comfortably. Carol turned on the crockpot that contained grated ginger compresses, took out the massage oils, and turned on a soothing tape. Chuck handed our carefully prepared birth plan to the nursing staff and arranged candles to improve the hospital's austere atmosphere. Mom and Alex rubbed my shoulders as I rocked back and forth on the only spot I felt comfortable—the toilet.

Then the nurse appeared. She hit the overhead light switches, blew out the candles, and ruined the mood we had carefully orchestrated for baby's arrival. (Can't have an open flame in the hospital.) She demanded I change into a hospital gown, and hooked me to the fetal monitor. Her ten-minute ultrasound strip required that I lay down on the bed. It was agonizing. The nurse's militant manner made me feel as if everything was falling apart.

Chuck pulled out Alexander's gift from the baby—a Nintendo Game Boy. Alexander was thrilled to have something to play with. He and mom went out to the waiting room for awhile as I meekly obeyed the nurse's orders.

About ten minutes later, our midwife, Kathleen, poked her head in the door. I almost jumped off the bed with joy. Now she would become first in command. More importantly, she was the midwife I had hoped would be on call. I loved how she embraced the spirituality of pregnancy and birth. I had hoped she'd be there when we welcomed our little one into the world.

Kathleen quickly examined me and pronounced that I was dilated to a three. Three? THREE?!- There had to be some kind of mistake. This kind of pain I remembered around the time they tell you, "You're dilated to nine. Any minute now. You're doing great Jody. It's almost over." Not three as in, "You may still have hours of this to go—three?" How in the world was I going to make it without taking drugs?

Be brave, be brave, I chanted inside. I ripped off the fetal monitor straps and stood up. When the contractions hit, I'd squat or hang from the nearest victim's neck. I felt so sorry for everyone, but it was the only position that I intuitively felt would help the baby come down the birth canal. It was all so intense I couldn't talk. I was so glad that Alexander was out playing with his new video game.

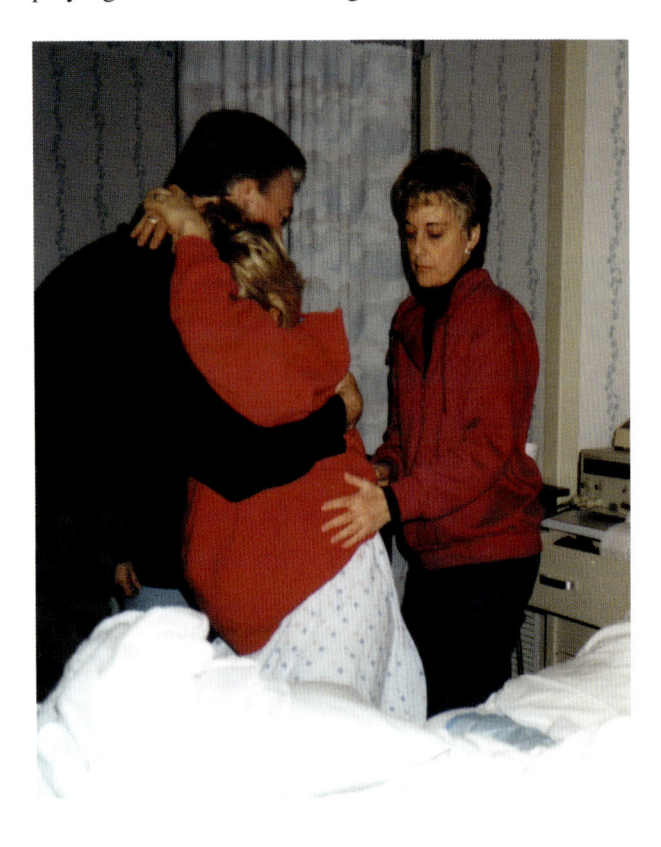

Kathleen watched a few contractions and sensed a shift in my progress so she rechecked my cervix. To everyone's surprise but mine, I had rapidly dilated to a full ten!

Now the excitement rose. Alexander and my mother came back into the room and began filming the delivery.

Because of the intense backlabor, there was no way I was going to lie in bed. I felt as if my tailbone would snap off with each contraction. Thankfully, Carol was there to push on my sacrum and rock me back and forth. When the contraction hit, I would lean across the birthing bed and hold on to the opposite side rails. Trying not to overdramatize the ordeal, I would bury my head in the bedding and beg Carol to push, while Kathleen urged me to do the same.

I had pushed twice during my labor with Alexander, so I hadn't planned on this. Soon, Chuck stood across the bed from me and had me hang around his neck as I pushed. I almost pulled all 220 pounds of him across the bed with every contraction. Carol kept pushing on my sacrum and O-O-O-ing with me. Kathleen, on the other hand, was patiently squatting at my feet in the catcher's position.

The baby's head finally crowned; the excitement was electric. Alexander took over the video camera. The nurse stood by the warming table waiting for the baby. Everyone was yelling "Push, Jody, push!" It took a good twenty minutes before the head was finally out. Thick black hair and eyes wide open. Alexander started yelling, "It's a boy! It's a boy!" He wanted a baby brother as much as I was hoping to give him a little sister to love.

I kept pushing until the tone in the room changed dramatically. I could tell by the whispers and the orders given that our situation was suddenly serious. The cord had wrapped around the baby's neck and she was turning blue. "Push the emergency button!" Kathleen instructed my husband. "We need a doctor."

Kathleen stood up and looked deeply into my eyes and said, "It is now time to push your baby out." It was clear that she meant—right now! I was completely on empty and I felt like collapsing in a pile of tears. Had Alexander not been there, I don't know if I would have been brave enough to keep pushing, because I honestly feared that it would break my back. But, I pushed and moaned, and in spite of myself, I let out one scream. At 4:01 A.M. Izabella was born! She was limp, blue and completely unresponsive.

Our birth plan had instructed the staff not to remove the baby from me or to cut the umbilical cord until it had stopped pulsing. Instead, Kathleen had to immediately cut the cord and Izabella was rushed to the warming unit. The overbearing nurse pushed Kathleen away in her attempt to make Izabella breathe by slapping the bottoms of her feet, roughly rubbing her head with a towel and jostling her around in a frenzy. Everything I had hoped to protect our baby from was suddenly happening. I collapsed over the side of the bed with the clamped cord, which was still attached to the placenta, swinging between my knees. A pool of blood was collecting at my feet. My mom, watching from the corner, was crying softly. Alexander calmly continued videotaping until Chuck took him and my mom into the hall. Everyone anticipated the worst. There was such a panic in the room, yet I felt completely removed from it. It was a strange combination of exhaustion and peace. Carol softly whispered to me, "Go to your baby." Her words seemed to hypnotically move me over to the warmer where Izabella lay waiting for me. As I looked down on my baby's little body, Carol said, "Call her."

STEP 3: Create a Birth Team

"Hi Izabella, at last you've come." She responded to my words by opening her eyes, taking a breath and smiling at me. She was so beautiful I wondered if, at that very moment, I was looking into the eyes of God. The nurse quickly took over and Kathleen canceled the call for a doctor. I went back to bed for the delivery of the placenta. Afterwards, Kathleen sutured a few tears, while the nurse continued to check Izabella's airways. Chuck rushed Mom and Alexander back into the room to welcome Izabella into the world.

Moments later, she was brought to me. Naked and creamy, Chuck placed her on my chest. She nuzzled in and began bobbing at my nipples—lifting her head from time to time to look into my eyes. We stayed that way for hours, only rising to move to the postpartum room where Alexander and Chuck were sleeping on a cot. Carol checked Izabella's head and spine and stayed in the room to keep an eye on her until just after the sun came up. After a few hours of sleep, Chuck and Alex headed for home.

When the day nurse came in that next morning, she found me dancing with Izabella to the music I had been playing to her for months—"Look What Love Has Done" by Mary Chapen Carpenter. The nurse appeared embarrassed to be witnessing such intimacy and left us alone for our dance. Later, she returned to take Izabella off to be cleaned up and photographed. When she returned it was official, a pink bow now stuck to the top of her head. I had a little girl.

In spite of the large age spread between our children, they have remained extremely connected. Alexander explains it like this, "When she was hanging upside down with her eyes wide open—she saw me first!"

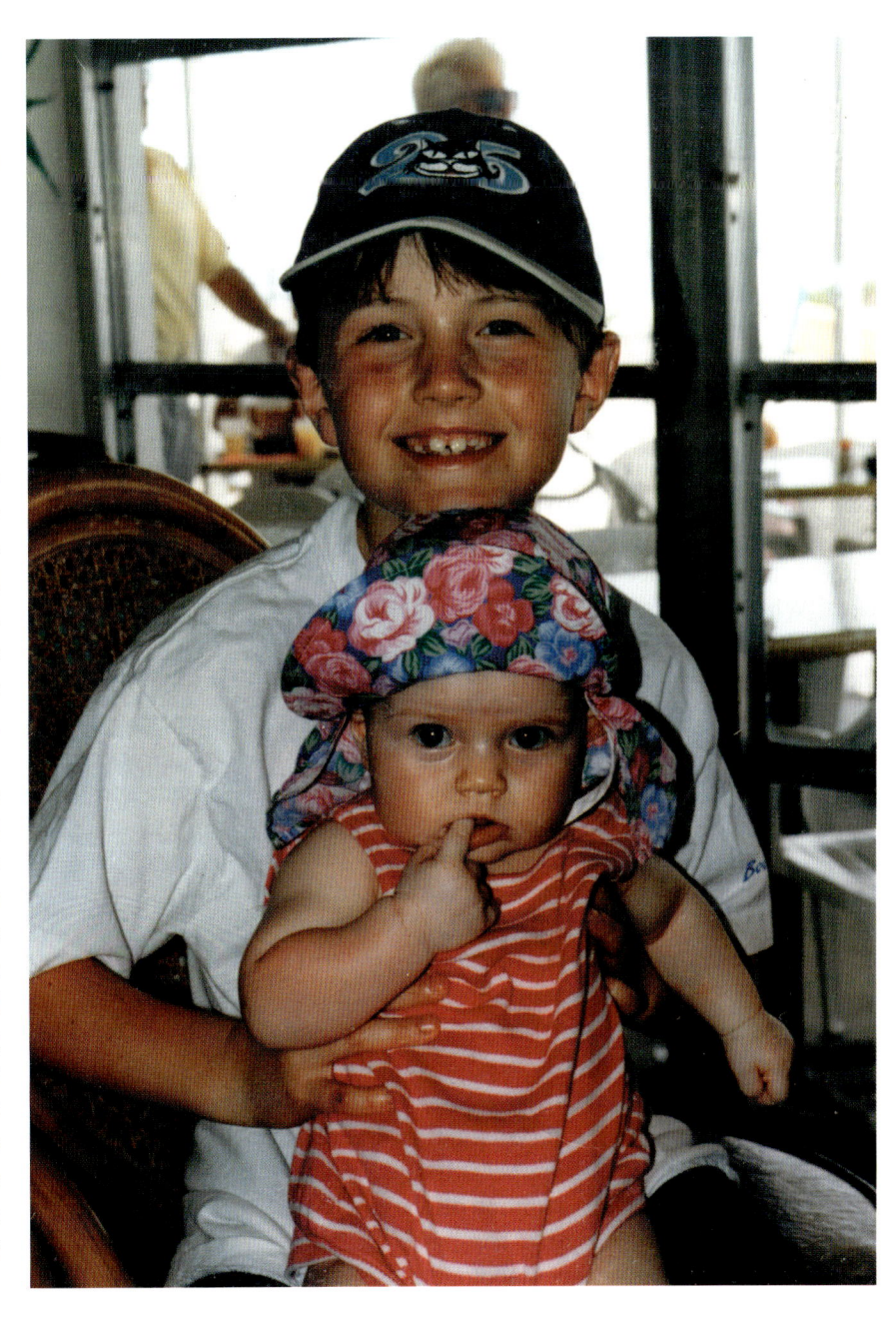

Hands Of Love

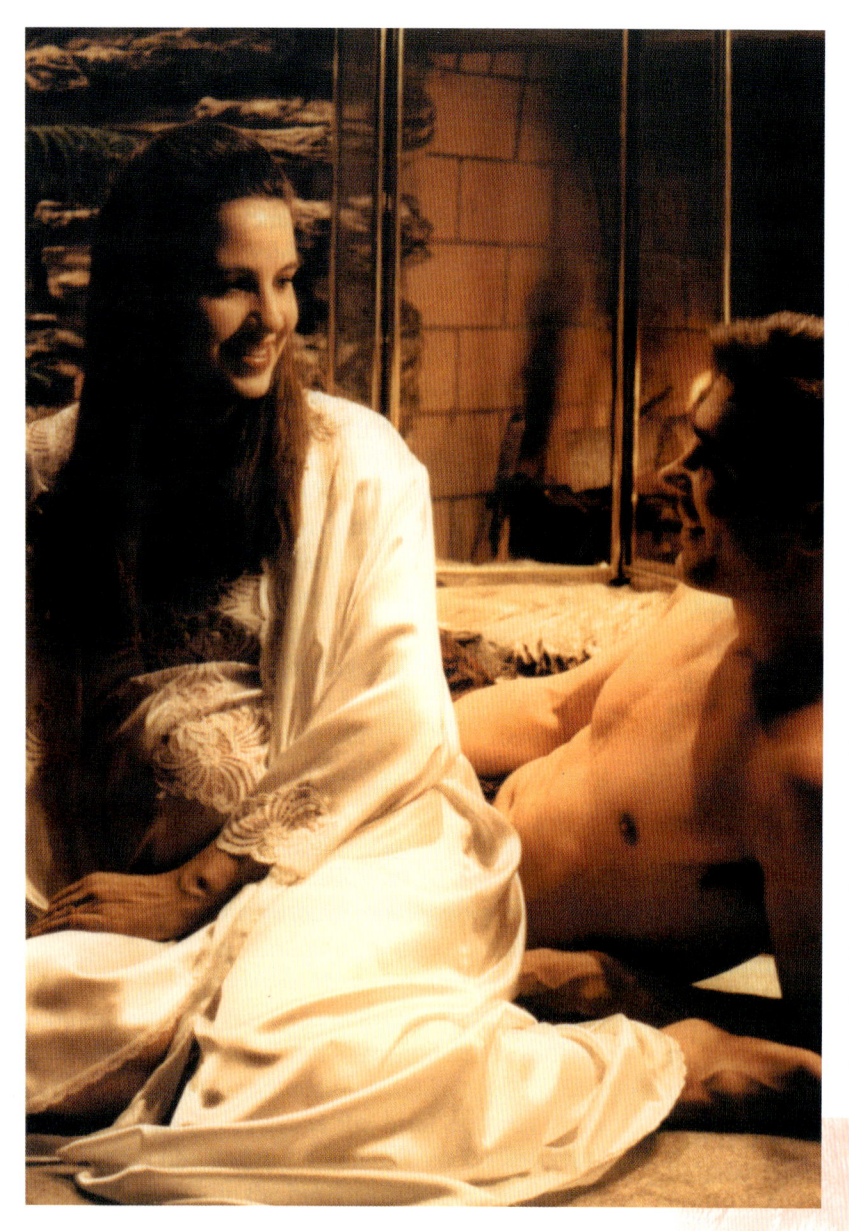

Just before graduation, I received a surprise invitation to join them for lunch. Murray blurted out their exciting news as soon as I arrived; Shannon was pregnant. They hadn't even told their family the good news, and they were already asking me to be a member of their birth team. I knew right then that these two were going to make wonderful parents.

During our lunch conversation, Murray seemed confident and sure about his decision to have a homebirth. Shannon, on the other hand, appeared reserved and apprehensive. Later, I spoke with Shannon alone. Although I fully supported Murray's plans for a homebirth, I wasn't sure if Shannon did. I had watched her eyes as Murray spoke with unguarded enthusiasm, and I listened to her unspoken words of fear. I felt I had to encourage her to thoroughly investigate all of her options and to follow her heart before finalizing any plans.

Only Shannon knew her limits. I encouraged her to follow her instincts and stay within those limits. She agreed to search deep within to find what was best for her and for her baby.

Birth is a Family Affair

First babies generally do not come into the world very quickly, and this birth was no exception. In Shannon's case, labor lasted approximately eighteen to twenty hours. To get a realistic picture of how she ended up delivering in her own bedroom surrounded by family and friends, I think it is only fair to begin this story by going back nine months.

As a husband and wife chiropractic team, Dr.'s Shannon and Murray Smith are passionate about three things: God, family, and chiropractic. I met them while they were still in chiropractic college. As students in my pediatric class, they were clearly devoted to each other and to the concept of pediatric chiropractic care.

SHANNON: *Initially, I had mixed feelings about the idea of a homebirth. I knew from all my previous training that I had to be comfortable with whatever arrangements we made, or my fear and apprehension could negatively effect the outcome of my birth. We interviewed many people before we made a decision about what type of birth attendant we wanted. In the end, when we agreed to have a homebirth, we hired both a midwife and an obstetrician. The OB was chosen because she already had a reputation for providing backup support to homebirth parents. She didn't hesitate to tell us she thought we were crazy, but she understood we intended to deliver the baby at home unless there were any complications along the way.*

STEP 3: Create a Birth Team

"Hi Izabella, at last you've come." She responded to my words by opening her eyes, taking a breath and smiling at me. She was so beautiful I wondered if, at that very moment, I was looking into the eyes of God. The nurse quickly took over and Kathleen canceled the call for a doctor. I went back to bed for the delivery of the placenta. Afterwards, Kathleen sutured a few tears, while the nurse continued to check Izabella's airways. Chuck rushed Mom and Alexander back into the room to welcome Izabella into the world.

Moments later, she was brought to me. Naked and creamy, Chuck placed her on my chest. She nuzzled in and began bobbing at my nipples—lifting her head from time to time to look into my eyes. We stayed that way for hours, only rising to move to the postpartum room where Alexander and Chuck were sleeping on a cot. Carol checked Izabella's head and spine and stayed in the room to keep an eye on her until just after the sun came up. After a few hours of sleep, Chuck and Alex headed for home.

When the day nurse came in that next morning, she found me dancing with Izabella to the music I had been playing to her for months—"Look What Love Has Done" by Mary Chapen Carpenter. The nurse appeared embarrassed to be witnessing such intimacy and left us alone for our dance. Later, she returned to take Izabella off to be cleaned up and photographed. When she returned it was official, a pink bow now stuck to the top of her head. I had a little girl.

In spite of the large age spread between our children, they have remained extremely connected. Alexander explains it like this, "When she was hanging upside down with her eyes wide open—she saw me first!"

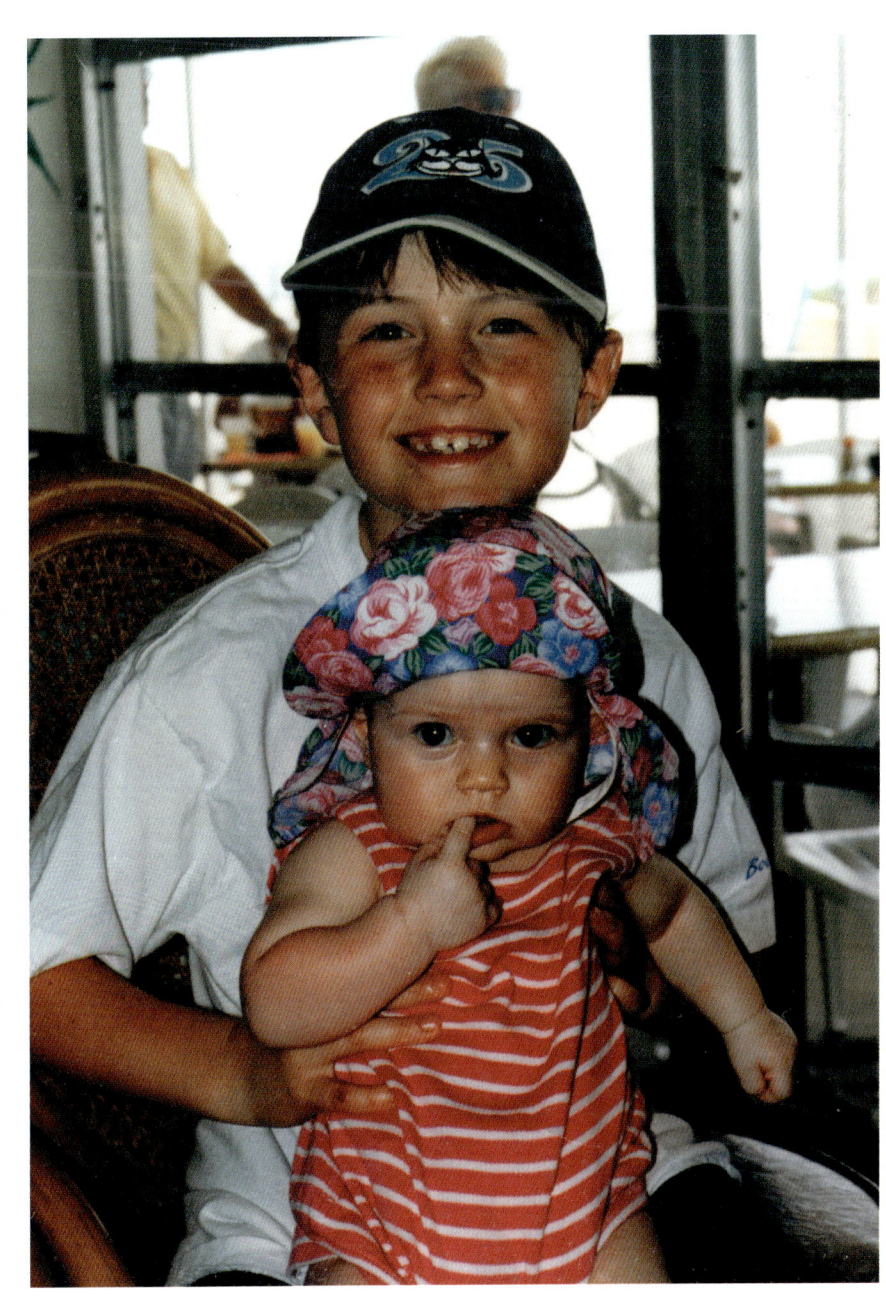

75

Recommendation #4: Welcome friends who wish to help you and themselves by witnessing the miracle of birth.

In ancient times, women were assisted during childbirth by others in the community. Having had a baby themselves, these women were handing down their cultural birthing practices from one generation to the next. Therefore, young women viewed birth as a rite of passage into womanhood.

That rite of passage changed its appearance when childbirth became a medical event. Birthing women were now taken into an operating room, where they delivered their babies in the presence of strangers. As a result, childbirth evolved into a mysterious event that the experienced woman barely remembered, and the uninitiated greatly feared.

Now, we find pregnant women and their partners trying to take the mystery out of childbirth by attending classes to learn how to give and receive the emotional and physical support that friends and family members used to provide. Some are learning that the best way to prepare for childbirth is to witness the experience firsthand.

When friends are allowed to assist in the physical support of a birthing mother, they are given the opportunity to eliminate their own fear of the unknown. With guidance, they can also provide the emotional support that often helps the birthing mother conquer her own fear of childbirth and deal positively with any unusual complications.

For example, here is the brief account of an experience I had with a woman who ended up having three neighbors join the birth team at the last minute. None of the women had planned on attending the birth, but each one was vital to the final outcome.

The early stage of Brenda's labor was long and slow. A chronic sufferer of headaches due to TMJ problems, Brenda had to endure jaw pain and headaches that were intensified with each contraction. Brenda's neighbors helped out by watching her two boys, cooking meals, and by trying to take her mind off the pain with jokes and conversation. I adjusted her spine, performed craniosacral therapy, and even photographed her in front of the fireplace in an attempt to distract her from the pain. We did get some beautiful photographs, but nothing I did took her mind off the jaw and head pain.

When it was time to go to the hospital all three friends made arrangements to join us. We had been together for so long at that point that they all wanted to stay until the birth was complete. Brenda's doctor decided to augment her slow labor with pitocin. While this worked to speed up the frequency of her contractions, Brenda now had to deal with the intensity of the artificially induced contractions along with the pain in her head.

Brenda's friends rallied around her when the contractions became extremely intense. They helped her husband, Colin, use cold rags to cool her down when her body began to sweat from the exertion of labor. I taught Colin and her friends how to help Brenda by using visualization to substitute the pain of labor for a similar sensation that she remembered as tough but pleasurable.

I asked Colin, to think of a time when Brenda had to exert a great deal of physical effort, while at the same time, experiencing emotional joy. Colin caught on immediately. As soon as a contraction started, Colin, who had Brenda cradled in his arms, would lean over her shoulder and speak softly into her ear. He spoke of a special time they had biking through a beautifully wooded park. Brenda listened to his voice and put herself back on the bike. Brenda's friends and I circled around her and listened as the two of them biked up steep hills and coasted down the other side. Colin reminded her of the beautiful scenery all around them, the breeze flowing through her hair, and the water that flowed along the side of the path.

When Colin took a break to go to the bathroom, Brenda's friends stepped in and talked her through the same visualization. Despite her pain, Brenda was able to relax her body and work with the baby as she turned the pain of the contraction into a similar sensation of exertion and relief.

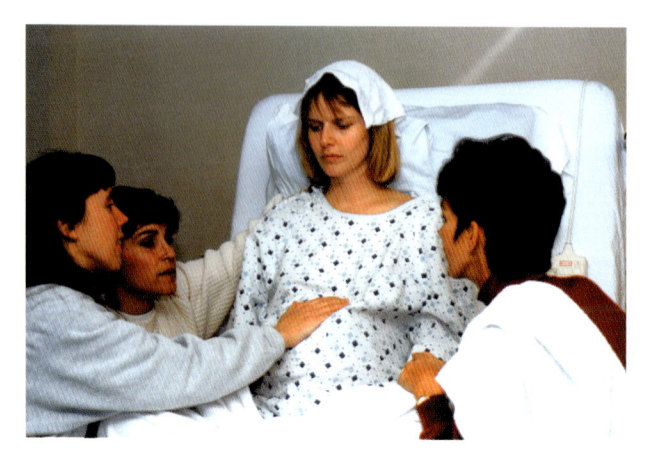

One of Brenda's friends had the most beautiful brown eyes you can imagine. To maintain her focus on the baby instead of the pain Brenda would stare into her friend's eyes. Brenda never broke her gaze

STEP 3: Create a Birth Team

throughout those final-pushing contractions. Finally, Justin made his way into the world without any other medical intervention.

The labor was hard on both Brenda and baby Justin, but with the emotional support of her birth team, Brenda succeeded in avoiding additional intervention that would have compounded the physical problems they both had endured.

~~

As you begin to form a birth team, it's a good idea to ask a number of people to be with you, but don't count on all of them being available at the time of delivery. Create your dream team, put the outcome in the hands of God, and trust that the right people will be there if you need them. I've rarely seen a birth team come together exactly as planned, but always exactly right for the situation.

If you have a long, exhausting labor, it's nice to have several people who can take turns resting and eating. Consequently, you will always have people with you who are fairly rested, moderately nourished, and emotionally supportive.

I'd strongly encourage you to welcome both men and women who express an interest in becoming a member of your birth team. With the current involvement we now envision for expectant fathers, they need real-life experience as much as women do. They, too, would benefit from helping at a birth before they are expected to assist the woman they love. You'd be surprised how many men have told me they would love to assist at a birth, but they are reluctant to ask because they don't feel they would be welcomed.

Trust me when I say that men can be extremely helpful when they provide support with the physically draining task of holding up a woman who wants to hang vertically from someone's shoulders.

Are you shocked at the thought of allowing a man to assist during birth? Ever consider having a male obstetrician deliver your baby? Is there a difference?

Now, I would like to share with you the story of two chiropractors, Dr.'s Shannon and Murray Smith. During the birth of their first child, they opened their hearts and their home to family members and friends. Their homebirth experience was the ideal—if there is such a thing. During her pregnancy, Shannon received prenatal care from a direct-entry midwife, from the obstetrician who agreed to provide backup support, and from me. Shannon and Murray wanted their first child to benefit from what each profession had to offer. My initial role was to help Shannon, but in the end it was to supervise and teach the other members of the birth team what to do.

Hands Of Love

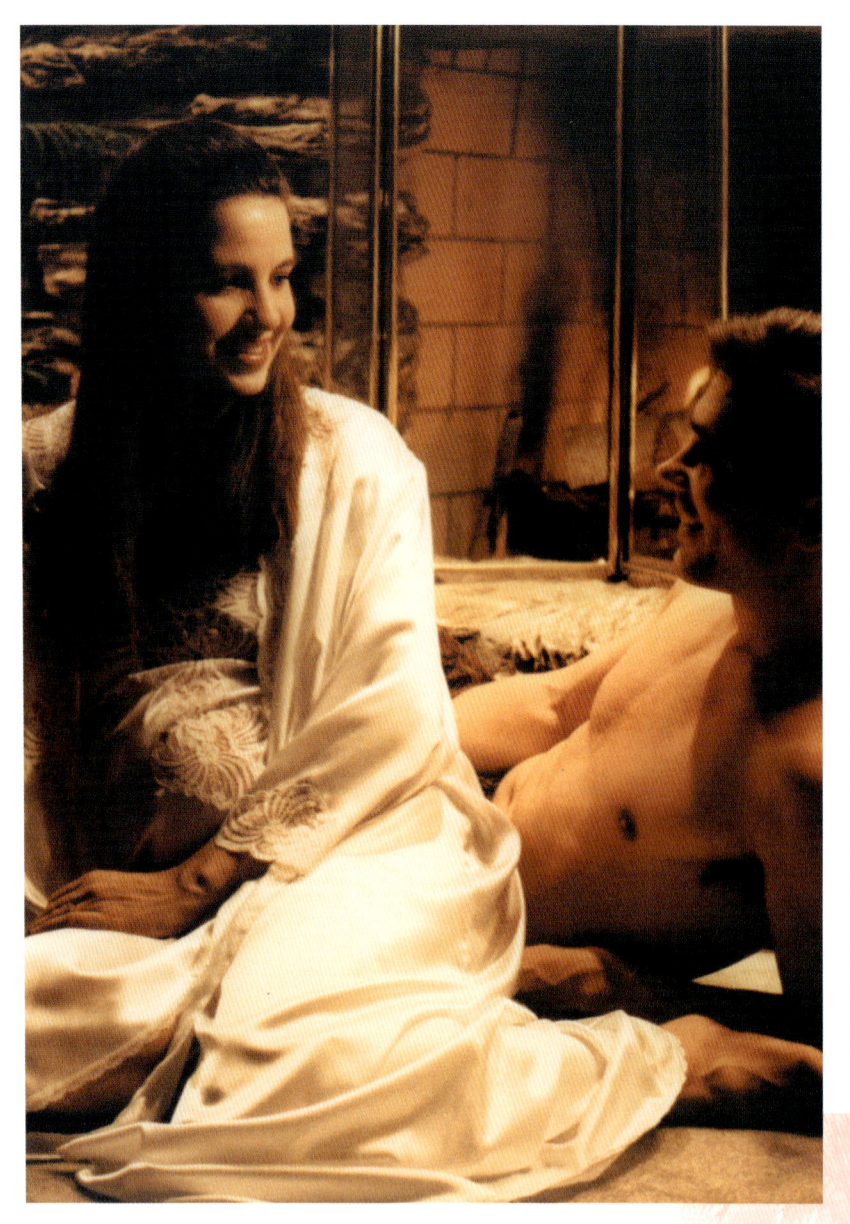

Just before graduation, I received a surprise invitation to join them for lunch. Murray blurted out their exciting news as soon as I arrived; Shannon was pregnant. They hadn't even told their family the good news, and they were already asking me to be a member of their birth team. I knew right then that these two were going to make wonderful parents.

During our lunch conversation, Murray seemed confident and sure about his decision to have a homebirth. Shannon, on the other hand, appeared reserved and apprehensive. Later, I spoke with Shannon alone. Although I fully supported Murray's plans for a homebirth, I wasn't sure if Shannon did. I had watched her eyes as Murray spoke with unguarded enthusiasm, and I listened to her unspoken words of fear. I felt I had to encourage her to thoroughly investigate all of her options and to follow her heart before finalizing any plans.

Only Shannon knew her limits. I encouraged her to follow her instincts and stay within those limits. She agreed to search deep within to find what was best for her and for her baby.

Birth is a Family Affair

First babies generally do not come into the world very quickly, and this birth was no exception. In Shannon's case, labor lasted approximately eighteen to twenty hours. To get a realistic picture of how she ended up delivering in her own bedroom surrounded by family and friends, I think it is only fair to begin this story by going back nine months.

As a husband and wife chiropractic team, Dr.'s Shannon and Murray Smith are passionate about three things: God, family, and chiropractic. I met them while they were still in chiropractic college. As students in my pediatric class, they were clearly devoted to each other and to the concept of pediatric chiropractic care.

SHANNON: *Initially, I had mixed feelings about the idea of a homebirth. I knew from all my previous training that I had to be comfortable with whatever arrangements we made, or my fear and apprehension could negatively effect the outcome of my birth. We interviewed many people before we made a decision about what type of birth attendant we wanted. In the end, when we agreed to have a homebirth, we hired both a midwife and an obstetrician. The OB was chosen because she already had a reputation for providing backup support to homebirth parents. She didn't hesitate to tell us she thought we were crazy, but she understood we intended to deliver the baby at home unless there were any complications along the way.*

STEP 3: Create a Birth Team

MURRAY: We had insurance that would pay only if we delivered our baby in a hospital, but we didn't want money to be a factor in our decision about location. After we interviewed two midwives, Jan and Jeannie, we knew that we'd pay whatever it cost to hire them as our primary birth attendants. Shannon was finally happy with my dream to have a homebirth.

SHANNON: During my pregnancy, I continued to receive prenatal care from both our OB and from our midwives. I also received Chiropractic prenatal care from Dr. Phillips. Sometimes, I would have up to three prenatal visits a week. Murray and I also read up on emergency childbirth, just in case we decided to go to the hospital at the last minute and risked delivery in the car. We became familiar with the hospital and designed our birth plan so that everyone involved would know what we preferred to happen during the birth. After making our decisions, we tackled the next step; we prepared our families to help them accept our decision to have a homebirth.

PAUL: (Shannon's dad) I had no problem with their decision. I asked one of the midwives what they would do in an emergency, or if the baby started to come out upside down. She said she'd call 911. I figured if that was all there was to it—then fine.

ANNA: (Shannon's mother) There are nine kids in my family and eight of us were born at home on the farm. Still, I had all four of my own children in a hospital, and I had mixed feelings for the safety of their baby.

SHAWN: (Shannon's older brother) I thought they had to be kidding. My children were born in a hospital, and I couldn't believe they'd consider a homebirth. I was skeptical and concerned that something might go wrong. It took awhile for me to accept their decision, but I didn't try to change their minds. I did ask a lot about the procedures used in a homebirth. The more we talked—the more comfortable I felt.

CHAD: (Shannon's younger brother) I thought it was cool and, since they were both doctors, I just figured they knew what they were doing.

As the weeks turned to months, and questions about "what if" kept coming, Murray got tired of explaining how they would handle any complications. One evening, at a family dinner, he shocked everyone (especially Shannon) when he cut the questions short by announcing, "If anyone in Shannon's family wants to attend the birth and witness it for themselves, they're welcome to come." To his surprise, all of Shannon's family took him up on the offer and said they would be there.

Finally, Shannon and Murray were comfortable with their decisions as to where to have the baby, who would be the primary birth attendants, and who would comprise the birth team. Now, they had to make decisions concerning routine screenings such as ultrasound sonography, lab studies to rule out diabetes, and the AFP test to rule out fetal malformations. Their chiropractic education included training in obstetrics so they were prepared to investigate each suggested test before making an informed decision. In the end, they chose not to take advantage of medical technology and relied solely on non-invasive evaluation tools such as auscultation, urinalysis, blood pressure etc.

Because of their extensive training, both Shannon and Murray were aware of the risk factors associated with any pregnancy, labor, and delivery. Shannon kept known risks down to a minimum by avoiding all alcohol and medications. They also stayed away from all smoke-filled environments. Shannon continued to follow a well-balanced nutritional program and faithfully took her recommended prenatal supplements. The pregnancy was uneventful and, based on her health history, Shannon's birth attendants agreed to honor her request to waive routine tests that she felt were unnecessary.

March 1993—The Time Had Finally Arrived

3:00 A.M.

Shannon's contractions were irregular, but strong enough to keep her awake all night. She sat up reading, *What to Expect When You're Expecting*, for last minute advice about the impending delivery.

> A common mistake made by first time mothers is to sit up all night when they are in early labor. They usually tire out when the baby finally does make his way into the world. Can you blame them for being so excited? It feels like Christmas Eve!

When dawn approached, Murray phoned everyone on the birth team and asked us to change our schedules for the day. Jenny was Shannon's best friend and the first to arrive at their home.

JENNY: *As a nursing student, I had already been required to watch two births in the hospital. After those experiences, I decided that I would never have children. I never wanted to go through what I watched those women endure during labor. When Shannon told me she was investigating the possibility of a homebirth, and wanted me to be there, I couldn't believe it. After what I had witnessed, I felt no one should risk having a baby at home.*

Eventually, when I saw how excited Shannon and Murray were, I softened my attitude and agreed to join their birth team. When I arrived, around 11:00 A.M., both of them appeared so relaxed and content with their decision that I, too, relaxed and started enjoying myself.

I was treating a patient when my receptionist stuck her head in the room and said, "Dr. Carol, Dr. Smith called. His wife is in active labor." I quickly started making preparations to have my patients notified and to have an associate take care of anyone who choose to come into the clinic that day.

> To be a doula requires that you be in a position to drop everything and go at a moment's notice. You have no idea if you will be gone for three hours or three days. Thankfully, I have always been able to do that. When I first started practice, patients would call and reschedule on the day that someone went into labor. It was uncanny. When others were notified that I had to attend a birth they, too, would happily reschedule.
>
> My patients often felt they were contributing to the birth, and my pregnant patients couldn't wait to hear how it went. When my practice consisted of too many patients to cancel, and reschedule, I had a resident and several interns who would take over and treat patients for me. I have always felt that God knows exactly how to plan things so we can continue to fulfill our destiny.

When I arrived, Shannon was in the early stage of labor, but her contractions were strong and steady. I immediately adjusted her spine to normalize nerve flow to her uterus and performed craniosacral therapy to insure that the pelvic musculature was relaxed and prepared for the delivery. We could tell when a contraction would start because Shannon would begin to make the O-O-O-ing sounds that I had taught her. When she starting making those sounds, Murray, Jenny, and I would stop whatever we were doing and join Shannon as she worked through the contraction.

I showed Jenny how to put her hands very gently over the baby and suggested that she visualize soft downy white pillows for the baby to pass through. I explained that the soft O-O-O-ing sounds would help Shannon center on the baby and relax the muscles of the pelvic floor. We all chimed in with Shannon and our voices sounded like one. All attention was on Shannon as we worked to help her focus all of her awareness on the baby and the contractions.

STEP 3: Create a Birth Team

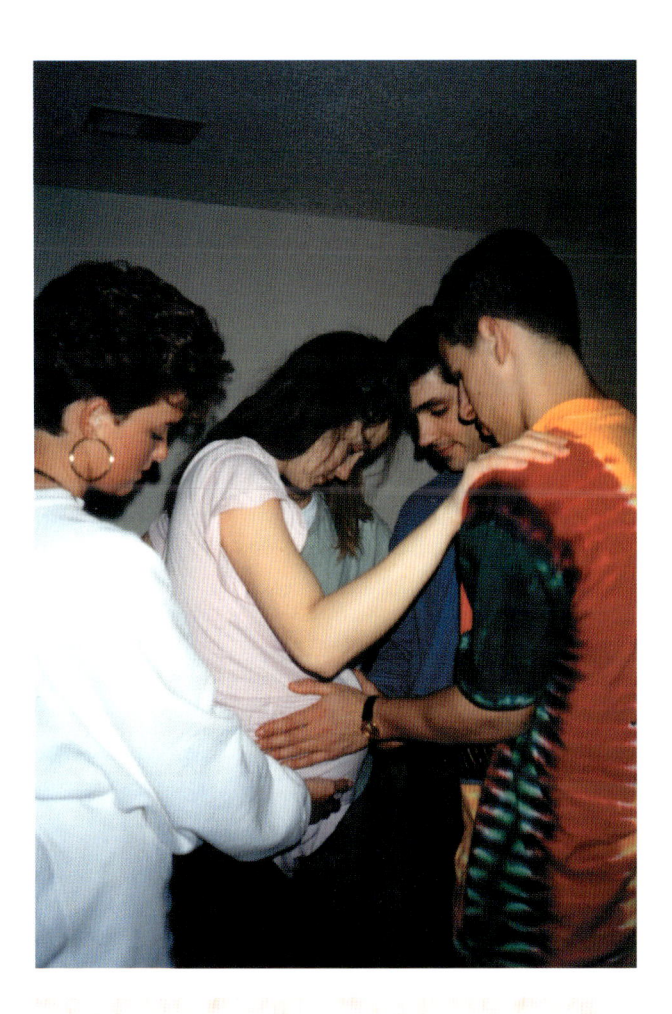

JENNY: *This was not at all like I'd expected. I couldn't help but wonder how long it would remain this calm.*

It was winter in Minnesota, but the sky was crystal clear, and the sun was unusually warm. Since we were staying home, we decided to go for a walk around the wooded neighborhood. Jenny was a bit surprised that we'd consider leaving the apartment, but everything we did surprised her.

I wanted Shannon to be as physically comfortable as possible so she wouldn't be distracted from the sensations of labor; before leaving for our walk, I adjusted her spine and performed craniosacral therapy to balance the membranes surrounding her brain and spinal cord. We wanted all systems to be working in unison and this was the best way I knew to accomplish that.

As soon as I was finished treating Shannon, Murray grabbed the video camera and we all headed out into the winter sunshine. The ground was covered with fluffy white snow from our recent storms. The afternoon sun blended with the crisp air making it delightfully warm on our face and hands. A Minnesota winter makes you crave this kind of day. We rejoiced in the moment as we walked and talked about this being a perfect day to have a baby.

We laughed and joked as we walked, but every three minutes Shannon would stop, wrap her arms around the neck of the nearest person, close her eyes, and lean her cheek on the welcoming shoulder. After taking a deep breath, she would begin to exhale with the familiar, long, soft O-O-O-ing sounds. One person would capture this moment in the middle of the street on the video, while the other person stood beside the hugging couple. The person on the side would gently place their hands on Shannon's hips, back, or pregnant belly. All three of us would then slowly sway with her as she used gravity, motion, vibration (a result of vocalizing the O-O-O-sound), and visualization to gently slide her baby down into the birth canal.

With my hands barely touching the baby, I could tell Shannon was working with her body, and not against it. I could feel the contraction sweep around from behind and come forward into my hands. When I felt the contraction peak, I would quietly encourage her to send her energy down the front of her abdomen. I would then rejoin everyone else in the O-O-O-ing and encourage Shannon to exhale as long as possible to keep the contraction going, and then to take a long deep cleansing breath and do it again.

Between contractions, Shannon laughed and told us a funny story she had learned from her new neighbors. The year before, when we had walked these same streets with Shannon's friend who was in labor, the neighbors had been watching. She learned they had been calling from house to house telling each other to look out into the street. "Is that woman in labor?" they asked each other. Now, here we were again... hugging in the street. We laughed as we wondered if they were peaking out their windows watching us.

Somehow, when a woman is in labor, you don't care what the neighbors are thinking. You just concentrate on that baby and how you want to help the mother be as relaxed as possible. Besides, it is fun to hug a pregnant mom freely and openly.

81

Shannon, Murray, Jenny, and I walked for over an hour before we headed back to the apartment. We then decided it was a good idea to relax the muscles surrounding Shannon's pregnant uterus since this might make it easier for the cervix to dilate.

Shannon was settled comfortably in her rocker, with a soft wool blanket covering her legs. To relax her pelvic floor muscles, I knelt down beside the rocker and placed my left hand on the small of her back with my right hand over the baby. I touched her abdomen light enough to take the tension out of the muscles. Shannon's muscles quickly relaxed and softened with the slight pressure I applied to the lower part of her abdomen. As I worked on the pelvic diaphragm, Shannon closed her eyes and continued to rock and O-O-O... through her contractions. This technique takes a little practice, but it's incredibly effective.

It had been approximately twelve hours since the early onset of labor. Shannon rested and rocked her baby as she began to slip away into a place deep within her mind; a place that took her away from the people that surrounded her. She surrendered to the power within that was taking on a life of its own. We all sat quietly around Shannon; soft music filled the room as we played the musical score to the movie *Somewhere in Time*. The melody of that tape helped all of us surrender to the flow and time-honored pace of labor.

As Shannon and I worked together, Jenny busied herself by picking up the video camera and capturing the moment on tape. After photographing Shannon in the rocker, Jenny turned and focused the camera on the wedding picture sitting on the coffee table. We agreed that the picture would be a beautiful addition to the birth story! Murray was in the baby's room completing a big birth certificate he had created for all the members of the birth team to sign.

4:58 P.M.

Shannon's mom, Anna, and sister, Carrie, arrived with a pot of warm, homemade soup. Anna was prepared to start feeding everyone. Shannon and Murray had gone off into the bathroom for some quiet time together and a warm bath to ease the aching in Shannon's back.

> Once, while looking at my large collection of birth pictures, my daughter, Wendy, remarked, "People sure do seem to spend a lot of quiet time together in the bathroom when they're in labor." She's right. Birthing mothers do gravitate to the bathroom. I think it is because they are small, dark, and quiet; they have warm running water for relaxing baths and showers—and only a few people can fit in the room at one time.

While Shannon and Murray had their quiet time together, I took advantage of the opportunity to explain to Anna and Carrie how they could help Shannon stay focused. I explained that by placing their hands over the baby they would be directing their energy from their palm chakra's (one of the largest energy vortex's in the body) to the baby. Both Shannon and the baby would benefit from the warmth and relaxation caused by that energy transference.

> If directing energy seems odd to you, think of what parents instinctively do when their child comes to them with a minor injury. They cover the injury with their hands and say, "I'll fix it." Many times, that's all it takes.
>
> There are toys that take advantage of electrical conductance of energy through our bodies to make them work. My favorite is the Lil' Rosy Doll that sings whenever you hold the positive and negative contacts inserted into her hands.
>
> We are electrical bodies. We can't see it, but like the energy frequency of your cell phone, it is there just the same.

I also explained to Anna and Carrie that if they joined in with the O-O-O-ing, they would be helping Shannon use sound to vibrate her uterus while relaxing the pelvic muscles. I also asked them to touch Shannon *as if* she were badly sunburned, so that no undue pressure would be applied to her sensitive abdomen. I suspect my comments sounded a bit strange, but neither Anna nor Carrie questioned my instructions. They simply nodded and followed my many suggestions.

After Shannon finished her bath, Murray came out of the bathroom, and Jenny went in. I encouraged her to stay close to Shannon and be prepared to help

STEP 3: Create a Birth Team

with the next contraction. Shannon wrapped a towel around her hair and put on a robe just as a contraction started. She immediately put her arms around Jenny's neck for support, allowing herself to drift into that deep place within her mind and body. Murray grabbed the camera to capture the moment. We couldn't help but chuckle as he whispered into the camera, "Oh, so this is what girls do when they go off to the bathroom together."

There's always room for quiet, lighthearted comedy during labor. After all, this should be a time of great joy and excitement. As long as it is respectful of the mother and what she's doing, it is fine to give in to the fun and excitement of the moment. But be forewarned, a woman in serious labor rarely has much of a sense of humor and dads have been known to get dirty looks after they've made funny, lighthearted comments. On many occasions, I have given a disheartened father a secret smile to soothe his hurt feelings. Luckily, Shannon missed Murray's cute comment.

5:29 P.M.

Murray, Carrie, and Jenny surrounded Shannon as they continued to direct energy from their hands to the baby. They encouraged Shannon with comments such as, "Doing well, Shannon, you're doing really well."

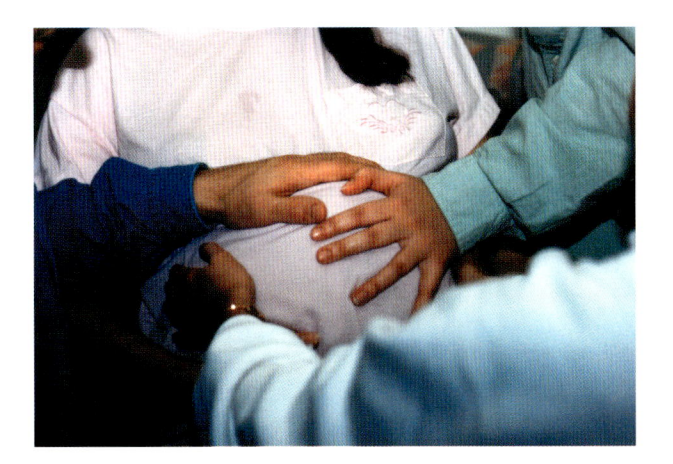

5:46 P.M.

After 14 hours of labor, Jan and Jeannie arrived and were welcomed into the apartment by Anna. Shannon responded by simply flashing a small, welcoming smile before she closed her eyes and went right back to the business of laboring. I quickly grabbed the camera and captured Jan's wave of hello while both Jan and Jeannie quietly laughed and unpacked their equipment. Before long, they had settled themselves in and began their work: watching, waiting, and recording vital signs. Later, the personal birth team would step aside as Jan and Jeannie took over the actual delivery.

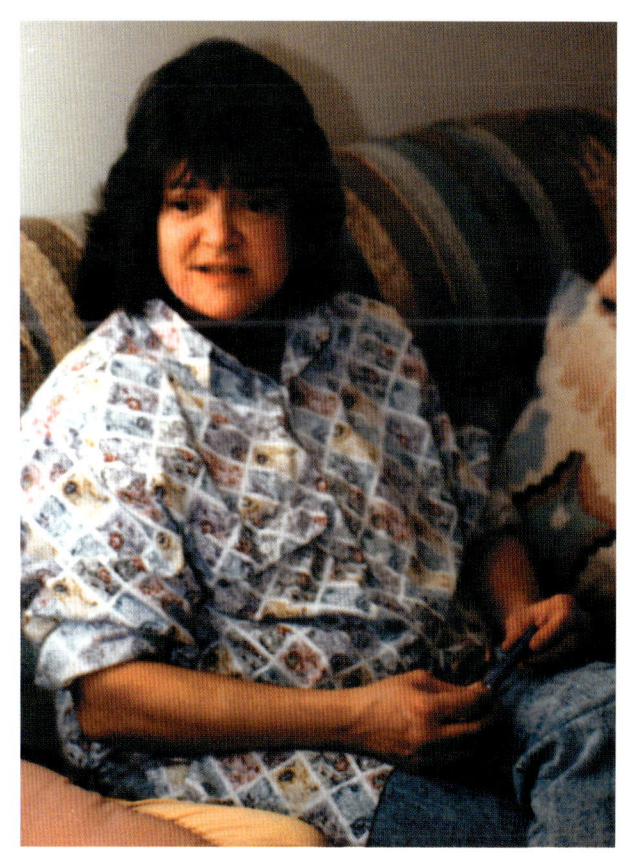

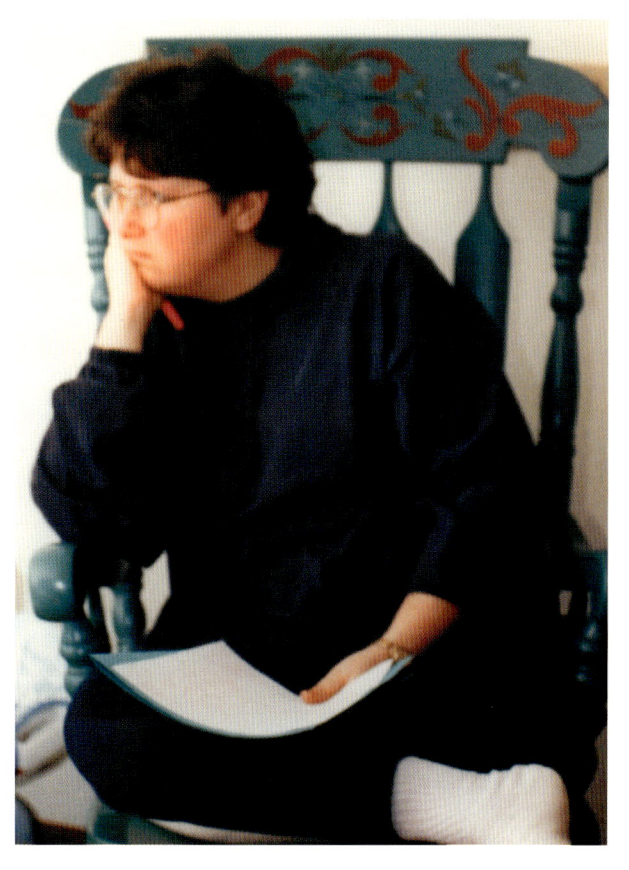

5:50 P.M.

Shannon's sixteen-year-old brother, Chad, arrived, took a seat on the couch, and began observing his sister and the people surrounding her. My role in this birth appeared to be changing from doula to teacher. I moved over and sat down beside Chad and filled him in on the *hows* and *whys* of what the others were doing. Within minutes, Chad knelt down beside his sister, placed his hands over the baby, and joined in with the now familiar O-O-O-ing. I was surprised that a boy his age would be so willing to accept this new and strange activity with such quiet resolve.

6:14 P.M.

Shannon and Murray stood up and spent a few minutes alone between contractions. Murray held her face while she rested her head on his forehead. When the contraction subsided, he kissed her softly as they waited for the next contraction. When Shannon's back began to ache, Murray rubbed an analgesic lotion over her muscles. He then placed warm cloths over the area until she felt better.

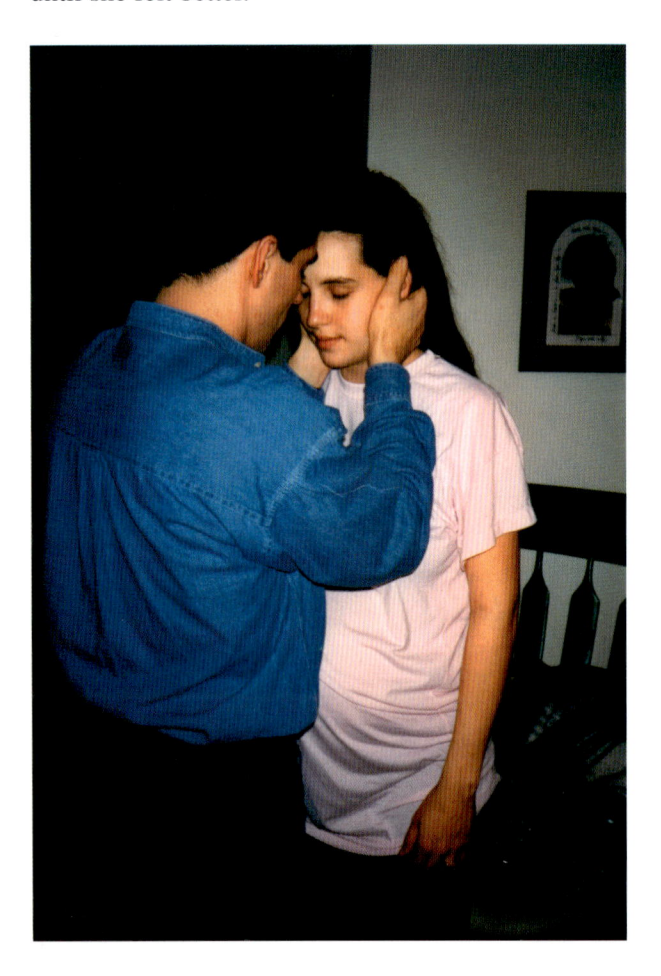

As I stated earlier, it's easier to conquer your subconscious fears if you begin as an observer of birth. Shannon had been given that opportunity when her friend, Marita, delivered her baby one year earlier. Shannon and Murray were both part of Marita's birth team, but Shannon's involvement was limited because she experienced a difficult emotional reaction to Marita's labor. Even though Marita's labor was uneventful, and without intense pain, Shannon responded negatively. Shannon had spent a great deal of time in the bathroom throwing up during Marita's labor and delivery; watching Marita labor seemed to have triggered the memory of her own birth and brought deep-seated emotions to the surface.

Shannon recognized how much that experience had helped her bring her own deep-seated memories associated with her own birth to the surface, so when her friend Lisa asked if she could attend the birth—Shannon quickly welcomed her on the birth team.

6:44 P.M.

Lisa arrived and I quickly filled her in on how to visualize the baby's descent through soft downy white pillows, how to synchronize her O-O-O-ing with Shannon, and how to place her hands gently over the baby. It was clear that everyone in the room was focused on the birth process, so Lisa joined in with quiet reverence and complete acceptance.

7:15 P.M.

Shannon's dad, Paul, arrived next. After waving a bottle of champagne toward the camera, he shook hands with the dad-to-be and gave his wife a kiss hello. After putting his packages in the kitchen, Paul quietly slipped over to watch. Anna motioned for him to join in. I chuckled as he put up his hand and said, "Wait. Wait. Give me a minute here. I can't just jump into this."

I stepped forward and gave Paul a quick explanation of what everyone was doing. He then knelt down to place his hands over the baby. He closed his eyes and quietly began to say, "O-O-O" ; he was right in sync with Shannon, Carrie, and Anna. Shannon responded to his presence with a quick glance and a small smile. She then closed her eyes and continued rocking her baby.

STEP 3: Create a Birth Team

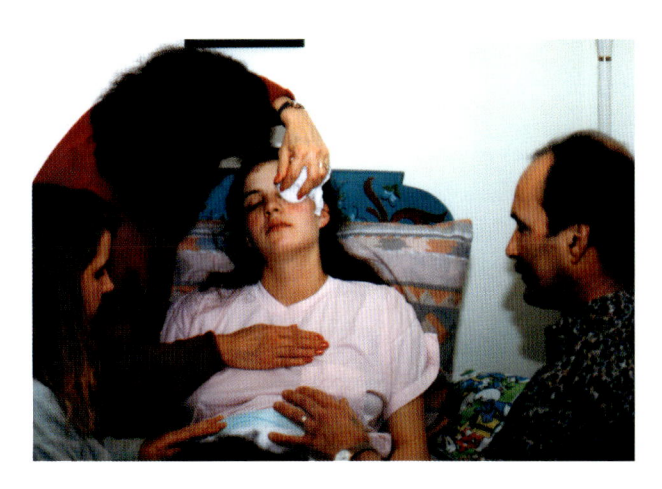

It is amazing how birthing can bring out the softest side of people when someone gives them a hint of what to do. To see all those hands barely touching Shannon, as they sent their love to the baby, was a sight I'll keep in my mind forever.

Throughout all of her laboring, Shannon continued to do simple things to stay relaxed and energized. She kept her face smooth, because she knew that a furrowed brow would cause her vaginal muscles to tighten up against the baby's head. She kept her hands relaxed, knowing a clenched fist would do the same thing. With each contraction, Shannon surrendered to the uterus tightening around her baby, as if she were giving the baby a snug but loving hug.

Shannon focused on allowing the contraction to build up in the front before she visualized the sensation moving gently downward toward the cervix. She would imagine the baby sliding into the canal and her cervix opening for the baby's head. I tried to help by lightly touching her forehead or hand when I observed tension in her body. That touch alone was enough to help her avoid tightening her muscles up against the baby.

Even though it seemed like it was taking an awfully long time for the baby to descend into the birth canal, Shannon never asked us what time it was. She never appeared impatient with the process, though inside I have to imagine she was. She seemed to know that if she remained focused and centered on the baby's journey, the birth would happen at just the right time. (Labor does have a way of wiping out the concept of time, unless other people have reason to bring it to the mother's attention.)

7:23 P.M.

Approximately, 16 hours after active labor had begun, Shannon's older brother, Shawn, arrived with a large bouquet of flowers, and a surprise date for the evening (Not wanting to miss the birth—or his date—Shawn brought her along). I wondered how his date felt about the peculiar change in their plans for the evening; I was sure she would never have another date quite like it. Everyone seemed to take her presence in stride as she took a seat off in the corner of the room. I had to assume that, for reasons unknown to us, God felt she should observe this labor. Shannon did not seem to know her brother had arrived. She continued rocking peacefully, with her mother on one side, her father on the other, while Murray knelt in front of her.

7:45 P.M.

Suddenly aware that the living room was full of people, Shannon and Murray slipped off to the bathroom for privacy and another hot shower. While they were gone, everyone ate, laughed, and settled in. The midwives went into the bedroom to finalize the delivery preparations. Shannon and Murray had already prepared the bed by covering their freshly washed sheets with a large sheet of plastic. The plastic was then covered with older sheets and blankets. After the birth, they would remove the top sheets and the plastic. Underneath would be their fresh clean sheets for the family bed.

I joined Jan and Jeannie in the bedroom and arranged some of the baby's stuffed animals so they would show up in the video and photographs taken during the birth.

Along with my duties as the family doula, I have always enjoyed being the family photographer. I feel that birth is a very special time and that photographs should reflect the true nature of the event.

In setting up, I focus on the background, because the family rarely thinks about it until later, when they show the pictures to everyone. A bare wall or sterile environment is rarely a picture you want to keep in the family album forever.

8:47 P.M.

Shannon and Murray were now ready to spend quiet time in the bedroom with the midwives and myself. Unlike so many other births I had attended over the previous decade, I now realized that my service as a doula was unnecessary at this birth. Shannon and Murray needed no assistance as they nestled together and tuned into each other and the baby. I generally play it by ear when I attend a birth and let the circumstances dictate the intensity of my role in the process. I knew my role at this time was to be their photographer—not their teacher, doula, or chiropractor. Shannon told the midwives she was content being alone with us for awhile. She asked the family to wait in the living room until it was time for the baby to arrive. Then, anyone could come into the room that wanted to.

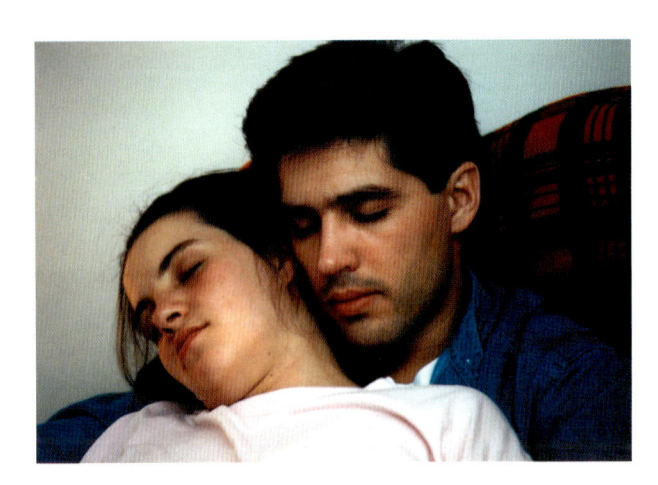

When Shannon decided to be alone for awhile, Shawn, his date, and Chad left—thinking they would return before the delivery. While Shannon was not willing to wait for her brothers to return, she did appear to be waiting for one more person to arrive before giving birth.

9:30 P.M.

Eighteen hours after labor had begun, a plane landed and Shannon's friend, Marita, hurried over to the apartment with her one-year-old daughter, McKenzie. It was hard to believe that exactly one year earlier I had been in this same apartment (Marita and Troy's at the time) with Shannon and Murray as her labor support team.

Marita let out a sigh of relief when she was told she was not to late. Before joining Shannon and Murray in the bedroom, Marita took time to let McKenzie delight us with her antics in the living room. Marita then slipped the worn out little-one into the new baby's crib in McKenzie's old nursery. To our surprise, she fell right to sleep without a peep of resistance. Shannon may have been subconsciously waiting for Marita to arrive, because the moment she entered the bedroom we saw Shannon rapidly progress to the pushing stage of labor.

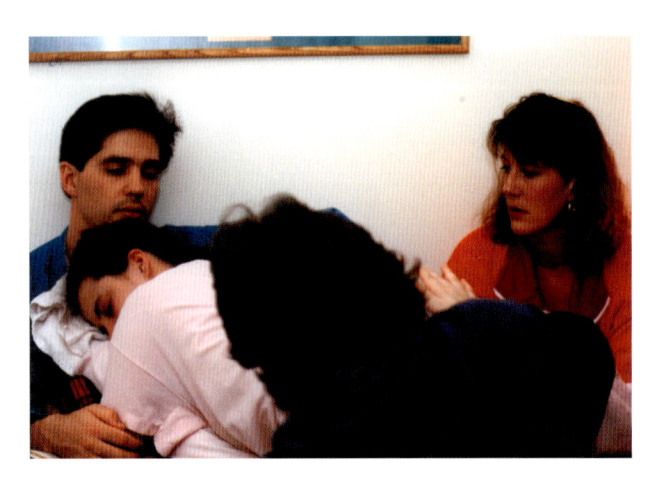

10:49 P.M.

Family and friends slipped quietly into the room as Jan informed them that the baby was crowning. Shannon decided to switch her position so she was lying on her left side with her head resting on Murray's arm. Murray lay behind Shannon while Marita sat in front. Both spoke words of encouragement, praise and guidance as Shannon began to ease the baby out.

10:51 P.M.

The baby was descending quickly. Shannon could barely be heard as she took a deep breath, tucked her chin to her chest and quietly pushed downward with the involuntary desire to help the baby get through the canal. Jeannie kept telling Shannon she was doing just fine and to be prepared to stop pushing when she told her to.

10:56 P.M.

Jan and Jeannie suddenly asked Shannon to slow down the baby's descent by saying," Pah-h-h—Pah-h-h." If the baby descended too rapidly, Shannon's tissue might have torn. I suggested that Shannon visualize a butterfly floating in front of her mouth and to softly blow it away. Wanting to avoid a tear, Jeannie supported the perineal tissue around the baby's emerging head, as Jan squirted a mixture of

STEP 3: Create a Birth Team

almond and vitamin E oil over the perineum. They encouraged Shannon to avoid pushing, by continuing to use her muscles to allow the baby to slowly descend through the birth canal. The heart tones continued to be stable, so they knew it was safe to encourage Shannon to go slower and allow the baby to rotate her body safely through the canal without any assistance from them.

As soon as Jan told Shannon that they could see the eyes, someone handed Murray a small compact mirror. Murray was restricted from moving to get a better view of the birth because Shannon had her head on his left arm. Stretching out his right arm in an attempt to get the tiny mirror down low enough to see the baby's head, Murray's eyes bulged with excitement as he continued to tell Shannon what a marvelous job she was doing. Verbal suggestions floated without faces into Shannon's consciousness.

"You're doing really well, Shannon. Puff the butterfly in front of your face, Shannon. Pah-h-h—Pah-h-h. Slow-Slow-Slow. Shannon, just slide this baby out. Keep breathing—you're stretching nicely—really slow now—let her slip right on out. The baby's fine—we can see the eyes—keep breathing nicely."

At the foot of the bed, Jenny could not contain herself any longer. This was not at all like the births she'd witnessed in the hospital. I laughed lightly as I heard her softly exclaim, "Oh, my g-o-s-h-h-h!"

10:59 P.M.

Shannon now had the entire head delivered. As we stood and watched, we all held our breath. The baby's head was in a perfect position with the back of the head just behind Shannon's pubic bone. The face became more and more purple as we waited... and waited. Jan and Jeannie remained calm (at least on the outside) while they supported the head and waited for the shoulders to begin their rotation out of the canal. Unfortunately, they were stuck.

11:01 P.M.

Twenty hours had now passed since the onset of labor. As we continued to wait, Marita whispered in Shannon's ear, "Oh, Shannon, you are doing just great! Shannon, you are making this look too easy. Let her slip right on out, Shannon."

> In other births, I have seen birth attendants rush this portion of the delivery process. Using manual force, they would assist the baby in rotating and bringing the shoulders out of the birth canal. In reality, only the baby knows how their body is lined up with their head and only they know what they need to do to safely roll their body out.

11:02 P.M.

Words of encouragement, guidance, and comfort continued to flow from Murray, Marita, and the midwives. As Jeannie slipped her fingers inside the birth canal to nudge the baby's shoulder into position, I realized that Shannon's leg was restricting the baby's movement. One of us asked Paul to lift Shannon's right leg up a little to give the baby a little more room to roll her shoulders into position. It worked.

Jeannie instructed Shannon to give a little push forward. After several little downward grunts, we watched in amazement as the baby began to spiral her body through Jeannie's hands as she supported Shannon's perineum.

Hands Of Love

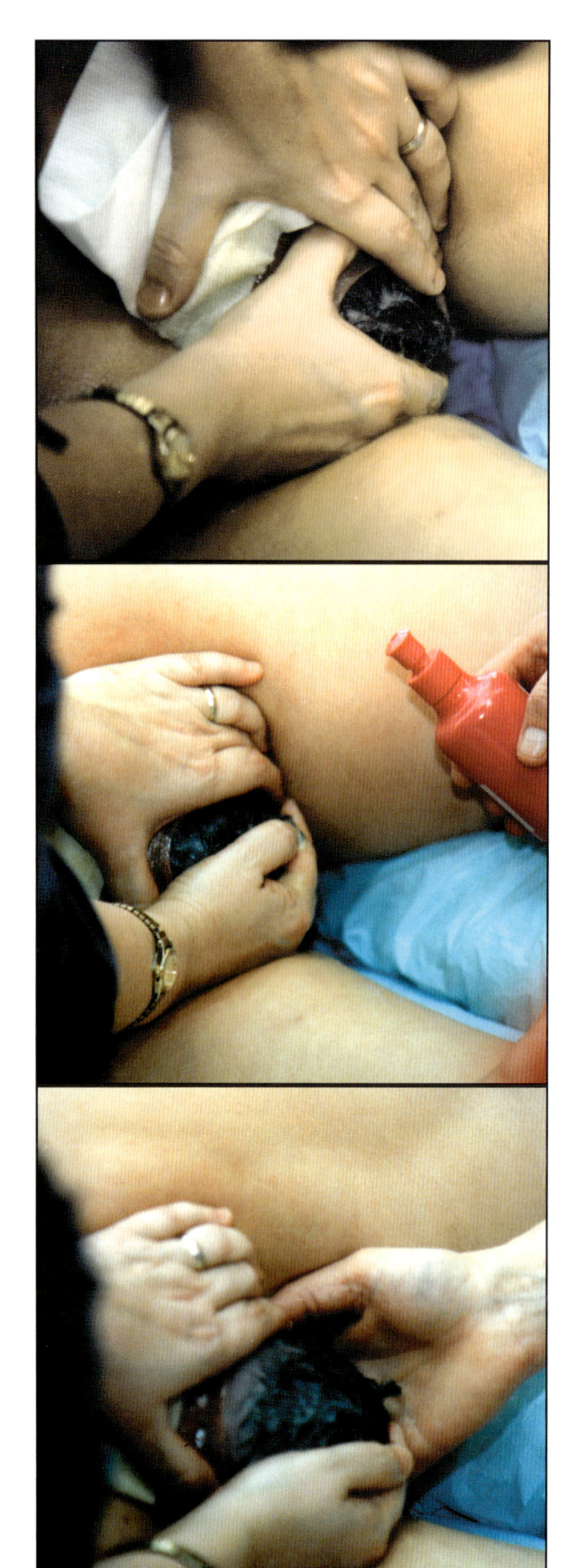

All the rest of us watched in awe, cried softly, and did what we could to capture on film the baby's rapid roll out of the canal. The baby rolled through Jeannie's hands and felt the welcome embrace of Jan's hands as she lifted her up to Shannon.

> Unfortunately, the mother who does all the work of birth rarely witnesses the miracle of her child's birth. Therefore, I carefully filmed most of the labor and delivery. I wanted to make sure that Shannon saw what a wonderful job she had done. She may have been experiencing a sense of chaos within, but the rest of us were in awe of her calm exterior.

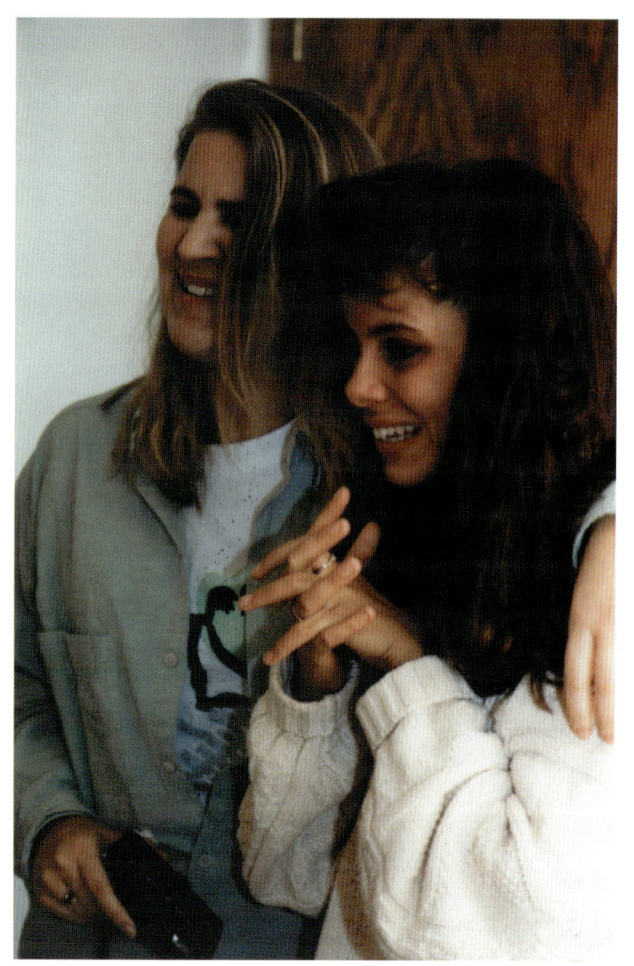

11:03 P.M.

All of a sudden, the room exploded with laughter, tears, and voices all talking at once. Shannon, on the contrary, was silent. She appeared happy, content, and fully focused on the newly born child resting on her belly. She couldn't bring the baby up

STEP 3: Create a Birth Team

very far because she was still attached to the placenta by an extremely short cord. Jan explained to Shannon that the short cord probably slowed the labor process. Any faster and the placenta may have been pulled away from the wall prematurely, resulting in fetal distress and heavy bleeding.

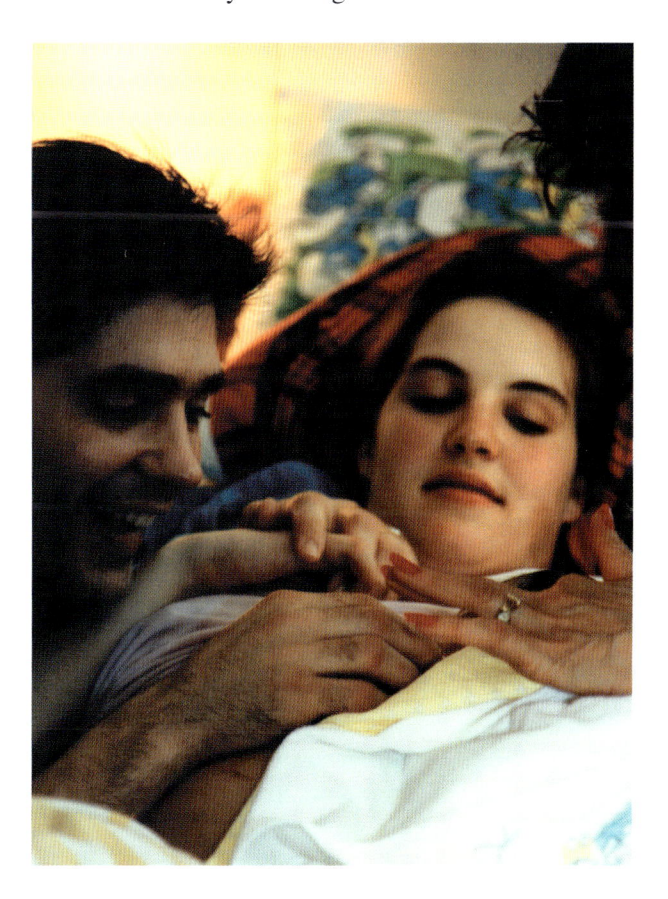

Suddenly, Marita asked if this was a girl or a boy. No one knew as she was already covered with a blanket. Murray spoke up right away with, "Hang on! I get to open this present!" Murray lifted the blanket with one hand and the baby's little leg with the other. He laughed with excitement and shouted, "Hey, my little Hannah!"

After covering Hannah back up, Murray planted a kiss on Shannon's forehead. He then looked up at the midwives and jokingly said with a huge grin, "Better double check that."

> If new parents are unaware of the sex of their unborn child, it's always fun to let them discover in their own way if they have been given a boy or a girl. Some parents don't even care as they rejoice in the beauty and uniqueness of their newborn. Eventually, we encourage them to reach under the blankets and find out for themselves. (It must be a great feeling to know you are loved and accepted no matter what gender you are.)

After Jan explained to Shannon why she couldn't pull Hannah up any higher, Murray started stroking Hannah's arm and cooed, "Oh, Honey. Are you okay? Are you okay? Did you have a little trouble coming down?" Meanwhile, Shannon continued stroking Hannah's hair and talking softly to her as all new mothers do.

> I have observed hundreds of women while they've held their newborns right after birth. What I've witnessed is that the mothers will innately begin stoking their baby's head in a pattern remarkably similar to the protocol I would use to realign the cranial bones. This natural reaction to realign the bones that were altered by the forces of labor is often hindered when someone places a hat on a baby's head to keep the heat in.
>
> Research with premature babies has shown that the hat wouldn't be necessary if the baby were placed directly against a mother's breast and then covered with warm blankets. A mother's breast temperature changes to either warm her baby up or cool him down, provided he's directly against her skin. Hats and warmers are unnecessary if a mother is given the chance to do what comes naturally with the body she has been blessed with.

All of a sudden, Shannon's mom and dad just had to reach in and touch their daughter. They stroked Shannon and the baby as they dealt with the charged emotions of the moment. Murray looked up at Paul and Anna with love and pride. As he held each of their hands he shouted, "Hey, Grandpa—Grandma!"

Marita turned her attention from the baby to Shannon. Marita whispered, "How are you, Shannon? Are you tired? You made it look like it didn't hurt at all." Shannon softly smiled at Marita and said she was fine, she was not tired, and yes, it did hurt!

> **SHANNON:** *Despite being surrounded by many people, I was not aware of anything except the baby and the words I heard from Murray, Marita, and the midwives. Later, after Hannah was born, I looked around and thought how wonderful it felt having so many of the people we loved surrounding us. Afterwards, the only discomfort I had was when Jan pulled on the cord to see if the placenta was beginning to disengage—it wasn't.*

11:27 P.M.

It was almost thirty minutes since Hannah's birth, yet Shannon still hadn't delivered the placenta. Jan suggested that they give the baby to Murray so Shannon could sit up and use gravity to disengage the placenta. Murray jumped up, pulled off his shirt, and waited excitedly for Hannah to be placed in his arms. As she was lifted from Shannon's chest, Hannah shocked everyone by letting out a loud-pitched scream. She was terrified. Murray quickly removed Hannah's blankets, placed her against his bare chest, and curled up on the bed next to Shannon. We put a warm blanket over the couple and with a sigh of relief, Hannah suddenly became quiet again.

11:35 P.M.

Shannon was lifted up to her knees by Jan and Jeannie. I got around behind her and placed my hands around her hips. With gravity, and slight pressure placed against the sacroiliac joints (the joints formed by the union of the sacrum at the base of the spine and the pelvic bones), Shannon completed her birth by delivering the placenta. Now, she could lie back on the bed with her husband and baby, and bask in the joy of the moment. No tears—no stitches. The rest of the family worked around them as they removed the top sheets and plastic from the bed so Shannon, Murray, and Hannah could settle in against the many pillows placed up against the wall.

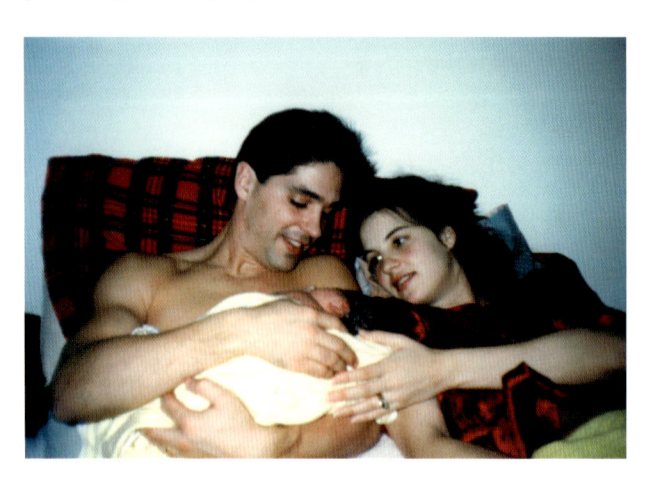

11:45 P.M.

It was now time for the midwives to get the *all important* height and weight measurements so the rest of the family could be called with the details. Before starting the pediatric exam, Jan examined the umbilical cord and placenta. During a homebirth, and in some hospital births, this inspection is shared with the family. It is often fascinating to see the sac lifted up for all to see and explore. The umbilical cord looks like the trunk of an ancient tree as the blood vessels, which look like branches, spread out across the placenta forming what we call the *tree of life*. It is an amazing sight to see.

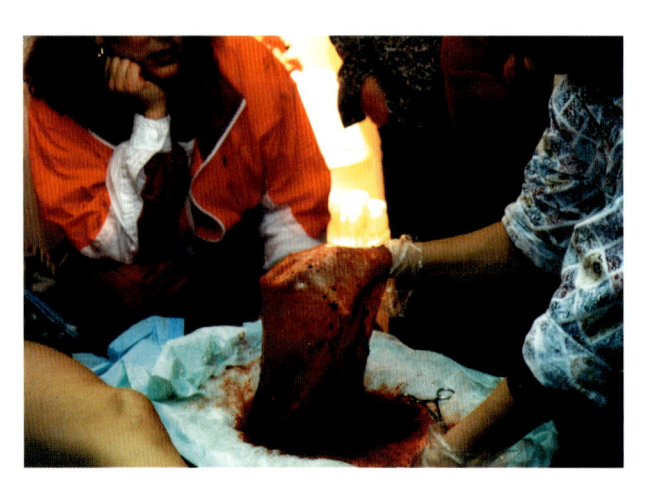

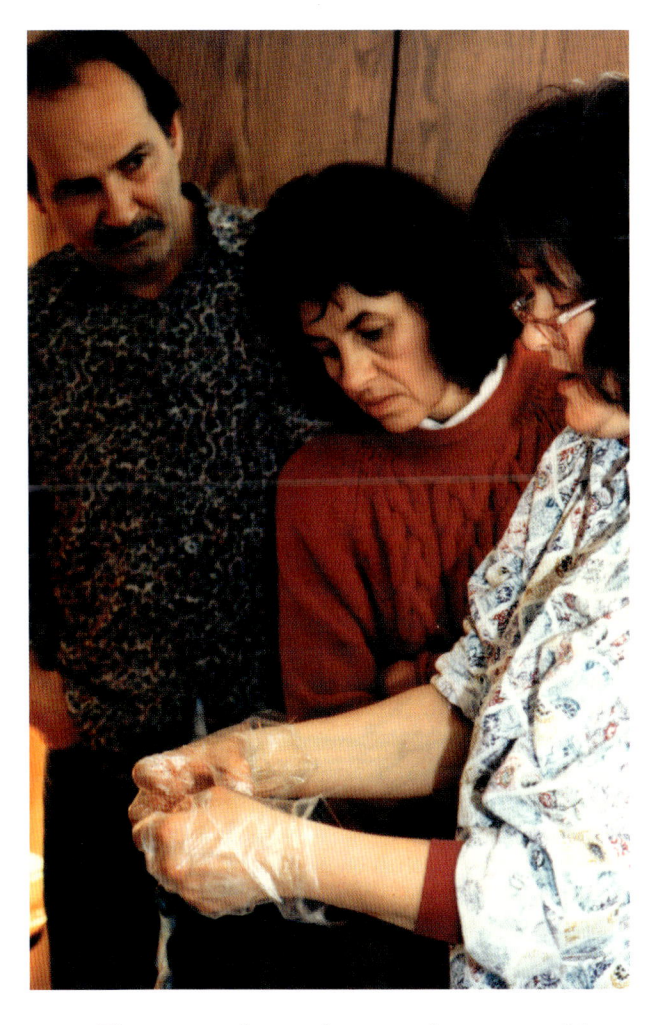

STEP 3: Create a Birth Team

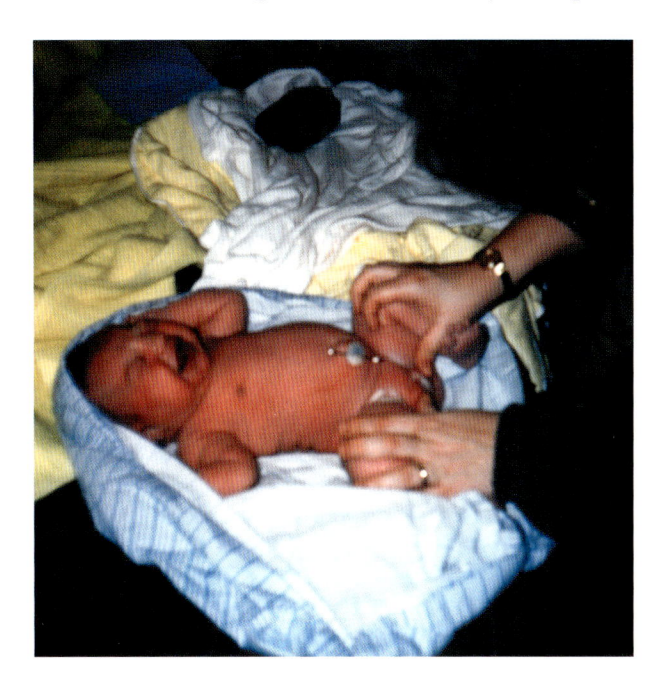

Hannah ended up weighing in at nine pounds—two ounces. Marita spoke with amazement as she announced that, not only did Shannon deliver almost exactly one year after she did, but both baby girls were born around 11:00 P.M. and they had identical height and weight measurements.

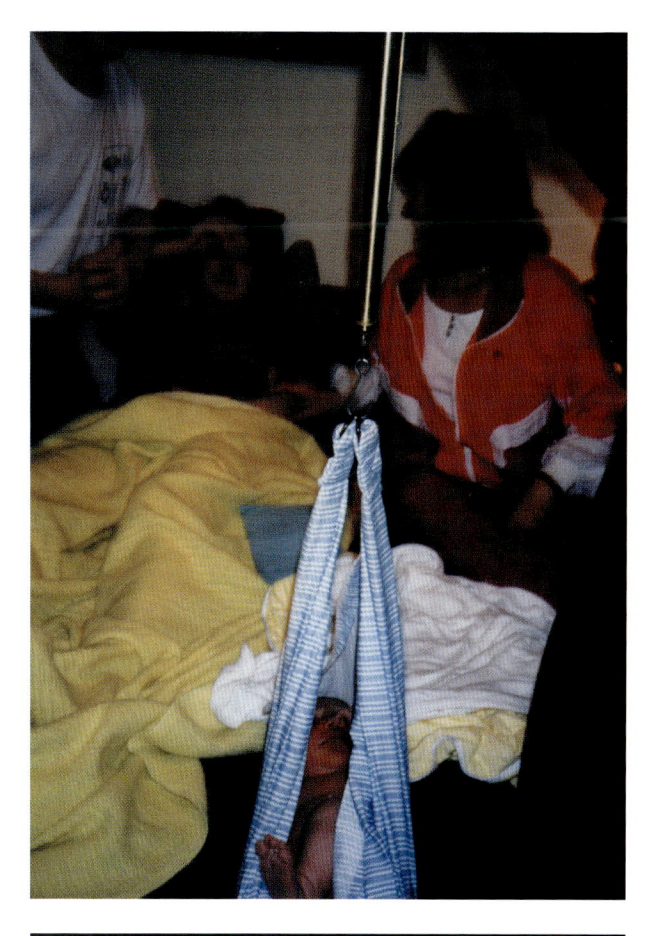

The exam of a newborn rarely occurs without tears as the baby is moved away from the mother. Jeannie was sensitive to that and kept Hannah as close to Shannon as possible. She performed her newborn exam with extreme gentleness, efficiency, and speed.

Even with the best of births, a newborn can suffer from structural misalignments either from their in utero position or as they maneuver their way out of the birth canal. The pain that can result from these misalignments may not show up for days because the baby received the mother's endorphins, a substance that raises the pain threshold and is released by the brain just before delivery. If the structural misalignments are left uncorrected, the new family may have a difficult time during the first month as the newborn cries from pain during most of her waking hours. Luckily, Hannah rested in the hands of two parents well trained to evaluate and correct those misalignments.

Hands Of Love

After Jeannie completed her exam, Hannah was wrapped up and held by Marita as the midwives turned their attention back to Shannon. They wanted to make sure that Shannon was able to eat something nutritious, so both of them stuck around while Shannon consumed a large bowl of homemade soup.

Little Hannah had such an easy birth that Shannon and Murray waited several hours before they evaluated Hannah's head and spine for any possible problems. She was fine.

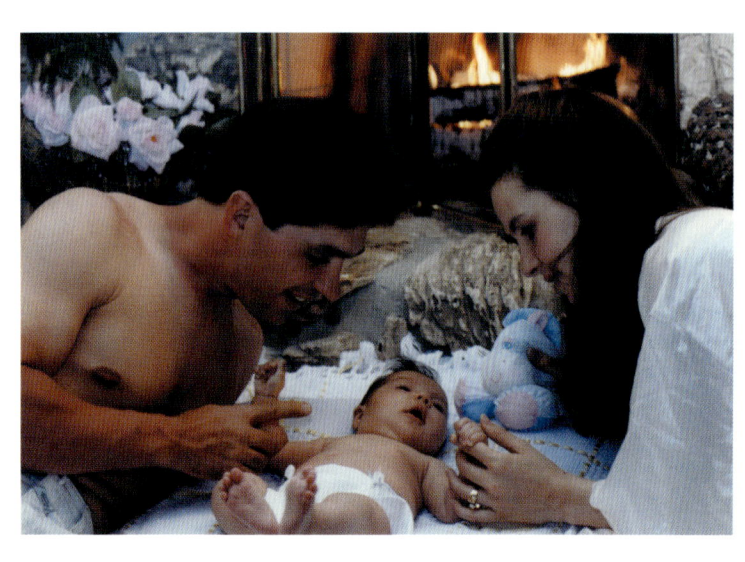

Jan and Jeannie continued to visit the new family for several weeks after the birth. Grandma and Grandpa were also right there to baby-sit or help whenever they could. Having been there for the whole labor and delivery, both grandparents developed a bond with Hannah that only grandparents who are part of the birth team can understand.

Having just graduated from college, Shannon and Murray spent their first five months with Hannah full-time. They both passed the Minnesota State Board exam and received their licenses to practice chiropractic in Minnesota. Hannah went with them on their search for a new town, a new home, and a clinic where they could begin their practice.

Within two years, a second baby, Holly, was also born at home. This time Shannon and Murray had to do it alone; Holly came flying out inside of her water sac only one hour after they called Jan and I. We were still on the road trying to get there when Holly made her rapid appearance. Again, Shannon had difficulty releasing the placenta. An hour after the birth, I arrived, adjusted her sacroiliac joints, restored nerve flow to the uterus, and the placenta disengaged.

Two years later Shannon and Murray delivered a son, Gabe, with the help of a midwife who lived a lot closer than Jan. A few years after that, Shannon delivered a third little girl who decided to come late at night before anyone could arrive to help. It happened so fast Murray had to wake up Hannah and ask her to videotape the birth while he caught the baby. (She did a marvelous job I'm told.) Dr. Murray has taken over the care of all their patients in the Crosby, Minnesota practice, while Dr. Shannon now devotes her full-time to the care of their ever-growing family. Their children, growing up on the shores of Lake Reno, have remained healthy and strong as they bask in the light of a family's love.

STEP 3: Create a Birth Team

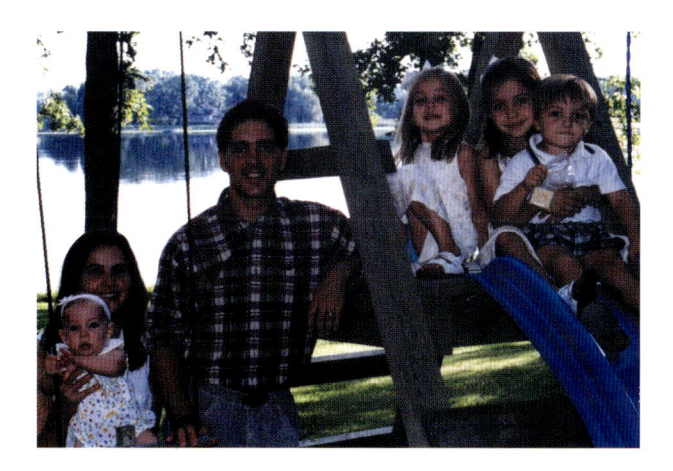

If you plan to have a hospital birth and want to bring in your own birth team, take a walk through your hospital first. See how big the rooms are. The size of your birthing room may be large enough to accommodate five people. It may be so small that even one additional person will be too much. Walk down to the nursery and ask a nurse if your hospital will put a band on the wrist of every member in your birth team, so they may accompany your baby into the nursery (most will not for security reasons). Ask if your hospital allows the birth team to accompany you into surgery if that becomes necessary. If they can't accommodate your support team or honor your wishes due to hospital policy, it is better to know that in advance so you can mentally prepare yourself for those changes.

Next, construct a written birth plan so that both the medical staff and your birthing team are aware of your goals for the process of labor and delivery. When you write this plan, be very clear on what your intent is in having additional support. Are they there to nurture you or just observe? Are they prepared to assist the staff, or will they need instruction? What is each person's role on the team?

If it is made perfectly clear that your team is coming to assist you in having a gentle and compassionate birth, and not to protect you or to make decisions for you, the nurses will not become defensive and territorial. Make sure that members of your birth team also understand the limits of their involvement. If they should say something that causes the nursing staff to become defensive, they can turn a birthing room into a silent, or not-so-silent, battleground. Remember, if you choose to birth in the hospital, you must expect the medical team to follow the protocols set down for them by the administration. You may not be able to have everything you want.

Here are a few guidelines for creating a birth plan. They were written by Amy Gilliland, one of the most respected doula educators in the DONA (Doulas of Northern America) organization.

1) Start out with a general statement introducing yourself, your philosophy and possibly your reasons for choosing your hospital or birthing center.
2) Use positive language whenever possible.
3) In general, it is more positive and descriptive to state what you do want rather than what you don't want. "To avoid an episiotomy or tearing of the perineal tissues, please use warm compresses and help me to breathe the baby out slowly."
4) Be specific. "I want to be free to move around during labor as I choose," rather than "I want an active birth."
5) Don't try to cover everything—only those areas most important to you. The reader can get bogged down in detail and your main message can be lost.
6) Use organizational headings that help to guide the reader. Here are a few suggestions. During labor—First Stage; During labor—Second Stage; Infant Care; Supporting Breast-feeding; Emergencies. You may or may not want to title the introductory paragraph.
7) Some parents wish to include sections on emergencies such as a cesarean operation, intensive care for their infant, or the baby's death.
8) As you read what you have written, ask yourself "How do I feel reading this?" Put yourself in the place of a hospital staff member and/or doctor.
9) Ask your caregiver to review the birth plan and sign the document. You may also wish to sign it along with your partner and doula.
10) If you are planning a homebirth it is wise to prepare both a homebirth plan and a hospital birth plan. It is especially important if you will be arriving at the hospital after a complication at home. In some areas it is unwise to reveal your homebirth arrangements. You may wish to discuss this further with your midwife or doctor.
11) When completed, use a highlighter pen to call attention to the most important phrases.

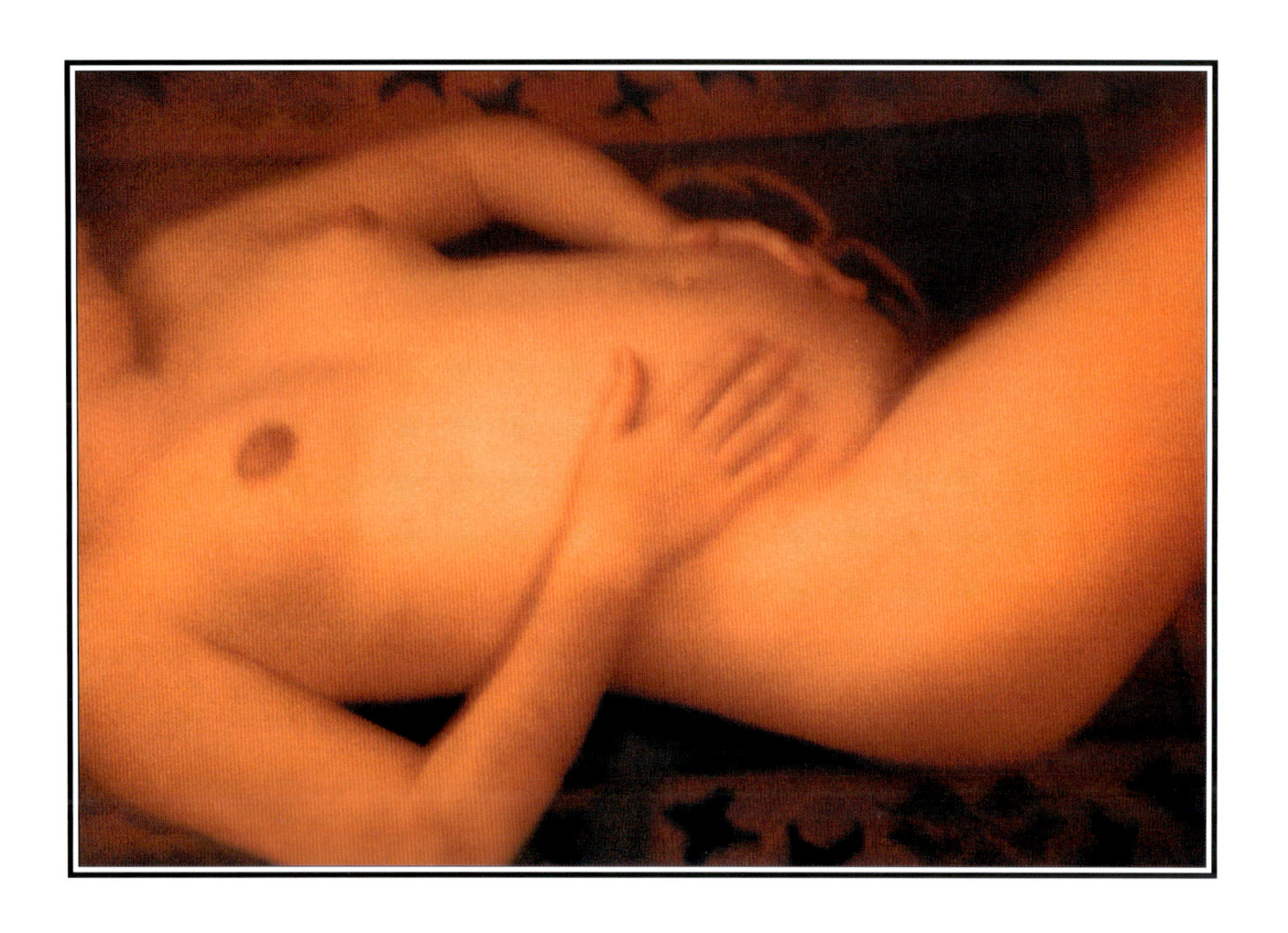

"So God created man in his own image, in the image of God He created him; male and female He created them."

Genesis 1:27 (NKJ)

Part Two

Respect The Human Body

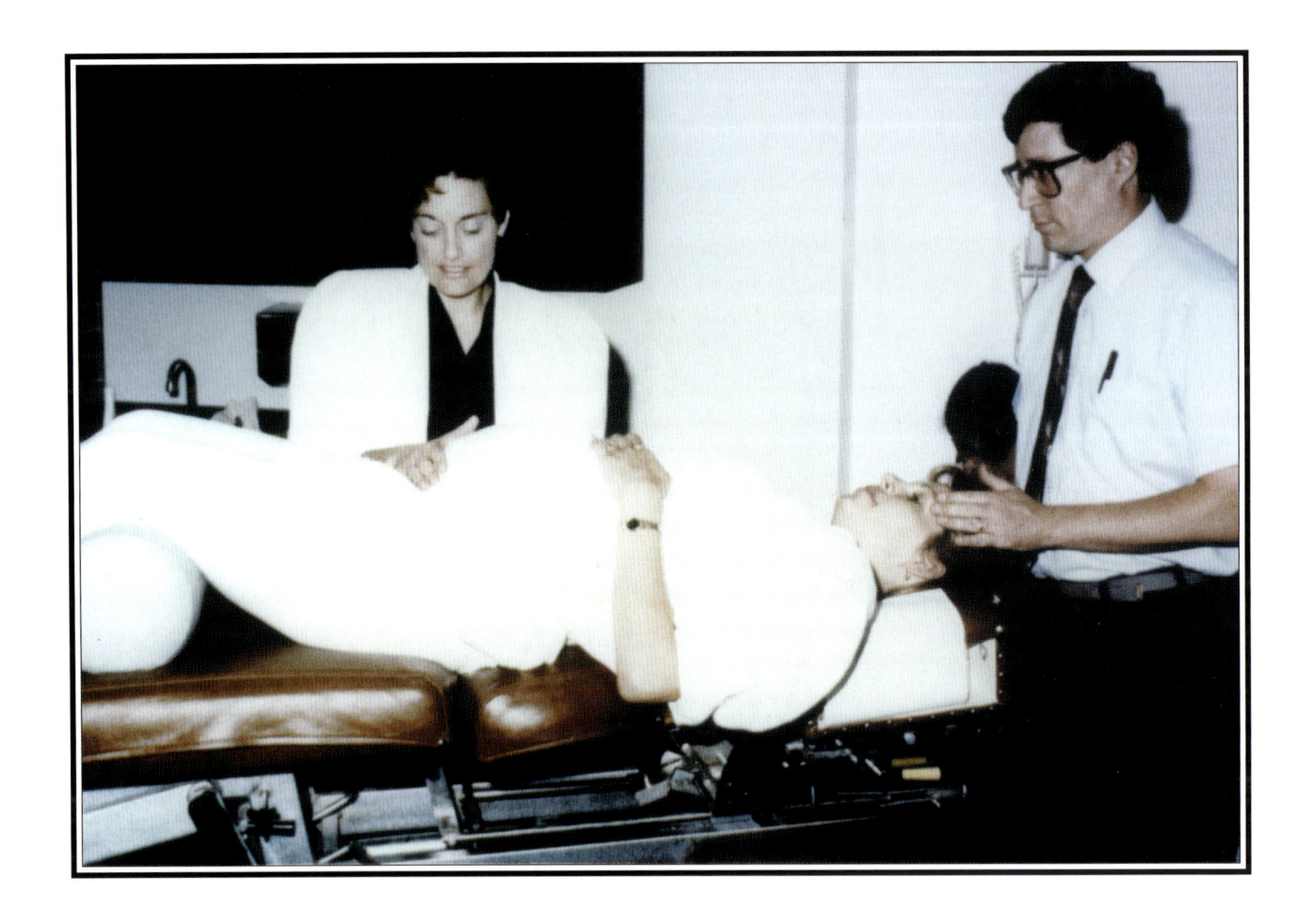

Pregnancy is beautiful; it should be a time of physical comfort and emotional joy. Chiropractic prenatal care can help a woman feel vibrant and energetic by removing any interference to this natural state of health.

STEP 4
Seek Relief for the Discomforts of Pregnancy and Birth

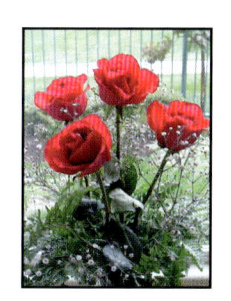

Once you have completed Steps 1 – 3 of this pregnancy plan you should have the peace of mind that all of the players are in position. By this time your baby has grown from a tiny seedling to a fully formed human being. There is no doubt in your mind that he is in there. Late at night you may lie awake wishing he would take a break and let you get some sleep. At other times, it is fun to just lie there and enjoy the soft rolling of his body. You may wonder if he has taken up boxing and is practicing for the pee wee Olympics, or maybe he decided to be a gymnast and is gearing up for the big event. Whatever it is he is doing in there, it is comforting to know he is fine and able to move freely. But, what happens if he can't?

Life Inside the Womb

Nestled in a twilight water world and wrapped tightly in a bed of pulsating, undulating soft tissue, your unborn child is subjected to continuous sensory input that stimulates the receptors responsible for touch and hearing. Free to swim, turn, roll, and play as much as he would like, your baby trusts that his home will remain open, expansive and accommodating to his playful moves.

Should your baby's environment become restrictive, due to distortions within your body, he will be confined to whatever position he can get into. Sometimes the restrictions become so severe he can no longer roll and play. His ever-growing body will then place undue force against your internal structures, causing you pain and discomfort that can last for days, weeks, or even months.

If the confinement is severe, I find mothers coming in for chiropractic care with symptoms that range from a wide variety of musculoskeletal complaints to unexplained emotional anxiety. I have learned to listen to what a pregnant mother *feels* and to read between the lines. Sometimes, the problem is clearly a structural imbalance within her body. At other times, her symptoms are a warning that the baby is terribly uncomfortable. I also find that a baby will try any way possible to let his mother know that he needs help. If he is stuck, he will punch and jab at her in an attempt to free some part of his body. Sometimes he can no longer punch or kick due to the in-utero constraint, but a careful examination of the mother's abdomen can reveal the abnormal position.

Chiropractic adjustments and craniosacral therapy are effective tools to free your baby and reduce the subsequent discomfort you may feel. This is accomplished by balancing your pelvis (and associated musculature) to assist the uterus in resuming a balanced, upright position.

> You might be asking, "What is it about chiropractic care and pregnancy?"
>
> I always have to laugh when my patients get up off the table and exclaim, "How in the world do other women get through pregnancy without adjustments?" Looking back on the severity of my own problems during pregnancy, (pre-chiropractic) I, too, wonder why other women put up with the many uncomfortable feelings that may crop up during pregnancy, labor or delivery when chiropractic care can make all the difference! Maybe, they just don't know?

If you don't know how great chiropractic prenatal care is, it is time you learned. To explain how this profession can help alleviate many of the complaints that pregnant women come in with, I'd like to take you on a journey into the world of the pregnant woman. Let's begin with the concept of balance.

The Importance of Balance

A new mother must provide her unborn child with a home that serves as an ever-expanding playground, a full-service cafeteria, and a warm comfortable cradle, all in one package. Few people are aware that to achieve this there is an incredible balancing act going on within a mother's body during every moment of her pregnancy. To accomplish this act, a mother must fine-tune all of the systems and structures within her body. Any imbalance within a mother's body can result in a deviation away from her normal state of homeostasis (physical stability) and toward a state of dysfunction, discomfort, and/or disease. Here are a few things you must know about the design of a woman's body if you are to appreciate it's remarkable ability to grow and deliver a child.

The Uterus

First of all, the uterus is not a free-floating home for the baby. It is anchored tightly into the bony pelvis by eight distinct ligaments. Imagine for a moment that the pear-shaped uterus is a hot air balloon; surrounded by a large and majestic mountain range, the balloon would be tethered to the ground to insure that it does not float up and away. Well, evenly spaced ligaments also anchor the uterus to the pelvic floor. If our imaginary balloon handlers were to misjudge where to anchor any particular stake used to secure the ropes in the ground, the balloon would tip—making it difficult, if not impossible, for someone to enter or exit the basket. The same thing could happen to the uterus causing the cervical portion, the cervix, to tip away from the center of the vaginal canal.

The Ligaments

When the ligaments on the front of the uterus contract more than the ones in the back, the uterus will be pulled forward. The forward pitch of the uterus can result in pressure being applied to the delicate nerves and arteries that supply the muscles of the groin and upper thigh. When this happens, a mother will suddenly stop walking and complain of pain in her groin or the muscles in front of her leg. If the uterus maintains this forward shift, the baby can be pressed down against the cervix. Mothers complain of extreme cervical pressure and feelings that the baby may *fall out*.

This pressure will cause the mother's brain to receive a message that the baby is fully-grown and ready to exit the canal. The result may be premature labor. With bed rest, the uterus drops back, and the contractions stop. When a mother gets up to go to the bathroom, the uterus falls forward and activates premature labor again—despite the use of drugs to stop uterine activity.

If the ligaments in the back contract more than ligaments in the front, the uterus will be pulled backwards. Often identified as a tipped uterus, this will usually correct itself as the baby grows and pulls the uterus upright. If it does not self-correct, the mother may experience back pain during pregnancy and/or delivery; she may complain of lower abdominal pressure and cramping.

Should the ligaments on one side of the body contract more than the other side, the uterus will be pulled sideways, which off-centers the baby and results in maternal rib or hip pain as the baby presses on those structures.

The Muscles

The mother's pelvic floor muscles are also performing a balancing act. If the muscles in the front are too tight, the mother may complain of pubic bone pain or cramping just above the pubic area. It may also be difficult for her to urinate. If the piriformis muscles on both sides of her bum are too tight, she will complain of discomfort that feels like a band of pain across her entire lower back. If the piriformis muscles are contracted on one side only, the muscles on the other side are stretched down on the large sciatic nerve. This will cause sciatic pain that shoots down that leg. Consequently, the problem is on the side OPPOSITE the side of pain.

You see it's all about balance. Chiropractors are helpful during pregnancy because we are experts at restoring balance to the bony skeleton and normalizing the tone of the muscles. When balance is restored to these structures, interference to the normal flow of the life force through the nervous system and the vascular system is reduced and a mother feels much better.

There are many common situations that may cause an imbalance to occur within the structures of the body, such as when a pregnant mother carries a sibling on one hip. She must contract one side of her gluteal muscles to arch the supporting hip upwards. Another situation is when a mother twists her body while taking a child in and out of the car. There is no ergonomically effective way to do this unless she has a large van. Another cause of imbalance is a job that requires repetitive twisting of the trunk muscles (i.e., computer monitors should always be placed directly in front of the body). Women also get their body

STEP 4: Seek Relief for the Discomforts of Pregnancy and Birth

twisted while sleeping, if they don't use pillows to support their back and elevate their leg. Previous physical injuries from accidents and sport activities may also result in an imbalance in the body.

Restoring balance to the structural framework and the muscular components of the body will result in a balanced uterus, which can contribute to a comfortable pregnancy and a happy mother/baby couple.

I could share thousands of stories of women who have come into my chiropractic practice with a variety of complaints such as extreme leg pain, heartburn, back pain, or premature labor. In the majority of these cases, they received a few adjustments and the complaints resolved quickly and permanently. Their stories would be short and to the point. Instead, I think it would be more helpful to share the story of a mother whose pregnancy was complicated by several factors. This is a mother who chose to ease the discomfort associated with carrying two babies by incorporating other modalities into her typical medical prenatal care.

Pebbles and BamBam

After years of medical treatment for endometriosis, Deb and Keith were finally successful at conceiving a child. They had no idea, however, how their life would be turned upside down by that pregnancy. I became involved with Deb as her chiropractor, doula, and friend.

I met Deb when I presented a lecture on chiropractic-doula support at her Minneapolis Bradley birthing class. Keith was unable to attend the class, so Deb brought Mary, her friend and labor support person. Never having seen a real birth herself, Mary was also preparing herself for the upcoming delivery.

After hearing my lecture, Deb began to wonder if she'd benefit from chiropractic care. She'd spent years dealing with endometriosis and had never realized that her gynecological problems might have been due to nerve interference to the reproductive system. After the class, Deb discussed her situation with me and scheduled an appointment for the following week. Keith was four hours away remodeling their newly purchased home, so it was a few weeks before I had the opportunity to meet him.

KEITH: *I was skeptical when I joined Deb for her second visit to Dr. Carol's office because I had been led to believe that chiropractors were witch doctors who would sprinkle magic dust on your back and charge you a lot of money, or worse yet, injure you. At the time of Deb's second visit, I had just seen two medical doctors for a pinched nerve in my back. Their only solution was pain medication. After Deb's appointment, I told Carol about my own back problems. She arranged for me to be evaluated and adjusted that same day. The pain was gone immediately after the adjustment and it has never come back. That experience changed my long-standing opinion of chiropractors.*

DEB: *I went through years of hormonal treatment and five surgeries for painful endometriosis. We eventually gave up on a medical approach to the management of my pain and were told not to get our hopes up for conception, due to the severity of the scar tissue. Consequently, Keith and I were extremely surprised and happy to finally get pregnant. We immediately made major changes in our lifestyle to accommodate this new and exciting journey into parenthood. I gave six months notice at my job, we put our house up for sale, and we bought a log home on the North Shore of Lake Superior. I had dreams of putting my baby in a backpack and spending hours hiking in the woods. I knew I would be nursing, so all I needed would be a few diapers and off we'd go. I had our new life all figured out and it seemed like a dream come true.*

When I was six weeks pregnant, I began having unusual pelvic pain. Since I had such a long history of endometriosis, I was quickly scheduled for a transvaginal ultrasound. It took the nurse only a few minutes to pull the ultrasound head out of the birth canal and say, "I have something exciting to tell you." We had no idea what she meant.

The nurse announced, "There's two." We had no idea what she could be talking about when we responded, "Two what?" She laughed and said, "Two babies." Keith turned as white as a ghost and I burst into sobs. The nurse had assumed we'd be happy. She had no idea how devastated I was. In that brief moment, all my dreams were shattered. All we ever wanted was one healthy baby and a peaceful life together in the North Woods.

We had planned to find a midwife and have a perfect low-tech birth experience for our baby. Twins! All of the possible complications associated with a multiple birth rapidly flashed through my mind. I continued to sob and asked the nurse if I would be required to have a c-section. She said, "Yes, you probably will, so you might as well get used to that idea." I was still crying when they took us into another room to meet with the obstetrician.

Unlike the nurse, the OB did not assume that we were happy with the news of having twins and asked us how we felt about it. I explained that I was devastated. She expressed how happy she was that we were reacting that way. The obstetrician explained that she's always concerned when a couple's initial response to the news is one of pure excitement. To her, that kind of reaction usually indicates they're not being realistic about the situation, and might be setting themselves up for problems down the road.

I asked for her opinion about the likelihood of having a cesarean. Unlike the nurse, the OB said, "No, your chances of having a normal vaginal birth are very good." Her caring and accepting attitude helped me as I continued to deal with the worry and sorrow that surrounded my heart.

Relatives and friends were not as understanding as the doctor had been about my concerns. Many people thought I should feel blessed. After all, Keith and I had endured years of medical treatment in our attempt to preserve my fertility. All along, we had accepted the possibility of having a life together without children. Now, they wondered how I could feel bad about having twins.

During our initial appointment, I was warned that discovering twins so early on in the pregnancy meant there was an increased chance that one of them might not survive. I was told it is fairly common for women to miscarry a twin and not even realize it. For a short time in the beginning, I couldn't help but wish that one of them might choose not to come into the world at this time. I was angry, unhappy, bitter, and irrational.

At 12 weeks, I had another sonogram. There they were—two real-live babies. Their feet were kicking. Their little hands were moving. I was sure they were waving at me. Suddenly, I knew. I wanted both of these babies. At times, I felt angry because they were coming at the same time, but I wanted with all my heart for both of them to live.

When I realized how much I wanted both babies, I also realized I needed to take especially good care of my health, so I scheduled myself for massage therapy and started interviewing various doctors.

KEITH: *I heard the nurse say there were two babies, but I didn't want to believe what I was hearing. When I could speak again I said, "You don't see anymore do you?" I was frightened to death that she'd discover a third one. I also knew immediately this was going to really complicate our lives, as the pregnancy would now be more difficult. I think it took me about a week to adjust and accept the idea of having twins. It helped me a lot to accept the reality when we saw them on ultrasound and nicknamed them Pebbles and BamBam. BamBam was the baby high in the uterus and Pebbles was the one down below. Ironically, that is how they came out—Pebbles first and then BamBam.*

DEB: *I started prenatal care in Minneapolis since I had to continue working there, but I wanted to find a good obstetrician near our new home. By the end of the pregnancy I would be able to join Keith in Two Harbors, but the idea of being three or four hours away from my doctor was not ideal. It seemed wise to eventually switch all care to the nearest city of Duluth, Minneapolis. I tried to get an appointment for a consultation with an*

STEP 4: Seek Relief for the Discomforts of Pregnancy and Birth

obstetrician who was known to accept multiple pregnancies. His receptionist absolutely refused to let me speak to him until I had a prenatal appointment with his nurse practitioner. Keith and I hated jumping all the hoops, but we finally agreed to meet with the nurse so we could get an appointment with the obstetrician. As we expected, the nurse was unable to answer our specific questions about the obstetrician's delivery protocol for twins.

Consequently, we were finally allowed to meet with the doctor. I felt he answered our many questions adequately. Keith, on the other hand, felt that the doctor was agitated with us for asking questions. Then, as we were leaving, the OB said, "You know, you should expect that your second twin will have learning disabilities." We were dumbfounded. When we asked "Why?," he said the placenta commonly deteriorates too fast for the second one to get enough oxygen.

We'd read everything we could get our hands on about twins, but we never read anything about the placenta deteriorating at a fast rate. As we walked out of the office, Keith looked at me and said, "We will NOT have our babies with him!" I went straight home and called my doctor in Minneapolis and asked her if she'd continue to be my doctor. She agreed, but only if I would agree to move back to Minneapolis for the last four weeks of the pregnancy. I would have moved back for the whole pregnancy in order to protect our children.

When Deb and Keith decided they wanted to have the babies in Minneapolis, they had to make arrangements for someone to be with Deb in case Keith couldn't get to the hospital on time. They asked her best friend, Mary, to provide labor support. She was a good friend and had offered her home to Deb during her last month of pregnancy so she'd be close to the hospital. Deb attended birthing classes in Duluth with Keith and in Minneapolis with Mary. This brings the story full circle, to the point where Deb and Mary attended the Bradley birth education class that I was guest lecturing in.

At that time in my career, I had started reducing the number of births I could attend and began encouraging people to let me train their friends and relatives to provide doula support. It was becoming difficult to attend one to two births a week and keep up with my practice and teaching. After meeting with Deb and Keith, I put my concerns aside and asked them if I could join their birth team. I had never seen two babies born at the same time and I loved the attitude this couple had about protecting their babies.

To my delight, they said yes. They also agreed to let my extern, Eileen, assist me in providing chiropractic-doula support during the delivery. Mary was as excited as we were about the way the birth team was evolving. At one point, she shared with me that she was glad to know that an experienced doula would be assisting her—"It is one thing to go through the class with Deb, but another to be the only support person at the delivery if Keith doesn't make it." Keith was also happy that Eileen and I were going to be attending the birth. He felt more secure knowing that if he should miss the birth due to a snowstorm, the rest of us would be with Deb and their babies.

Deb and Keith agreed to make the four-hour drive down from the North Shore every two weeks to see me. At each visit, I would give Keith pointers on what he could do if she started having discomfort or pain due to the position or size of the babies. I gave him written instructions on how to relax the pelvic floor muscles and showed him how to do some of the work. All that training paid off when Deb's truck was rear-ended while sitting at a stop light.

Deb told me she was looking off to the side with her foot on the brake when another vehicle struck her truck and drove it forward about eight feet. At the time, she was extremely upset and fearful, but appeared to be physically uninjured. Thankfully, the babies seemed quiet and Deb felt no sign of impending labor. She got back in the truck and went on to her destination, feeling relieved that nothing serious had happened and that she and the babies were all right.

The next day, Deb began to have serious complications. She was unable to lift her legs to climb the stairs. They tingled and felt extremely weak. Her symptoms continued to get worse throughout the day. When Keith arrived home, he lifted Deb into the truck and took her straight to an emergency room. The babies were checked out and showed no signs of distress. Deb was told to go home and rest.

I received a frantic call as soon as Deb and Keith arrived home from the hospital. Duluth was too far away for a house call, so I suggested that Keith read the information on how to release the pelvic floor muscles. I explained to him that Deb had her body slightly rotated on impact. Her lap belt stabilized her pelvis and her harness stabilized her left shoulder.

Consequently, I was sure that the impact had caused the free right shoulder to torque forward and to her left, causing a twist in the muscles of her torso and diaphragms. The weight of the two babies and all of their amniotic fluid would increase the amount of torque applied to her musculature. I went on to explain that the tight muscles within her pelvis could constrict the structures that supply blood and nerve flow to her legs. This would result in the symptoms she was describing.

Keith was willing to try anything. He read the information on transverse fascial release of the pelvic diaphragm (the same procedure I use to relax the pelvic floor muscles during labor) and proceeded to try it. To their surprise, it worked. As Keith gently performed the maneuver, Deb could feel the tension subsiding. It wasn't long before her symptoms started resolving. As Deb's muscles continued to relax, the tingling in her legs stopped and she fell asleep.

The next day was Saturday. Deb was able to drive herself to Minneapolis and I spent two hours restoring balance to the rest of her body. The symptoms never returned; we all believed that Keith saved those babies because he was willing to step out of his comfort zone and do something unusual to reduce her discomfort.

DEB: *During the last part of my pregnancy, I suffered from carpal tunnel syndrome, gastroesophageal reflux (excessive burping up of stomach contents), premature contractions, tremendous swelling of my legs and feet, heartburn, and pain in my hands and feet. The chiropractic adjustments really helped relieve most of the symptoms except premature contractions. They would always subside but only for about one week after an adjustment. During the ninth month, it would only help for about three days. But with regular treatment, the contractions were minor and my cervix didn't change until the ninth month; my doctor held off giving me medication to reduce the contractions until then.*

I don't believe I could have gone full term without the chiropractic and massage visits, and I seriously think the comfort provided by treatment was critical to my being able to carry the babies to fullterm.

While chiropractic adjustments and medication helped me avoid premature delivery during the ninth month, nothing helped relieve my problems with reflux. If I laid down for even a few minutes, my stomach contents would come up and I would start coughing as it went into my lungs. For the last two months, I did everything in a seated or semi-reclined position. Dr. Carol even had to perform chiropractic adjustments with me in a semi-reclined position. I slept each night alternating between lying on my side in a recliner and sitting up on the couch. (I never slept for more than one hour at a time.)

Initially, we were doing whatever we could to avoid having pre-term babies. The last thing I wanted was to have two babies living in the special care nursery instead of at home with us. By the end of my ninth month, I was begging to know when the OB would induce me. The chiropractic care helped relieve most of my discomfort, but I simply didn't think I could take it anymore.

My doctor finally said she was willing to stimulate the hormones and possibly activate labor by reaching inside of the cervix to strip my membranes. She agreed to do this the week before the due date, but insisted that I be scheduled for a non-stress ultrasound before she did the procedure—I guess she wanted to make sure the babies could handle the tight squeeze of a labor contraction.

I don't know why they call it a non-stress ultrasound. It is extremely stressful to be strapped to a machine, told you have to push a button every time you feel the baby move, and you're expected to distinguish one baby from the other. If one of the babies did not pass by moving the appropriate amount of times, I had to go back in two days for another ultrasound—more stress!

STEP 4: Seek Relief for the Discomforts of Pregnancy and Birth

During pregnancy, my babies were exposed to a transvaginal ultrasound, five regular ultrasounds, and weekly non-stress ultrasounds for two months. On one occasion, I was told the babies did not "pass the test" and I stressed! For the follow-up test two days later, I used a technique Dr. Carol taught me to wake the babies up and get them moving.

Just before going in, I drank a big glass of orange juice to get the babies charged with energy. Then I talked to them and told them they had to wake up, and move, or we'd have to stay on the machine a long time. I warned them; if they didn't move for mom, the nurse would make me use the instrument that made the loud noise against their ears—and that wouldn't feel very good. They listened, moved immediately, and I was allowed to get off the machine. They were both just fine.

From that point on, every time a nurse said one of the babies had an abnormal heart rate, or they were not moving around the right number of times, I would mentally tell the babies what they had to do—and they would!

It was almost Christmas, my due date was around the first of January, and I didn't want to be pregnant any longer! I felt like it was time to get this show on the road. I had eliminated the medication used to stop premature labor, so I had regular Braxton Hicks contractions. Ironically, I had none of the usual indicators of impending labor. No bloody show. No leakage of water. After spending months successfully keeping me from having premature contractions, we were trying everything we could to get labor started.

We made love, had a friend's 12-week-old baby nurse on me for nipple stimulation, and walked the mall. Nothing worked. At the mall, people would always appear so shocked to see me walking around. They just couldn't resist stopping me to ask if I was overdue, or if I was carrying twins. At that point in time, I would usually snap at them. I was in no mood to carry on a conversation about why I was so incredibly big! Eventually, my abdomen seemed to be in one long continuous contraction that was impossible to time.

It was Thursday when my doctor finally reached inside and stripped my membranes away from the cervix. On Friday, I had another non-stress ultrasound. The nurse felt sure I would have the babies over the weekend and tried to cheer me up by saying that she didn't expect to see us back the following week. That was nice to hear. Saturday came and went. Nothing!

On Sunday, I woke up early, and to my excitement, I saw the release of the mucus plug! Finally, we were getting somewhere. I used a piece of litmus paper to test for amniotic fluid. The paper turned blue. Now, I knew my water was leaking out. We called the obstetrician and went straight to the hospital. They put me on a continuous fetal monitor, which showed I was having minor uterine activity, but they couldn't confirm that the water bag had broken. They sent us home, again. We were so incredibly disappointed. Keith unloaded the suitcase and stereo from the car. This was the third time he'd packed and unpacked our things. I was so upset I called Carol.

That evening we went over to Carol's house. (We had become good friends by now.) She had the lights down low, a fire going in the fireplace, soft music playing in the background, and a recliner. She had Keith lie down on the couch to get some much-needed rest; he hadn't had much sleep since he'd moved down from Two Harbors a week earlier. I was somewhat used to sleep deprivation, but he wasn't and it was taking a toll on him. For the next two hours, Carol worked on my terribly swollen legs and arms. She did polarity therapy, acupressure and craniosacral therapy. Finally, she adjusted my neck and sent us home. That night, I slept for several hours without waking. That was the most sleep I'd had in weeks.

On Monday, I refused to let Keith pack anything into the car when we went in for another non-stress test. This time, during the exam, the nurse pushed up on the baby's head and water gushed everywhere. I was right! My bag had broken and the baby's head was just plugging up the opening! Finally, my doctor said I could stay and have my babies. Unfortunately, we didn't have our music, clothes, or anything else we needed for the labor! We called Mary right away and asked her to stop and pick up some of our things.

As labor contractions got stronger, I tried using the O-O-O tone that we'd learned from Carol in the birthing class. Unfortunately, it just didn't work for me. I think it might have worked if my contractions had come and gone like they were supposed to. But these contractions never followed a normal pattern. Instead of building up and then relaxing, they were continuous and strong. It was as if I never stopped contracting.

Despite the intensity of my contractions, the doctor wanted to hurry the labor along by injecting pitocin. I refused. She agreed to wait, but since my water had broken on Sunday, she insisted on starting the pitocin within a few hours. It was time to call Carol.

When I told Carol we were in the hospital, she said that it would take several hours for her to get away from the clinic. A baby was coming in from out of town and he had to be treated before she could leave. I really wanted to wait until she arrived before allowing them to start the pitocin—but my time was running out. Finally, I got tired of putting the doctor off and I knew I couldn't wait for Carol any longer—I let them put in the IV.

1:00 P.M.
DEB: *As soon as they started the pitocin, I started throwing up. I refused to come out of the bathroom to be hooked up to the monitor; this angered the nurse. Then Keith tried putting the analgesic Carol had given us on my back, but I couldn't stand the smell of it. In fact, once he had it on his hands, I didn't want him anywhere near me. I kept shoving him away because the smell was so terrible. I'd always liked it before, but not now! Keith kept trying to wash it off, but I could still smell it. Another problem was that whenever I would lean up against him, he'd hug me really tight.*

I was extremely sensitive to smells, and my skin suddenly became very sensitive, too. I kept pushing Keith away because his efforts to comfort me just heightened my sensitivity. This was not going the way I had hoped. The contractions were nonstop and the pitocin just made me more uncomfortable.

3:00 P.M.
I could no longer cope with the pain and continuous contraction—I finally accepted a shot of Nubain. I really didn't want to take anything and struggled with my decision before I accepted the shot. When they assured me it would be like having a good stiff cocktail, I gave in.

3:15 P.M.
Finally, Carol and her extern, Eileen, arrived. I was hiding in the bathroom. All of a sudden, between the shot and Carol's presence, I was able to get myself centered and relaxed. All I wanted to do was to sit on the toilet and lean forward, resting my head on Carol's shoulder. Somehow, she just kept rocking me and that allowed me to go deep within myself.

If anything changed or anyone asked me to do something different, I would start to come out of my calm place within, and I would panic. I only felt pain if I started to lose my focus. Then, I would cry out to Carol, "Help me, I can't relax!" I remember her picking up my limp arm and letting it drop. "Does this look like a woman who can't relax?" I heard giggling from the doorway where Keith, Eileen, and Mary were quietly watching us. They were watching from the doorway because I didn't want anyone except Carol coming near me while I was in the bathroom. Keith ran interference so we could be alone and made sure the lights were kept off. Mary was extremely helpful and would get anything we asked of her, from ice cubes to hot rags.

STEP 4: Seek Relief for the Discomforts of Pregnancy and Birth

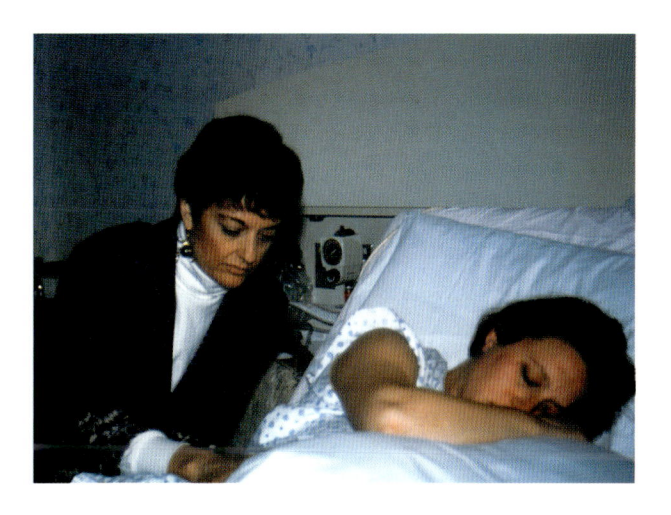

KEITH: *I felt really rejected by Deb. I wanted so bad to help her with the labor, but I just couldn't get the smell of that damn analgesic off my hands and I couldn't hold her right without making her mad. Finally, Carol explained that I was holding Deb too tightly and that her skin was extremely sensitive. Later on in the labor, Deb finally let me help. She would stand in front of me and put her arms around my neck. She would bend her knees and hang on my shoulders to let gravity help the babies move down. I planted my feet and held her up, even though it was absolutely killing my back.*

At some point, someone started rubbing the muscles that were starting to spasm in my back. That back rub was one of those hurts— but feels great feelings. While the massage absolutely saved me, I didn't bother to ask who was doing it. I think it was Eileen.

5:00 P.M.

I finally asked Deb to lie down. I wanted to do a pelvic diaphragm release so I could relax her pelvic muscles. That really helped move her toward complete dilation. Finally, the nurses came in and brought us all scrubs. Since Deb and Keith had presented the doctor and nurses with a copy of their birth plan, no one questioned the fact that we were all going into the delivery room with Deb and Keith. We took turns changing in the bathroom. While one person changed, the rest of us continued working with Deb. When she began to show signs of involuntary pushing, I gave her some last minute advice.

I told Deb I would coach her through the second stage by encouraging her to let the baby slide rather than telling her to push it out. (The word push sometimes sounds negative, where slide is the same action—just a lot easier on the baby.) When she felt the urge to push, I wanted Deb to take a deep cleansing breath of oxygen, tuck her chin to her chest, round her pelvis up toward the ceiling, and hold that breath as I counted to ten. I encouraged her to follow her instincts first, and our coaching second.

DEB: *I was glad they didn't try to move me to the delivery room any sooner than they did. I suspect that would have been awful. It would've broken my concentration and increased my pain.*

When I did begin to push, I wondered why we weren't moving to the delivery room. I thought that you pushed once or twice and out came the baby... so shouldn't we get going?

When I got to the second stage of labor, I was extremely excited to finally be able to DO something more active to get my babies out. I no longer had to focus so hard on riding out the contractions; I no longer needed to concentrate on staying in control; I didn't even care where I was or who was around. They could have put me in the middle of the street for all I cared... I was delivering my babies!

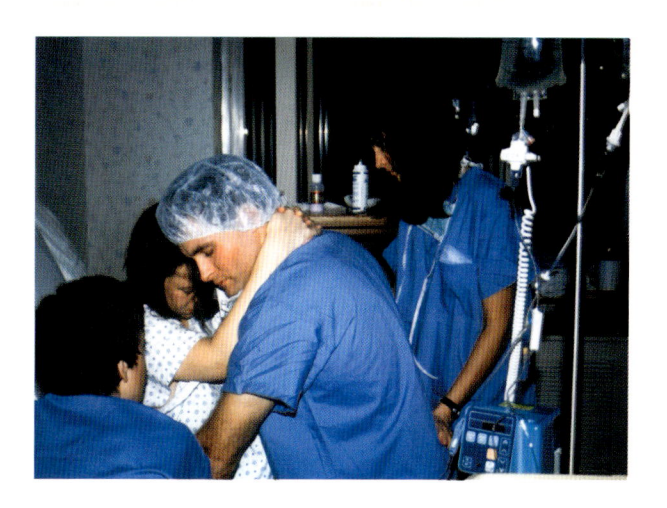

Hands Of Love

KEITH: *Moving Deb to the delivery room was like a disorganized parade. Mary, Eileen and I gathered the portable stereo, tapes, camera, and several rolls of film. Carol stayed close to Deb as they moved her entire bed to the delivery room. We had already told them that we didn't want her transferred to a delivery table, so they pushed the whole bed into the delivery room, along with two baby warmers, all the medical equipment to do a C-section, and the ultrasound monitor. Somewhere in the process of moving from the labor room to the delivery room, Mary, Eileen and I were separated from the parade. We lost Deb.*

There we stood. We had on our scrubs. Our arms were loaded down with everything we needed for the delivery room—and we didn't know where to go. Suddenly, a nurse rescued us and sent us in the right direction. As we entered the operating room, I quickly had the lights dimmed and I turned on the tape we'd been playing throughout the labor. We were organized but the room was incredibly small for the number of people in attendance.

Carol, Mary, Eileen, and I crowded around Deb while the nurses stood back with the two neonatologists who were observing. They seemed to be ready to step in if Deb had problems, but for the time being, they let us just carry on as we had in the labor room. Mary tried to take pictures, while Carol continued to encourage Deb to keep sliding our babies down. I stayed as close as I could and held Deb's hand.

> Dr. Leboyer in his book *Birth Without Violence* suggested that we dim the lights in the delivery room to spare the baby any unnecessary pain. Somehow, I think his concept has been misunderstood. Now, room lights are often dimmed for the comfort of the mother (which is good), but a large spotlight is then pointed directly into the emerging face of the newborn. The newborn must then adjust from the light of a twilight world to a glaring spotlight no more than two feet away. I once video taped a newborn covering his eyes with his forearm as he screamed from the intensity of the light shining in his eyes.

The beautiful voice of Prudence Johnson singing lullabies filled the room. The delivery room lights were dimmed to block out the ominous presence of machines and emergency equipment. More than seven staff people stood in the background. After getting everything set up, we all turned our attention to Deb and the little crowning head. At the foot of the bed, the obstetrician sat between Deb's legs. Shining over her shoulder was the biggest, brightest spotlight they could point toward the baby. The medical staff stood in the dim light, providing Deb with the illusion of privacy while little Pebbles gradually worked her way down the canal toward the bright light.

Deb pushed for about 20 minutes before Pebbles (later named Becca) slid into the doctor's hands. She was passed immediately to the neonatologist for evaluation, leaving Deb and Keith unable to see or touch her. Deb was frightened and worried when Pebbles only let out one tiny cry. Silence filled the room for several minutes before Deb expressed her concern. A nurse wrapped Becca up and brought her right over to the bed. Deb and Keith held her and cried as they marveled at her tiny face. She was fine.

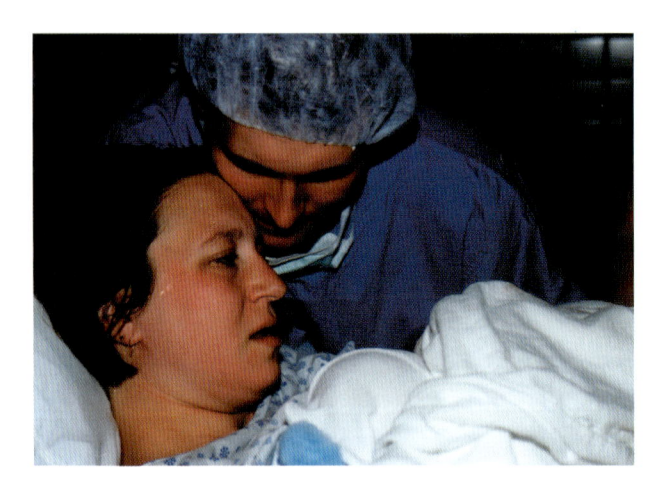

All of a sudden, Deb held Becca out to the crowd and shouted, "Somebody take this baby!" BamBam was coming.

Mary quickly took Becca from Deb and handed her to a nurse. Mary and Eileen followed the nurse as Becca was rushed to the nursery. The birth team had previously agreed that Eileen and Mary would stay with the first baby, while Keith and I stayed with Deb.

STEP 4: Seek Relief for the Discomforts of Pregnancy and Birth

The OB examined Deb and said her cervix had reduced itself to seven centimeters after the first baby delivered. She now had to dilate quickly up to 10 centimeters for delivery. Unfortunately, BamBam was still high in the uterus and was not coming down as quickly as they wanted him to. A nurse then climbed up on a stool and began to apply pressure on Deb's abdomen to push BamBam down.

The monitor, pushed up against Deb's bed, began to register signs of fetal distress. The baby's heart rate was dropping and not coming back up after the contraction. Everyone's focus seemed to gravitate to the monitor and away from Deb. I started to get nervous as I watched the nurse look with distress toward the OB. The room was beginning to feel charged with the energy of people preparing to go into action at any moment. Suddenly a nurse said, "We have to get this baby out!" I looked down at the face of the OB and knew I had to do something quick if we were to avoid an emergency cesarean.

The OB sat next to me. We both faced Deb and the fetal monitor. Suddenly, I threw caution to the wind and decided it was time to risk looking foolish. I turned my back to the OB, rested my hand on Deb's knee, and softly asked her to look at me. I looked right in her eyes and said in a soft, but firm tone, "Deb, the heart rate is dropping. I want you to go inside and talk to the baby. Ask him to bring it back up."

I looked at the monitor and told her to bring the rate up to a value about five beats above the existing one. I continued giving her numbers about five increments above the registered level until the baby's heart rate was in a safe range.

Deb couldn't see the monitor, but she grasped the gravity of the situation. To everyone's surprise, she closed her eyes and quickly brought the baby's heart rate up into a stable and acceptable range. We repeated this twice with each successive contraction. I then humbly turned around toward the OB, shrugged my shoulders, and said, "I just find that it works." When the next contraction resulted in the same drop in heart rate, the OB surprised me by jumping in and saying, "Now, Deb, I want you to bring the baby's heart rate up to..." I turned the coaching over to her.

Within 20 minutes of Pebble's birth, BamBam was delivered safely and without intervention. In fact, after Pebbles cleared the way for him, BamBam popped out while the OB was distracted; Keith had to dive in and catch him. He had turned upside down (face up), but had no trouble getting out. Deb said it was the strangest sensation to have him inside of her one minute, and gone the next. His cord was so short that he couldn't be brought up to Deb's breast. As soon as I saw that BamBam was fine, I took off for the nursery and left Keith and Deb alone to get acquainted with their little boy.

I entered the nursery and told Mary that BamBam was born safely. She took a few more pictures before rushing back to the delivery room. I found Eileen standing next to the warmer. She had one hand over Pebbles head and one on her chest. I watched as Eileen tried unsuccessfully to calm her. Pebbles had been screaming ever since her removal from the delivery room. I finally told Eileen I would try and calm Pebbles and asked her to go back to the delivery room and help Deb.

Fortunately, the hospital staff was extremely cooperative and allowed us the freedom to float between the nursery and the delivery room as we continued our role as doulas.

I laid my hands on Pebbles and gave her permission to go ahead and cry all she wanted. I told her how much I understood her frustration at being separated from everyone and that it was okay to cry. I also assured her that she never had to do this again in this lifetime. This finally calmed her down.

Pebbles stared into my face and tried to blink away the thick, clear antibiotic a nurse had mistakenly placed on her eyes. Unfortunately, Deb and Keith's request to hold off on applying the eye cream or giving her a vitamin K shot during the first hour after birth had been overlooked.

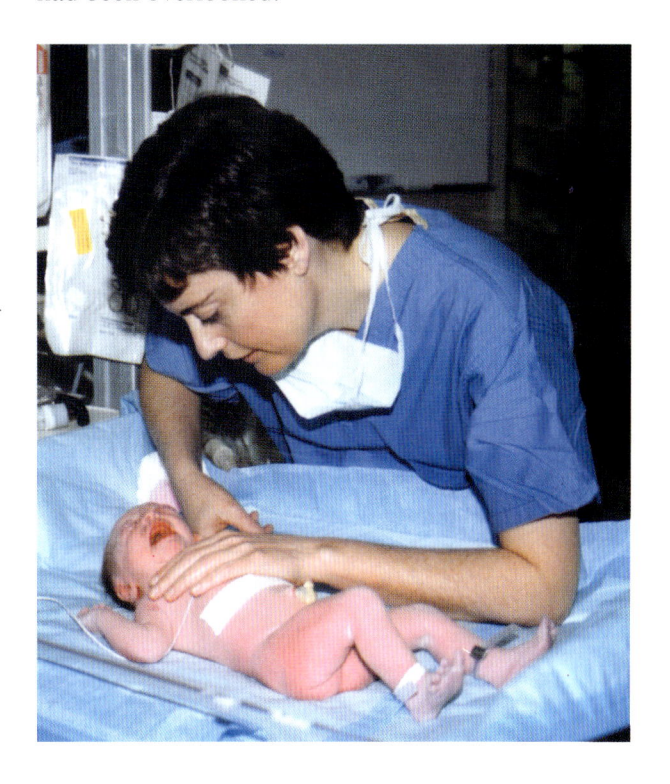

Pebble's little eyelids continued to flutter as she attempted to clear the cream from her eyes and look at me. A few minutes later, she seemed to have cleared enough of the cream to focus on my face. This kept her quiet for a few minutes. She must have realized that I was not her mom, because it wasn't long before she started screaming again. Soon afterwards, Keith arrived with BamBam (later named Erik), who was screaming just as hard as his sister. I asked the nurse if the twins could be put in the same warmer. "Sure, but just for a few minutes."

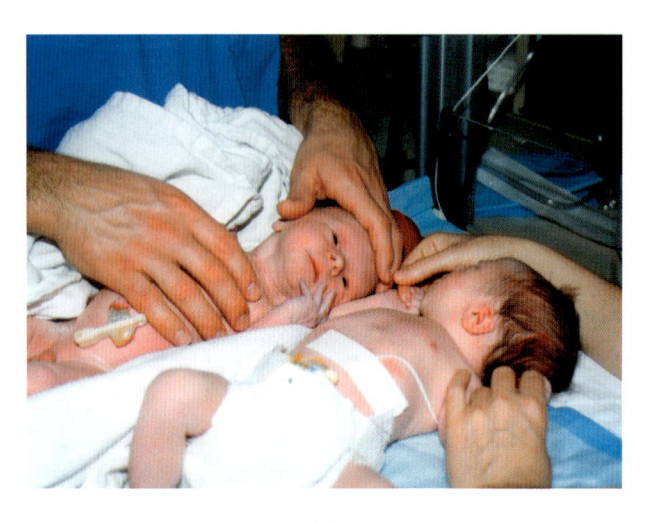

I dropped the side of the warmer down and Keith set BamBam down on the edge, his head resting on Pebbles arm. They immediately turned toward each other. They stopped screaming and stared into each other's eyes. A sense of calm suddenly came over both of them as they obviously recognized each other. BamBam held on tightly to Keith's fingers as Pebbles held on to mine. They stared silently and intently at each other for several minutes. Sadly, the nurse requested that BamBam be moved to another warmer for his newborn physical.

Keith lifted his son to move him to another warmer. Both babies responded immediately as if they were being physically torn apart. It broke my heart to watch them cry. I knew they felt both the loss of their mother's presence and their companion of nine months. Keith did his best to try and keep his hands on BamBam as he received a physical that involved squeezing his genitals to make sure the testicles had descended, pricking his heel for a blood sample, getting a shot of Vitamin K, and having an antibiotic placed over his eyes. I watched Keith cringe and I worried about his obvious anxiety. I finally had Keith come and stay with Pebbles. I felt he needed to bond with her too. This was a good time for me to try and calm BamBam.

DEB: *Suddenly everyone from the birth team was gone from the operating room except Eileen. She returned from the nursery just as Keith and Mary left with BamBam. It felt so wonderful to have Eileen there with me as she reached out and held my hand. I was not upset about being separated from the babies, because I knew they were with Keith, Carol, and Mary. I was feeling good and had just started to come out of my dazed state when the OB asked me to slide my bottom way down to the edge of the bed. She wanted to suture the vaginal tears I received when BamBam came flying through upside down.*

Before I had a chance to respond, a nurse from across the room yelled out, "She can't do that!" When asked why not, the nurse replied, "Because she's had an epidural!" I guess seeing how calm I had been during the delivery, she thought I'd been medicated. Everyone informed her that I hadn't had an epidural. I guess it surprised her that someone could deliver twins without one.

All of a sudden my body began to shake. I held onto Eileen with all my strength. The tremors were so strong they scared the daylights out of me. I can't tell you how glad I was to have Eileen there with me. I don't know what caused the tremors, but they continued for weeks after the delivery and scared me every time. I suppose it had to do with the sudden change in hormone levels.

After I was moved into my maternity suite, Keith brought Pebbles to me. BamBam remained in the nursery because his glucose was low. Carol, Mary, and Eileen had all left by this time. I wasn't happy at all with the nurse's decision to keep BamBam in the nursery. I hadn't seen him since the birth and I didn't like the idea of him being alone. The staff wouldn't let me have him until almost midnight, so my anxiety level was very high for the next 2 – 3 hours.

Outside of that initial experience, the hospital staff was just wonderful. They brought in a cot for Keith and let us take the babies out of the warmers and into bed with me. Keith was absolutely exhausted and proceeded to pass out

STEP 4: Seek Relief for the Discomforts of Pregnancy and Birth

cold. Nothing woke him up—not the babies, not my yelling at him, not the nurses, or the cleaning people. He didn't wake up when the doctor came in to check on me, when our breakfast tray arrived, or when we had visitors. He finally woke up with my father looming over his bed checking to see if he was alive. Keith slept like this for several nights that first week.

Sleep deprivation and stress may have taken its toll on Keith those first few days, but it was not long before both of them felt the impact of having two new babies. The next few months were exhausting, but they worked together as a team to get the job done. Deb nursed around the clock, while Keith did the chauffeuring. Many times, Keith was barely able to pull himself out of his state of deep sleep to get a baby for Deb to nurse. Before falling back to sleep, it was his job to carry the one she had been feeding back to the crib. Before he knew it—it was time to do it all again.

I laughed as they told me Deb woke up one night screaming, "Where's the baby?" They tore the bed apart looking for the missing baby. When the bed was stripped of all covers and found to be empty, they made a mad dash to the cribs. There they were... sleeping like angels. Who took the baby back? Deb and Keith often wondered if they were losing their minds along with their sleep.

Getting the kids changed and fed was not all Deb and Keith had to contend with during those early months. Erik (formally known as BamBam) was extremely fussy compared to Becca (formally known at Pebbles), and at times, he cried for hours on end. He spit up excessively after each feeding and rarely slept. Since Becca had none of these symptoms, they assumed it was not related to what Deb was eating, but more to a biomechanical problem within Erik. After all, looking back at their birth, Becca had a nice gradual descent through the birth canal. Erik, on the other hand, found himself asleep one minute, being shoved downward the next, and then had a rapid flight out of the birth canal. Also, it's possible Deb's unrelenting reflux was due to the abnormally high position Erik maintained in the uterus. Who knows what type of physical stress he endured in his cramped position above Becca?

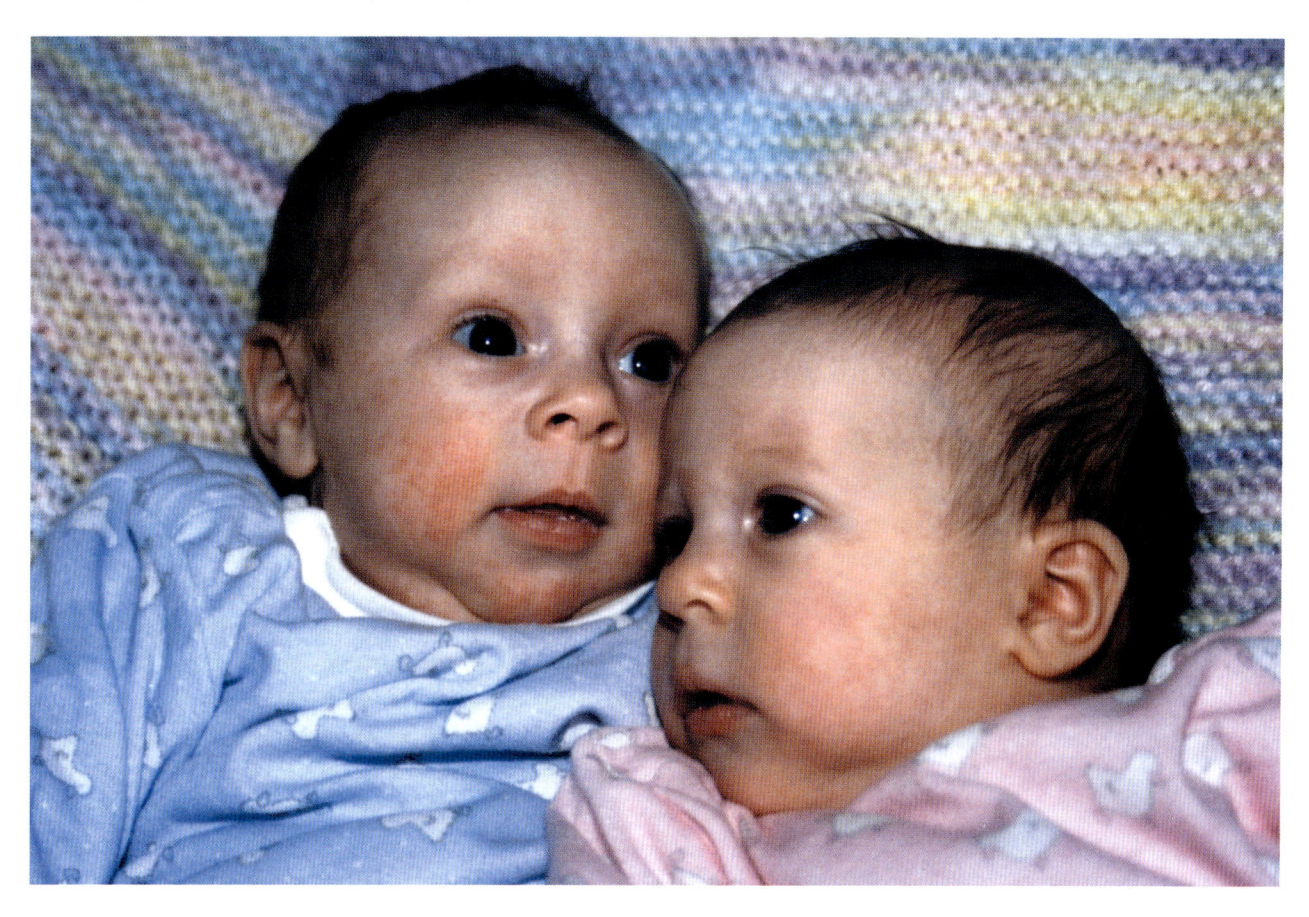

Deb: *We want to stress how valuable the chiropractic care was for the babies right from day one. The difference in their mood and behavior was extreme. Carol taught us how to let them suck on our finger to smooth out the bones at the top of their mouth, and how to relax a ligament at the base of Erik's spine to relax his muscles and ease his discomfort. We would do these things everyday, and that seemed to calm him down between trips to Minneapolis for treatment. After a visit to Carol's office, we always saw an immediate improvement in his disposition, and he stopped spitting up.*

Also, the doula support was so valuable for us that I have since helped my friends by providing them with the same support. One family I helped had a horrible first birth when they were alone at the hospital. After I provided doula support with the second birth, the husband adamantly proclaimed, "Everyone should be forced to come to the hospital with one or more doulas to help the husband!"

I was so pleased to learn that Deb had helped another woman in labor. All I have ever asked of the families I have helped was to have them offer the same assistance to someone else in labor. If we all help each other, birth may again be viewed as a natural and normal occurrence associated with life on this planet.

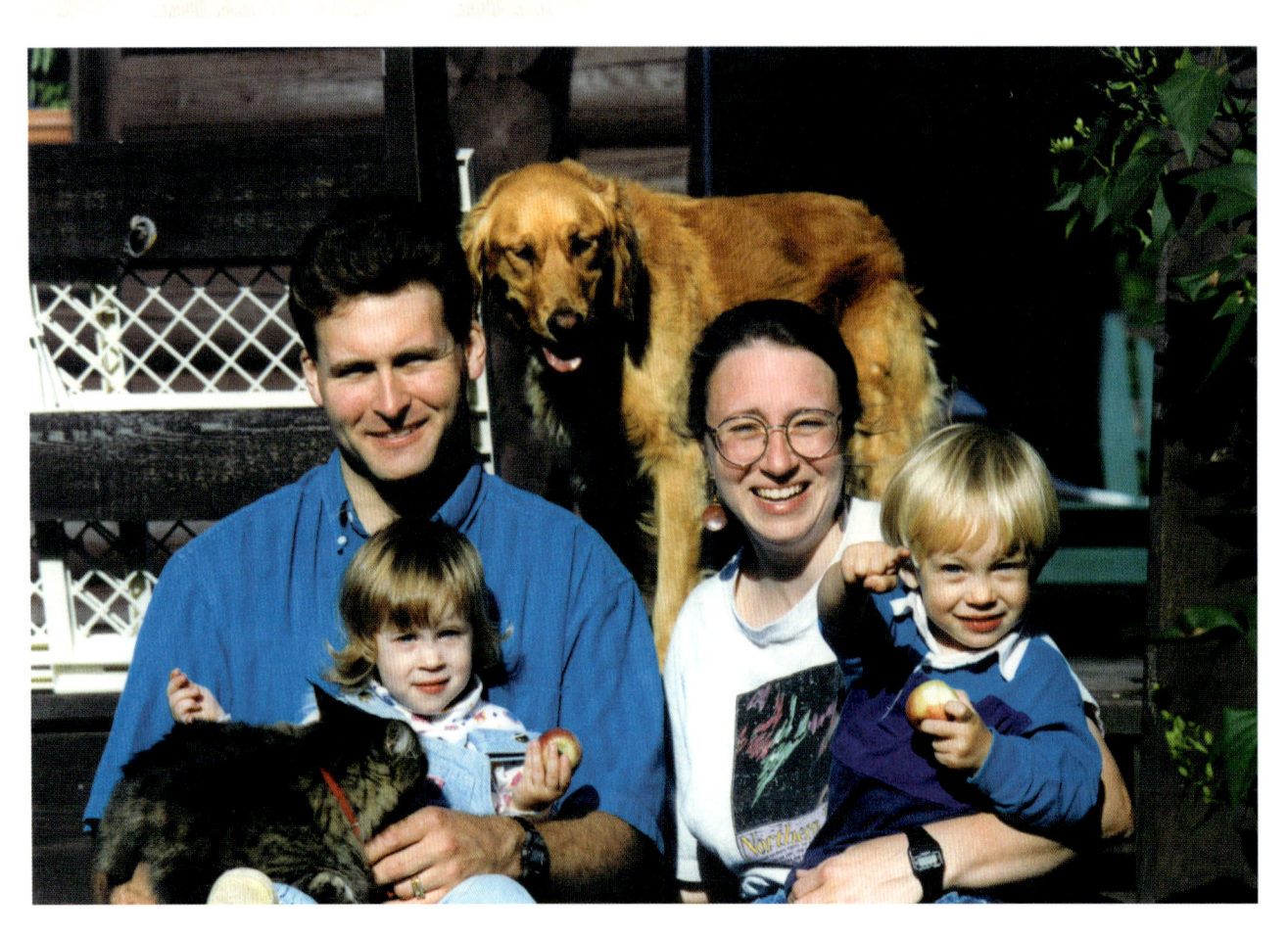

STEP 4: Seek Relief for the Discomforts of Pregnancy and Birth

In–Utero Constraint

Did Erik's constricted position high in Deb's uterus contribute to her reflux? Did that same constriction contribute to his problems after birth? To understand the answer to those questions, you must journey inside a woman even further and look at the intricate design of her body. Let's investigate the muscles that cross the body and divide the lung and heart compartment from the abdominal compartment. Then we can look at the structures that traverse through those muscles.

The muscles that make up the ceiling of the abdominal cavity are referred to as the respiratory diaphragm, and the muscles that make up the floor of the cavity are referred to as the pelvic diaphragm. These two diaphragms work as supports for the rib cage and pelvis, while they anchor the muscles that run up and down your body. Together, they provide a protective environment for your baby's first home. As these muscles cross your body, they afford passage for the structures within your body that are responsible for a baby's survival. These include: the aorta and inferior vena cava (blood vessels that provide blood flow in and out of the heart), the esophageal sphincter (where the esophagus flows into the stomach), the urethra, the colon, and the cervix or prostate. These muscular diaphragms form a strong support system for your baby. Balance and a proper tone within their fibers is crucial to your child's descent out of the womb.

The uterus can expand freely, and evenly, if the ligaments and muscles surrounding the uterus are balanced. If the respiratory diaphragm is too tight (hypertonic) there may be a restriction in blood flow to and from your heart. And, your abdominal organs may not move upward as the uterus grows. Increased tension in the respiratory diaphragm may also result in a malfunction of the esophageal sphincter, thus causing heartburn and reflux.

If the pelvic diaphragm is too tight, it will be difficult for the baby to force the cervix open. A hypertonic (tight) diaphragm may also alter the way a baby maneuvers through the birth canal, as those muscles are instrumental in guiding the body during birth.

Abnormal tension within the muscles or ligaments surrounding the uterus will result in uneven forces being applied to the home of the unborn child. It would be as if he is trying to grow up in a balloon that has an odd shape. He must accommodate the space available to him—no matter how cramped his world becomes. This will affect the tone of his own muscles, the alignment of his joints, the strength of his ligaments, and most importantly, the formation of his cranium.

Erik had difficulties with digestion during his first months of life because he wasn't in a position in utero, in the womb, to properly line up his body mechanically for optimum function of the craniosacral system. That's a fancy term for saying he was squished up into the corner of the uterus and wasn't able to get his head against the cervix which would have allowed him to mold his cranium properly. Multiple births can be hard on babies!

I was able to alleviate his discomfort by reducing the interference to his normal nerve flow.

To summarize, Erik's in-utero constraint resulted in a combination of problems that contributed to his irritability, indigestion, and reflux. First, his head was not pressed against the cervix prior to delivery because Becca held that position. Therefore, he was unable to properly mold his cranium or align his spine to protect his brain and spinal cord. Second, when the nurse applied pressure to Deb's abdomen, Erik was forced into position before he could prepare for the descent. The third problem was his extremely rapid descent through the birth canal. When babies "fly through" they often have a problem with the function of the sphenobasilar joint, a joint formed at the junction between a bone at the back of the head and one in the front.

All of these factors contributed to Erik's cranial and spinal imbalance. Pressure on the nerves to his internal organs caused the problems he was experiencing after birth.

The best treatment for Erik's structural imbalance was chiropractic adjustments to realign his bony structures and craniosacral therapy to restore balance to his entire body. Together, these treatments resulted in a calmer, happier Erik.

> Chiropractic adjustments for babies are extremely light finger contacts that realign the bony segments and restore normal tone to all structures of the body. Craniosacral therapy is another gentle modality used by a wide range of healthcare professionals including massage therapists, chiropractors, osteopaths, medical doctors, psychiatrists, psychologists, dentists, physical therapists, and acupuncturists. This modality focuses on restoring balance to the membranes that encapsulate the brain and spinal cord. Both techniques improve sensory, motor, and intellectual function of the newborn.

(actual size)

Accidents happen to women that imbalance their body so severely that the uterus simply cannot expand properly to accommodate a growing baby. A mother may be totally free of pain and unaware of this happening until it is too late and she delivers a premature baby. The following story is of a woman, Yvonne, who had a motorcycle accident prior to the conception of her first son. Yvonne was thrown from her motorcycle as she sped down the highway. She somersaulted several times before landing in a twisted heap—shocked but apparently uninjured. Yvonne had no idea that her pelvic muscles were twisted and tight from the accident. A few months later, Yvonne conceived her first child. Unfortunately, the torsion within her pelvis restricted the growth of her uterus and her tiny growing baby was forced to fold in on himself rather than stretch out and play within the womb.

Cody was held so tightly within Yvonne's pelvic cavity that the pressure of his body against the cervix caused Yvonne to go into premature labor. At 24 weeks gestation, during an ultrasound, Cody began to exhibit signs of fetal distress. An emergency C-section was performed to save his life. Weighing only 500 grams (approximately 17 ounces), Cody lived for more than eight months in the Neonatal Intensive Care Unit of Children's Hospital before going home to his family. He suffered from growth retardation, visual problems, and delayed development.

Yvonne was discouraged from having another pregnancy because there was a strong possibility that her uterus would never be able to accommodate and grow with another baby. Fortunately, God did not agree with the recommendation. Here is her story.

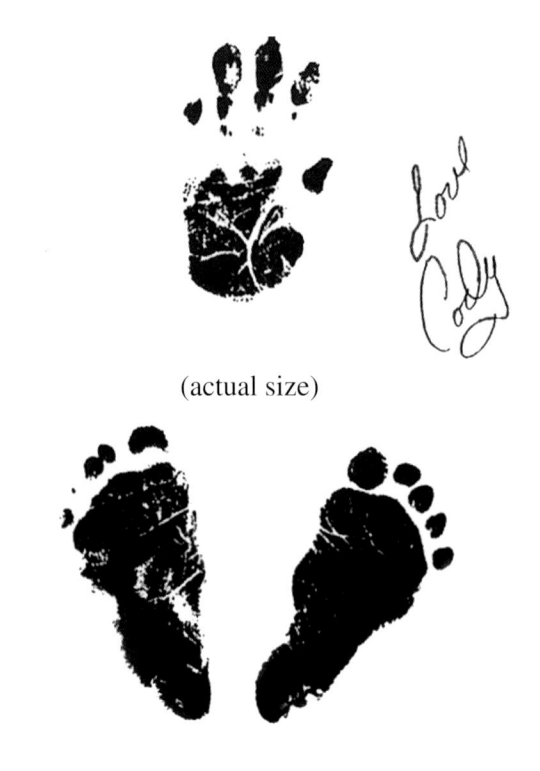

A Chance to Grow

Written by Yvonne

Travis John Huber was born November 12, 1991. However, the events which lead to his birth actually started back in early 1990. That was the first time Dr. Carol worked on me with chiropractic care and craniosacral therapy. After having my first son Cody at 24 weeks gestation, I wanted to prevent a repeat of his traumatic premature delivery.

During Cody's emergency cesarean, my uterus was unable to expand outside of my lower pelvis. It had to be cut both horizontally and vertically to free Cody. Consequently, I was discouraged from getting pregnant again. I was also warned that, if I did get pregnant, I would have to have another cesarean. I was high risk for a ruptured uterus because of the way they had to cut it open during Cody's birth.

After watching Carol work on Cody, I had her work on me. She relaxed my diaphragms and (to our surprise) I got pregnant again. After we found out I was pregnant, I saw her on a regular basis in an attempt to prevent another premature delivery.

STEP 4: Seek Relief for the Discomforts of Pregnancy and Birth

I had a difficult time finding an obstetrician who would accept me as a patient due to the problems associated with Cody's birth. I wanted to avoid excessive intervention, but I was eventually forced to receive my prenatal care from a neonatal specialist, a perinatologist.

Fortunately, my pregnancy progressed smoothly during the first three months, and no intervention was recommended. Suddenly, during my fourth month, I felt the baby drop downward. I wasn't in pain, yet I knew things weren't quite right when I started having contractions. I knew that if I called the perinatologist he was going to recommend total bedrest and drugs. I didn't want to do that, but I also didn't want history to repeat itself. In a panic, I called Carol instead. She suspected right away that my sacrum was the problem. She immediately instructed my husband on what to do. Mark was also a chiropractor so he was able to follow her verbal instructions and perform the standing adjustment she described. My uterus shifted upward. The contractions stopped and everything was fine. Mark continued using this adjustment in-between my visits to Carol's office.

With their help, my uterus expanded properly, and I was able to carry Travis to full term. I went into labor on my own and didn't even know it. During my last appointment with Carol, she informed me I was in labor and drove me directly to the hospital. I was surprised to find that I had dilated to four centimeters, with just minor menstrual cramps. Travis was delivered safely by cesarean section with Dr. Carol and my mom at my side in the operating room. (Mark didn't make it in time.)

We now have two wonderful boys and we're very grateful for the opportunity to raise both of them!

PREMATURE CONTRACTIONS

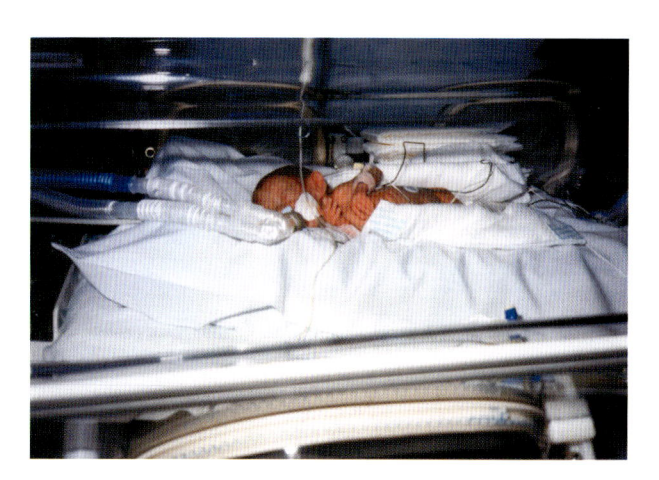

A Drug-free Approach to a Serious Situation

Premature contractions are one of the most serious complications associated with structural imbalance. The fact that you are contracting early on in the pregnancy is an indicator that either something is wrong with the baby, or with your body. There is no easy way to address abnormalities in your unborn child, but you can do something to correct a possible imbalance within your body.

If you're having contractions, your medical doctor will usually recommend bedrest and medication to relax the uterus. Unfortunately, these recommendations can result in other problems. Bedrest for several months will not prepare your body for the stamina required to deliver a baby. And the drug terbutaline will alter your normal physiology. The effect can be very uncomfortable for both you and your baby.

The imbalance in your body that may be causing your uterus to tip forward, forcing the baby to apply pressure to your cervix, can be easily corrected in many cases. The technique is quick, simple, and easy to teach to your partner, doula, or midwife. Before I show you how to do it, I want to share another story with you of a mother who dealt with this problem during all three of her pregnancies. She was also the patient responsible for teaching me how a mother can fix the problem herself.

The Chiropractic Advantage

Written by Leslie Lundgren

My first son, Lukas, was born 12 weeks premature. I went into labor at 25 weeks (full term is 40 weeks). My doctor prescribed terbutaline and put me on complete bedrest. At 27 weeks, after continued contractions and pelvic pressure, I had an abruption of the placenta (it separated from the wall of the uterus). I was hospitalized and given intravenous injections of magnesium sulfate. I continued to have contractions and Luke was born at 28 weeks, weighing only two pounds and eleven ounces. Luke now suffers from the effects of such an early birth with delayed development and cerebral palsy.

During my second pregnancy, I began seeing Dr. Carol Phillips along with my obstetrician. Around the 25th week, I again had contractions and pelvic pressure. I hadn't started dilating, but the baby had dropped. Carol worked on me and through a comfortable technique, performed while I was standing, something changed and I felt an immediate relief of the pressure and discomfort in the front of my body. Carol taught my husband how to perform this technique whenever I had contractions and we were able to prevent another premature delivery. I'm thrilled to report that our second son, Erik, was born on his due date at a healthy eight pounds and five ounces!

History repeated itself with my 3rd pregnancy, and again, chiropractic care and this technique helped control the contractions. I was able to carry my third son, Jack, right to his due date.

~~~

Both Leslie and Yvonne showed signs of having a structural problem before they felt contractions. Most women do, but they aren't aware of the warning signs. Here's a typical scenario. You're walking along feeling fine, when all of a sudden, you stop dead in your tracks because you suddenly feel extreme pressure in your groin or down the front of her legs. You'll grab something for support, bend forward, and start thinking, "What in the world was that?" The pressure against your cervix may give you the sensation that the baby is going to fall right out. You may feel a shooting pain down the front of your legs. A sense of weakness keeps you from taking a step; you fear that you'll fall on your face if you do.

Then, just as quickly, the pain is gone. You can stand up and walk without a problem. You may continue to feel the pressure against the cervix, but otherwise you feel fine—until it hits again. It may be sometime before you begin to feel a tight cramping sensation in the front of your abdomen.

All of these may be present, or you may feel just the contractions. At any rate, you shouldn't experience any of these symptoms. They are all early warning signs that the uterus is tipped forward and the baby is dropping down on the cervix. That pressure is stimulating the release of hormones which are causing the uterus to start contracting.

When you take medication, and lie down, the contractions usually subside. If you get up to go to the bathroom, they start up again. Logic will tell you that if the drug was working to reduce contractions they would work even when you get up to go to the bathroom. Obviously, lying down is what stops the contractions. In that position, the uterus tips backward and the baby moves away from the cervix.

I have found that the uterus will often tip forward in women who have had a traumatic injury to their sacrum; the added weight of the amniotic fluid and the growing baby applies stress to the unstable sacral segments causing them to buckle. I have found that a simple maneuver can be performed that will realign those segments. It appears that when the sacral segments are realigned the broad ligaments, which are attached to the sacrum, pull the uterus up and back into a more optimal vertical position. Anyone can perform this maneuver and help a mother and her baby.

The Buckled Sacrum Maneuver

To perform this maneuver, the mother stands several feet away from a wall, she places her feet in a stable position, extends her arms forward, and rests her hands against the wall. (I tell her to imagine that I am a police officer who is about to frisk her.) **(See Figure 1)**

Next, a partner, friend, or doula stands perpendicular to the mother with one hand in front, just above the pubic region, and one in back over the lowest part of her spine. With fingers pointed toward the floor, the hand in back applies slight pressure to the mother's low

STEP 4: Seek Relief for the Discomforts of Pregnancy and Birth

back and sacrum as the hand slides down the entire length of her spine. **(See Figure 2 and 2A)**

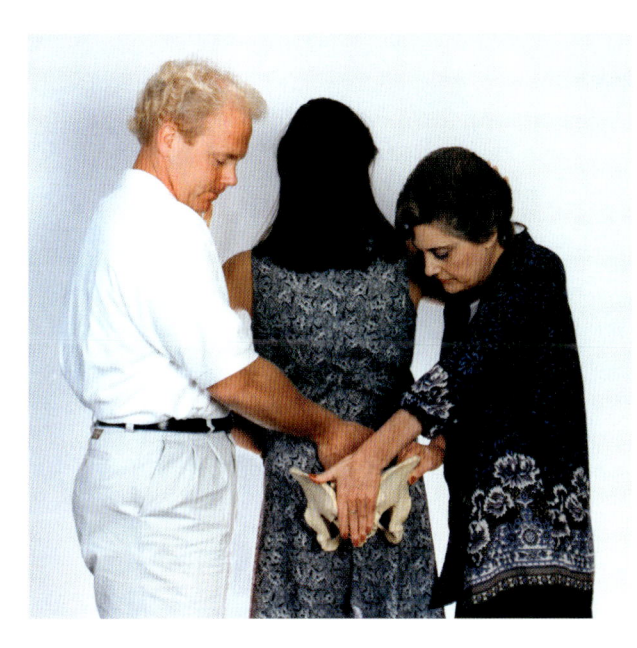

Figure 1: This is the position taken by a mother who is being treated for premature contractions.

If the palm of the hand feels any resistance to the downward motion, the partner is to maintain the downward pressure against the sacrum for several minutes, or until the buckled sacral segments smooth out and the hand slides down without resistance. The hormones of pregnancy, combined with pressure against the segments will cause the pliable sacrum to mold to the contour of the hand. This is an extremely

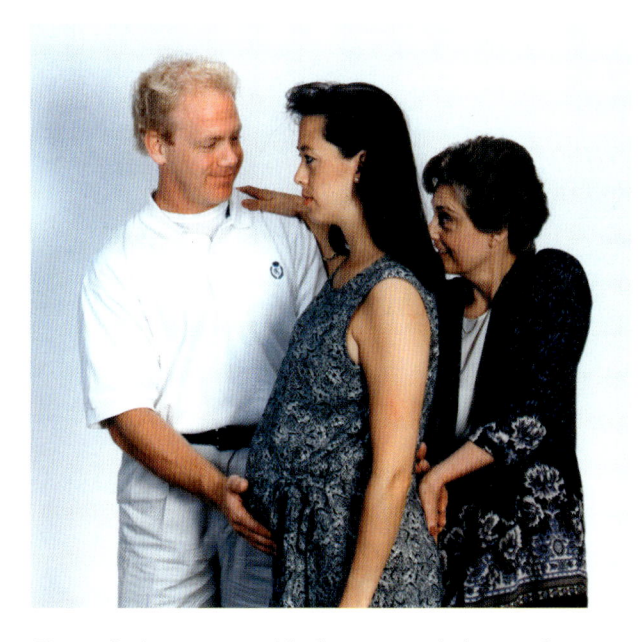

Figure 2: A partner molds the sacrum, balances the tone of the uterine ligaments, and alleviates premature contractions.

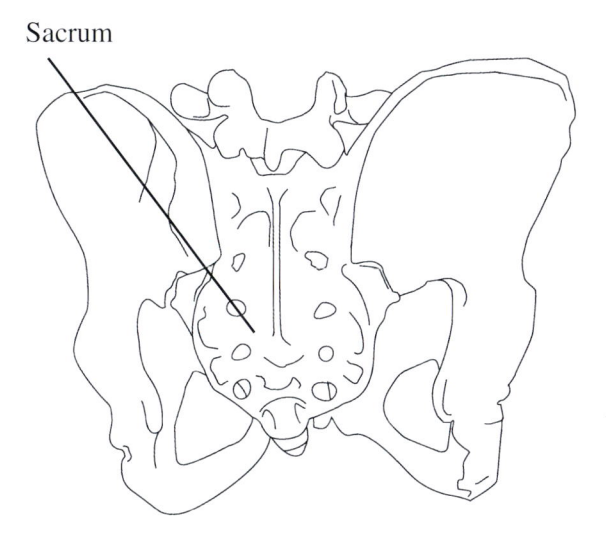

Figure 2A: The sacrum is the large bone that rests between the two pelvic bones (often called the hip bones). The sacrum should have a soft C-shaped curve to it.

gentle maneuver and no pressure is applied toward the baby by either hand.

When the sacral segments realign themselves, balance is restored to the uterine ligaments and the uterus no longer applies pressure against the structures located in the front of the abdomen. The mother usually has an immediate resolution of any thigh pain and premature contractions; the baby no longer feels as if he will "fall out" at any moment.

Women who remember a time when their feet flew out from under them before they fell on their bottom will be predisposed to this problem. Therefore, they need a way to address the problem themselves. My patients have taught me they can sometimes stop the contractions by lying on the floor with a small rolled hand towel about two inches high and four inches wide slipped under their low back. They will slide the towel downward until the buckled segment of the sacrum restricts it. The weight of a mother's body resting on the towel works beautifully to help the sacrum realign itself.

A mother, Heidi, once brought her five-month-old son, Christian, into the office with a diagnosis of congenital torticollis. This is a condition where a baby has never been able to hold his head up straight due to severe spasms within his neck and back muscles. Christian's pediatrician had been waiting for the condition to correct itself. When that did not happen, he wanted to schedule Christian for surgery to have the muscles in his neck severed. Heidi chose chiropractic treatment instead.

Heidi had spent her last three months of pregnancy on bedrest while she took medication to stop premature delivery. The medication failed to stop the contractions, but bedrest was helpful. Christian's bum was lodged deep beneath Heidi's rib cage, so she also suffered from severe rib pain that persisted for several weeks after delivery. During their initial chiropractic visit, Heidi's mother reported to me that she observed the doctor pulling so hard on Christian's head to get him out of the birth canal that she feared he would be "decapitated." (I'm sorry for saying that but that's what she said.)

Christian had a fairly speedy recovery after receiving chiropractic adjustments and craniosacral therapy. When Heidi started having contractions with her second pregnancy, she came in right away for prenatal care. This time, her symptoms were managed successfully without the use of medication and bedrest. I remember on one occasion receiving a tearful phone message from Heidi. She was so excited she just had to share her good news with me. "Oh, Carol, I can't tell you how good it feels to know I can stop the contractions and go on with my day. I don't have to go to bed or take the medication. It just feels so wonderful to be able to stop the contractions. I just had to tell you!"

I love that kind of a message. By the way, Danny was born without complications or intervention, as was her third baby—despite repeated episodes of premature contractions. Again, she was able to handle her pregnancy complication of pain and premature contractions without drugs or bedrest simply by incorporating chiropractic prenatal care.

A woman's body is exquisitely designed to conceive, nurture and birth another human being. During gestation, a woman and her unborn child will unite in an oceanic blend of energy and identity. Where one ends and the other begins no one knows.

—*Carol Phillips*

STEP 4: Seek Relief for the Discomforts of Pregnancy and Birth

Childbirth—A Miracle in Design

A baby will prepare for birth long before active labor contractions begin. During the last four weeks of gestation, provided her life is not consumed with other activities, a mother will spend many quiet hours connecting with her baby. Silently, they will get to know each other as they physically prepare for the journey of birth.

During the final stages of pregnancy, a mother will help her baby line up his body so that her muscles can slowly twist, turn, and maneuver him through her pelvis in a safe and natural manner. This will be a dance of power, strength, and agility—provided both are structurally balanced and not forced to perform the dance of birth prematurely.

When the time for birth is upon them, some women experience overwhelming excitement, mixed with sadness; they realize it will be the last time the two of them will perform as one. When the cord is cut, a child symbolically and physically becomes an individual—capable of independent thoughts and actions. Mother and child will be divided physically, yet, spiritually and energetically they will be one forever.

When preparing for a delivery, it is important that everyone involved in the birth understands the miraculous design of the human body. We need to learn how a baby slowly, gently, and with great precision, molds his head to accommodate his mother's unique shape. And, that a mother in labor moves her body in subtle ways to accommodate for her baby's position in the canal. When we learn how they dance together—each responding to the other's every move—we marvel at the miraculous journey of birth and develop a new and exciting respect for the human body.

As a mother in labor, you may find it difficult to know who is leading and who is following. There is one thing I have learned. Only your baby knows when he is ready to go out onto the dance floor. He may start the dance, but he relies on your agility, your grace, and your ability to ad lib once the performance has begun. Your baby has never moved like this before and may be reluctant to leave the safety of the womb. Therefore, be patient. He may start and stop several times before the final performance.

While the two of you weave your way into a new life together, relax in the knowledge that your birth team is off to the side ready to help, if you need them. You may rely on them for emotional, physical, and spiritual support, but deep inside, you will eventually realize this is your dance, your work, and your reward. You and your baby are a team, and together, you will be able to do what is necessary to complete the dance you have choreographed.

If you are an observer, and there are no complications, it is best if you minimize interference. Watch as the two of them blend into one harmonious pulse of energy and you will see a dance that very few people have the privilege of witnessing.

I will now take you on a journey through the birth canal. This journey will not only help you understand why some women experience excruciating pain during labor and others do not, but it will also help you see birth from a baby's perspective.

By the end of this step in our birth plan, you will have learned how to use body mechanics to help a baby line up properly—reducing or eliminating unnecessary pain during pregnancy and delivery. I hope this detailed description of the birth process helps you visualize an ideally choreographed birth.

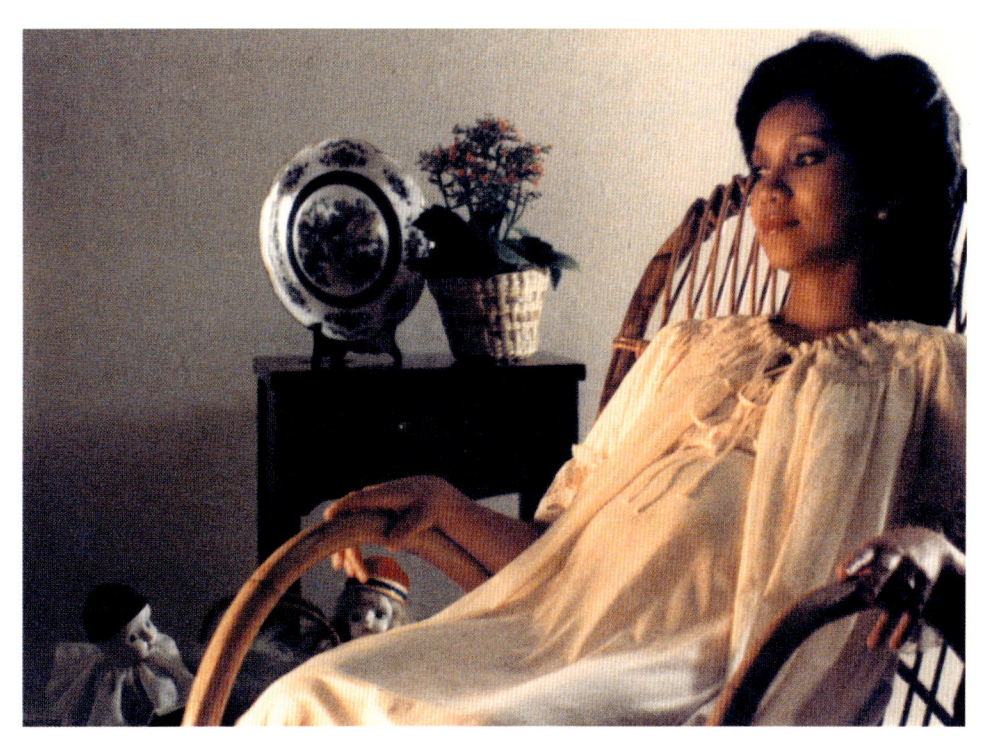

Preconception

Suppose you're a spirit preparing for a new life. You have decided to go inside your mom and investigate the new home God has created for you. You look up to the left and see fluffy white clouds (her stomach, spleen, and pancreas); these are organs capable of moving upward to give you more room when you grow from a tiny seedling to a big human being. You look up on your mom's right side and see a beautiful, purple mountain (her liver).

Wow! Look at that horizon! It's pulsating. It's pink, soft, and moves like an inchworm making its way around the world. You can't help but wonder if you'll be allowed to play with it (that's her colon). Looking down you see that your new home is resting on something big and round like a trampoline (her bladder). Maybe you'll be able to jump and bounce on it when you get bigger.

The Anatomy of Birth and The Dance of Life

A Baby is Formed

On day one, a single sperm out-swims every other competing sperm and joins with an egg that has traveled on a long dark journey to the site of their union. Together, they successfully beat the odds and unite to form a unique, powerful human being. Within a month, this minuscule human being will have a brain, a spinal cord, and arm buds. Soon, this baby will form a protective fluid encasement for his brain and spinal cord, the dura mater (**Figure 3**). He will then form a protective encasement around the dura mater in the form of spinal vertebra and cranial plates.

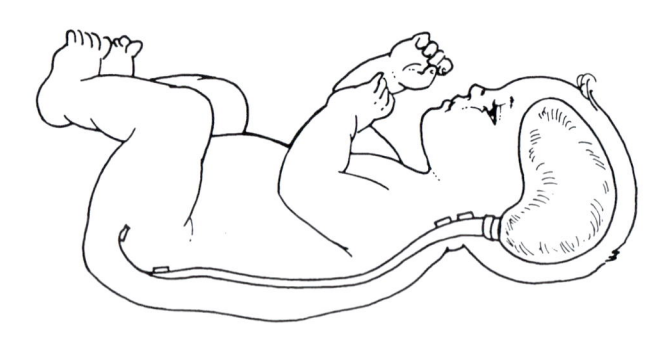

Figure 3: The dura mater forms a protective, nutrient-rich encasement around the baby's brain and spinal cord.

1st Trimester—Discovery

What a great place to play. You can float anywhere you want. You find yourself going back and forth between this new home and your spiritual home with God. As time goes by, He watches as you stay longer and longer with your mom. He smiles and knows that eventually you will get so used to the soft caress of the inchworm, to the fun of jumping on the trampoline, and to the tickling sensation of clouds on your back and bum that you won't want to be gone from her for very long. You will be called back time and time again, until you can no longer bear to be away from the rhythmic hypnotic sound of your mom's heartbeat vibrating throughout your soul.

STEP 4: Seek Relief for the Discomforts of Pregnancy and Birth

> One day, as you play in your new home, you realize the soft slippery rope you have been swinging on is starting to tickle your tummy with a sensation of warm thick nutrients moving to every part of your new body. When you open your mouth, you feel something warm move down into your throat. Strange new taste sensations make you smack your lips for more. Suddenly, thoughts form in your consciousness. . .
>
> *Amazing! That great tasting liquid just moved right on down my body and came out between my legs. This is great! I can drink it in and pee it out whenever I want.*

The dura mater serves as a shock absorber, provides essential nutrients to the baby's brain and spinal cord (also called the central nervous system), and forms the foundation for the growth of his cranial plates. The cranial plates will begin to form on the dura mater at various sites called ossification centers. The soft plates will grow and spread across the dura like ripples from a pebble thrown into a pond. They will continue to spread out until they are large enough to form a protective support and encasement (the skull) for the brain. (The individual cranial plates will continue to grow toward each other well into the second year of life. As they join to form moveable sutures, the remaining exposed dura mater (his soft spots) can no longer be felt.)

By the third month in utero, tiny graceful hands and feet will form to help your baby begin the acrobatic feats that will soon give you the delight of feeling movement. During the fifth and sixth months, he begins to hear voices, music, and loud noises.

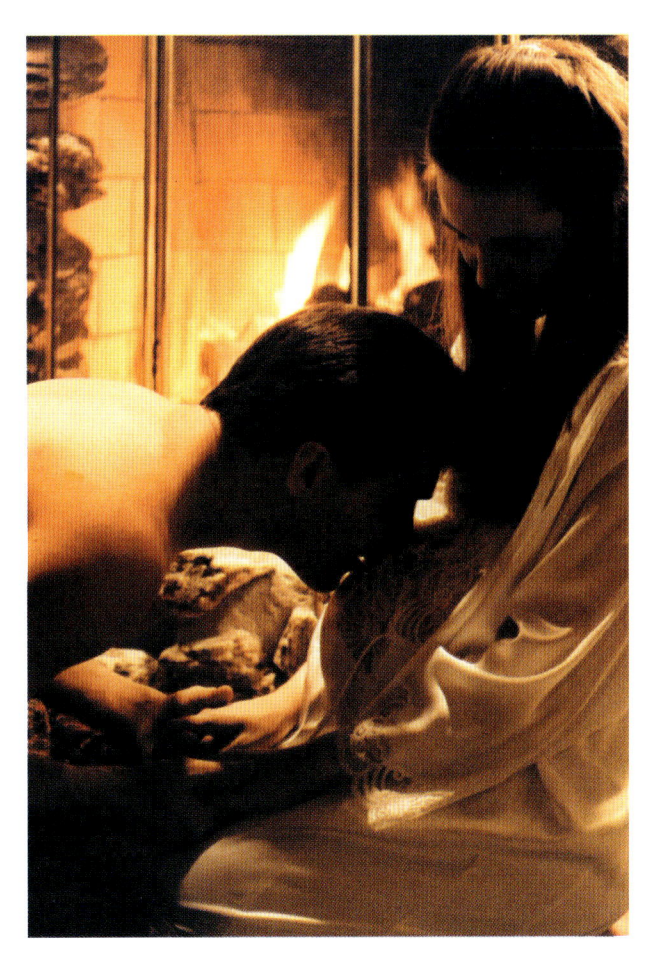

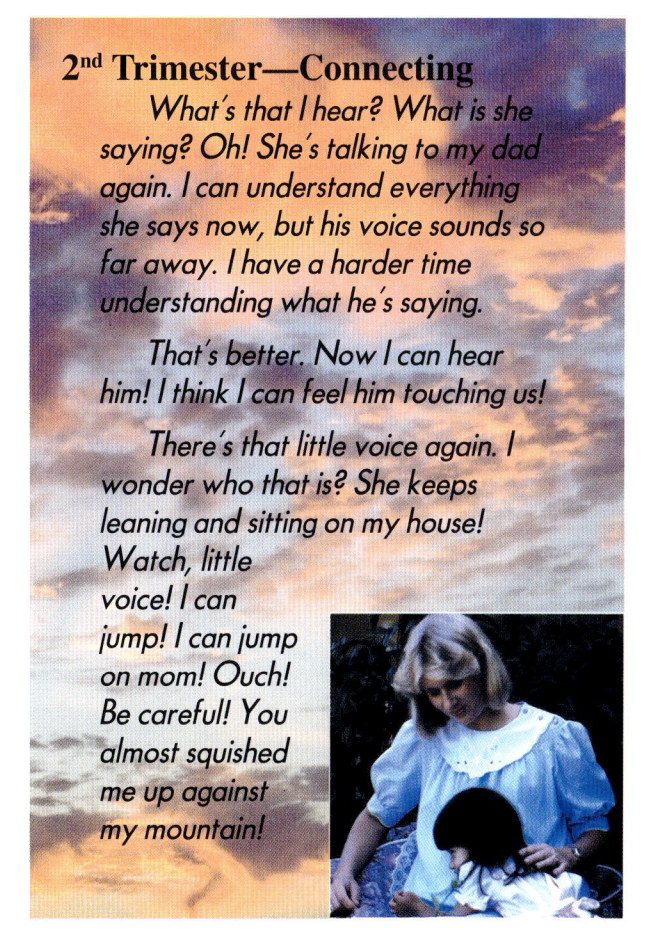

2nd Trimester—Connecting

What's that I hear? What is she saying? Oh! She's talking to my dad again. I can understand everything she says now, but his voice sounds so far away. I have a harder time understanding what he's saying.

That's better. Now I can hear him! I think I can feel him touching us!

There's that little voice again. I wonder who that is? She keeps leaning and sitting on my house! Watch, little voice! I can jump! I can jump on mom! Ouch! Be careful! You almost squished me up against my mountain!

3rd Trimester—Bonding

Mom. Hey, Mom, wake up! It's too quiet. Watch me! I'm doing a headstand! I can do headstands all the time now! It's getting too hard to jump with my feet because my head is so heavy. It now feels better to be upside down.

Gravity Will Help Him Turn Upside Down

During the seventh month, the volume of your amniotic fluid is reduced. This mysterious reduction in fluid gives your baby more room to grow, but eliminates his buoyancy. He is now influenced by the pull of gravity and his head, the heaviest part of his body, will be nestled down against the lower cervical portion of your uterus. The cervix is secured within your vagina by the concentric muscles of your pelvic diaphragm and by ligaments that secure it to the sacrum. The pelvic floor muscles guide your baby into your pelvis and through the birth canal.

It's Time to Guide Him into Position

During the last months of pregnancy, you will feel your baby tossing, turning, rolling and playing. Eventually, he will position himself with his back on your left side. Most babies will stay in this position because your softer organs (the stomach, spleen, and pancreas) will move up against the respiratory diaphragm and give him more room to stretch out. Your lungs and heart will move up to accommodate these organs, while giving your baby the room he needs for comfortable growth. There isn't as much room for his spine on your right side because of the location and consistency of your liver. The liver is harder and larger than the other organs and is not as accommodating for his growing spine.

Note: Should your baby be forced over to the right because of an imbalance in the ligaments that support the uterus, he will have to fold his body down to accommodate the reduction in available space. When he forces the liver up against your rib cage you may feel discomfort all along your ribs on the right. With his bum pushed over to the right, your baby's head will have to move over to the lower left quadrant of your abdomen. This could result in hip or leg pain as he presses on the canal that houses the nerves and arteries to the lower extremities. This is what happened to Heidi and Christian and it's the reason he was born with torticollis. (Page 115)

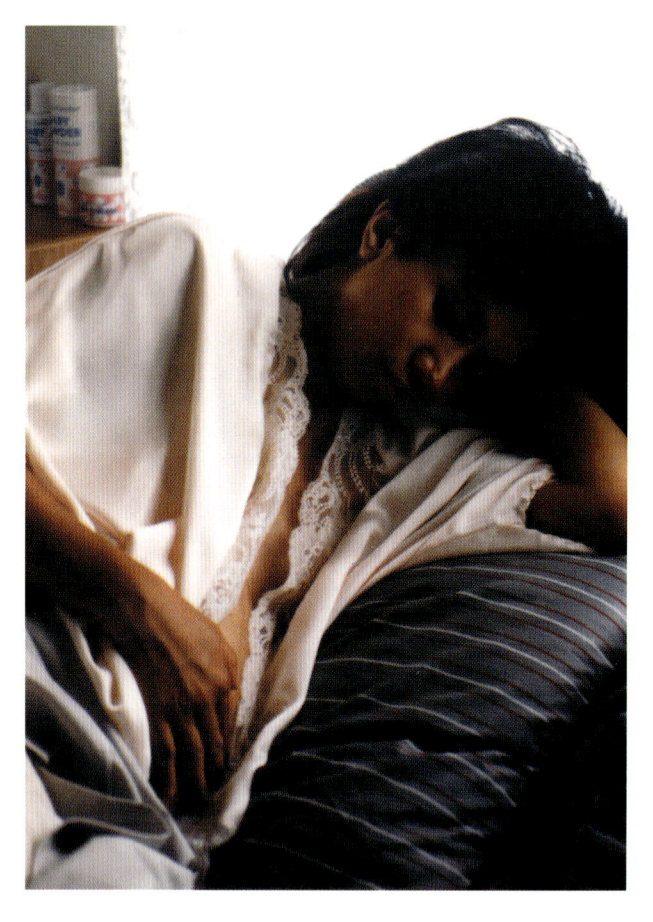

The Gift of Braxton Hicks Contractions

During the last month of pregnancy, the undetected, compressive forces of the uterus (Braxton-Hicks contractions) gently push your baby downward. Ideally, his spine is against the left side of your uterus and his elbows and knees are flexed against his chest. With his ankles crossed and feet extended, the top of his foot will now be pressed up against the top of the uterus.

Pressure applied to the top of his feet may fire proprioceptors, triggering a reflex that causes him to extend his leg and push his body downward (the placing reflex).

(After birth this reflex is tested by holding him upright against the side of a table. When the top of his foot is brushed against the side of the table he will take several steps as his leg moves from the flexed to

STEP 4: Seek Relief for the Discomforts of Pregnancy and Birth

the extended position. I think he was given this reflex so he could help push his body down deeper into the birth canal after each contraction.)

Your spine, the uterus, and your baby's spine should all be parallel. In this position, his spine will be forced downward with symmetrical pressure being applied to his head, which rests against the cervix. During these contractions, you should feel nothing more than a strong tightening of your stomach.

Braxton-Hicks contractions will prepare both of you for childbirth, because they activate neural pathways and stretch muscles. They will also prepare your baby for life outside the womb by helping the uterus massage his skin to stimulate his sensory receptors. If he is positioned correctly, the contractions will force his head to slowly and gently move into a flexed position. As a baby's chin moves toward his chest, the cervical vertebra will stack up and protect his brainstem from the forces of labor. With his head fully tucked forward, your baby will now have the crown of his head resting against the top of your cervix. This is called a vertex presentation.

Note: If you are experiencing painful pre-term contractions that seem to be occurring in rapid succession with the slightest provocation, you are most likely experiencing a hyperirritable uterus. A warm bath, in which you have your abdomen fully submerged, will usually stop or reduce the intensity of these contractions. Chiropractic care should be considered to reduce the pressure on the lumbar nerve roots. If contractions continue throughout the bath, try the buckled sacrum maneuver I showed you earlier. If they still continue, notify your birth attendant immediately.

When your cervix is centered properly within the pelvic floor muscles, your baby will be centered within the pelvic inlet. If he is on your left side, his face will be looking at your right hip. His spine will be parallel to your spine and his pelvic bones will be centered under the highest part of your respiratory diaphragm. In other words, his butt should eventually be resting directly in the center of your abdomen where the ribs meet at the center of the sternum, the xyphoid.

The Molding Process Can Now Begin

In order for your baby's head to fit through your pelvis, molding of the cranial plates must occur. Molding is the term used when the cranial plates are gently forced to overlap to reduce the size of the cranium. As the exposed dura mater also overlaps, it forms a protective encasement for the many blood vessels that supply blood to the brain. The forced reduction in the size of the cranium will result in an evacuation of some cerebral spinal fluid and blood down into the spinal canal. This will also reduce the size of the cranium.

In order for the dura mater to encase the entire brain and spinal cord, it descends down through the spinal canal and attaches firmly into the tailbone (coccyx). As a result of this attachment, your baby's spine will be forced to curl forward as his head is forced into flexion.

This curled position will allow his vertebra to stack up and form a protective wall around his spinal cord. This position will also open the spinal foramen (holes formed by the joining of each vertebra) and will prevent pressure from being applied to the spinal

---

You know, mom, I love listening to you. I love it when you rock me and sing to me. I love the way you keep hugging me tighter and tighter. Those hugs are helping me pull my hands and feet in close.

I love the stories you read to me. Maybe I'll be a writer when I grow up. And I love the music you play for me. Listening to that man play the saxophone made me wonder about being a musician. I don't know. Maybe I'll be a writer or a musician someday, but for now, I just love the way you show me all the incredible possibilities for my life.

Dad. Hey, Dad! Wake Up! Let's play that game again. You tap on mom's tummy three times and I'll try to kick my wall three times. I did it this morning. Remember? Remember?

Dad? Will you read me another story? Mom keeps going to sleep and I'm not tired. I haven't heard your voice all day and I'm just starting to understand you better.

nerve roots. Your baby's spine can now protect the central nervous system as the compressive forces of labor force him further into your pelvis.

The molding process begins when the left parietal bone at the top of your baby's head comes to rest against a lip of bone on the top of your sacrum, the sacral promentory **(Figure 4 and 5)**.

stress fibers will permit only a slight overlapping to occur in order to protect a large blood vessel, the sagittal sinus, which is housed between the parietal bones **(Figure 6)**.

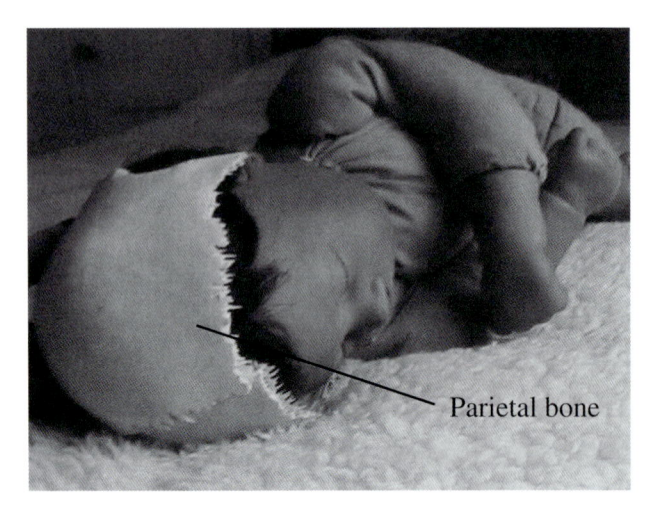

Figure 6: One parietal telescopes beneath the other to begin the molding process.

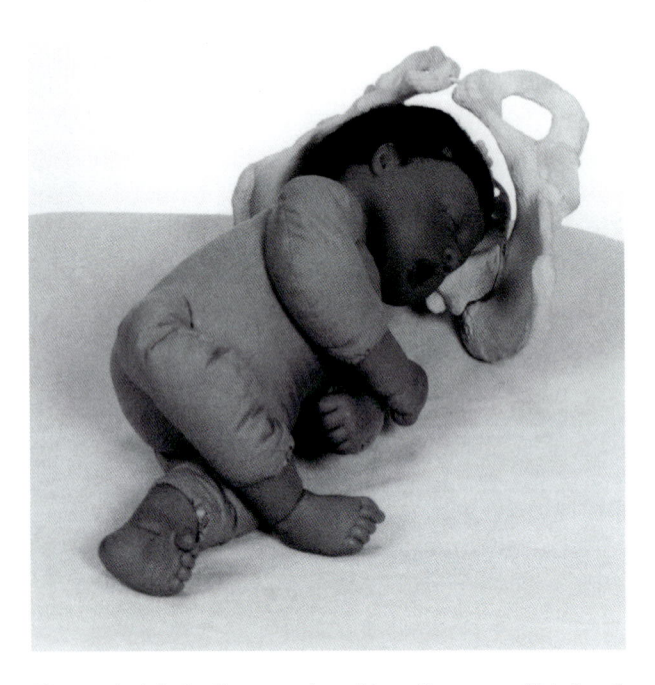

Figure 4: A baby lines up the widest diameter of his head with the widest diameter of his mother's pelvis.

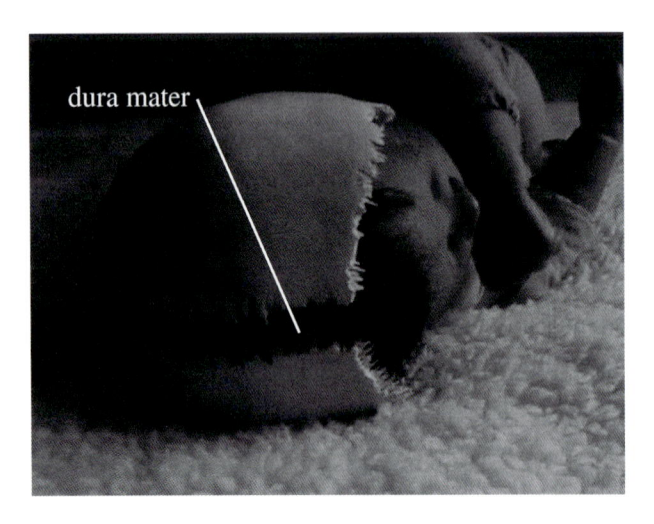

Figure 5: Unossified dura mater remains between the cranial plates to allow for molding.

The first layer of muscles, which are directed from the front of your pelvis to the back, will apply pressure to the right side of his head and force one parietal bone to slide slightly under the other. Dural

The Last Two Weeks

I'm getting tired of being squished in here. I'm trying to keep my bum up at the top so I have more room and I'm hugging myself as tight as I can, but it's getting harder and harder to move my hands and feet. I've heard your voices for so long; I can really imagine what you look like. Can I come out now? I rarely go back home anymore. God lets me stay almost all the time now. He says it's almost time for me to start my new life. We talked about our plans. We made a decision about what I need to do for the world. Mom, you really helped me with that decision. Your belief in me has helped me decide that I can make a difference in people's lives. God said I'll forget what He and I decided, but I'll slowly remember as I get older and older. He also said I'd never forget what you've taught me so far.

122

STEP 4: Seek Relief for the Discomforts of Pregnancy and Birth

Your baby can now slide down a little further against the cervix and so that his head will rest against a layer of muscles traversing from one side of your pelvis to the other. These hammock-like muscles will telescope the front of his cranium, the frontal bone **(Figure 7 and 8)**, and the back of his cranium, the occiput **(Figure 9 and 10)**, beneath the two parietal bones. The stress fibers that form the dura mater will protect the blood vessels by restricting the amount of overlapping that can occur.

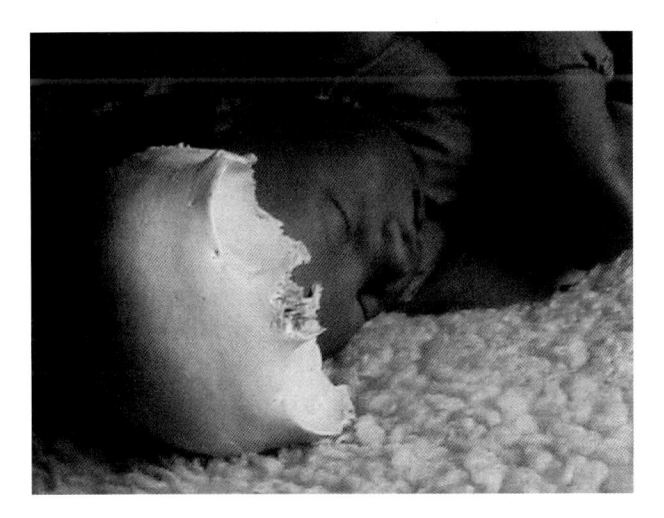

Figure 7: Frontal bone

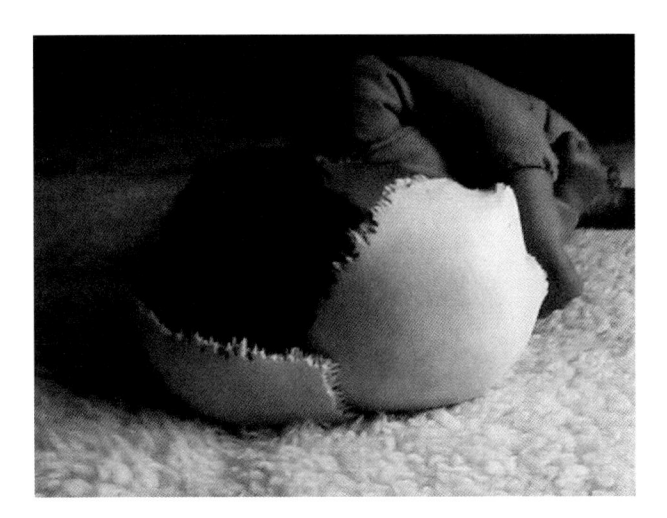

Figure 8: The frontal plate telescopes under and/or over the adjacent parietal plate to reduce the size of the cranium and protect the brain.

Prolonged contact of your baby's head against the cervix is called engagement and it will stimulate the release of hormones from your placenta. It's still a mystery as to how the baby controls the hormone release, but I think simple biomechanics has a lot to do with it.

The hormone, oxytocin, will activate stronger contractions, which are more intense than the Braxton Hicks contractions. Oxytocin will also regulate your contractions into a rhythmical pattern. Your cervix will continue to soften and thin out as it blends in with the wider part of the uterus. Your baby's head can now rest directly against the opening called the os. Continued pressure against the os will start a cascade of hormonal responses in both you and your baby—this will lead to the *active* stage of labor and delivery.

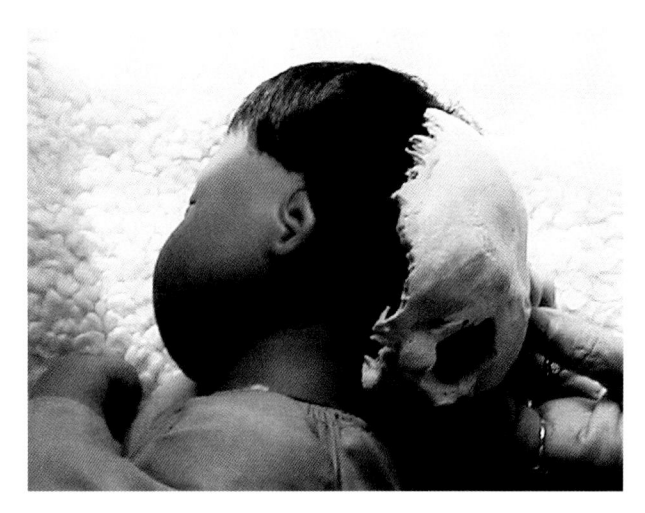

Figure 9: The Occipital bone

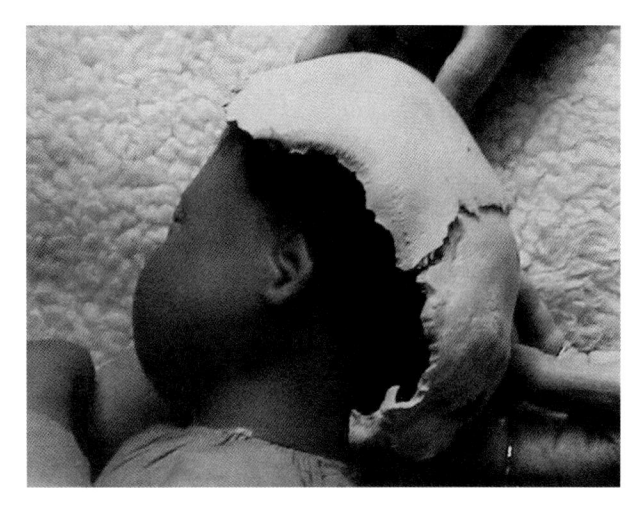

Figure 10: The largest segment of the occipital bone telescopes under and/or over the adjacent parietal plates to further reduce the size of the cranium.

The Last Week

God told me that you and I are going on a journey together. He warned me that it might be scary at times, and it might hurt, but He said He would never leave us alone. He told me that He created both of us so we could make the journey together; He gave both of us some powerful substances called hormones. Your hormones are more powerful than mine, because you're bigger, but together we have enough for both of us. He said our hormones work like rocket fuel to take us through birth together. Just you and me, mom! We'll still be able to hear other people, but at the end of our journey it will be just you, me, and God. He also said not to worry, he will give you enough endorphins (natural pain killers) for both of us, so we can do what we need to do.

A Few Days Before Birth

Imagine that it has been approximately nine months since you were conceived. Ideally, your arms and legs are now crossed and folded tightly in front of your body and your spine rests up against the left side of the womb. Your bum is curled forward and pushed up against the very top of your home and your neck is tucked so far forward that your chin touches your chest. Your head is now snuggled against your mother's cervix making it difficult to turn and look around.

Your mom's continual hugging makes it difficult to move any part of your body. Your skin feels tingly as she squeezes you. It feels like the mountain, clouds, and inchworm are hugging you so tight they are forcing you to drop down as far as you can go. The bottom of your home is beginning to stretch—decreasing the pressure on your head.

Labor and Delivery

Ideally, active labor begins when the top of your baby's head rests squarely on your cervix with the widest diameter of his head parallel with the widest diameter of your pelvic inlet. In this position, effacement and dilation will be symmetrical. Effacement is the thinning of the cervix. Dilation is the opening of the cervix. Gradually, his head will pass through the pelvic inlet. Now, with his body tightly flexed forward, your baby will turn his head and shoulders. He can accomplish this because the next layers of pelvic floor muscles are directed obliquely across your pelvis. They will now apply pressure to the side of his head and against the temporal plates (**Figure 11**).

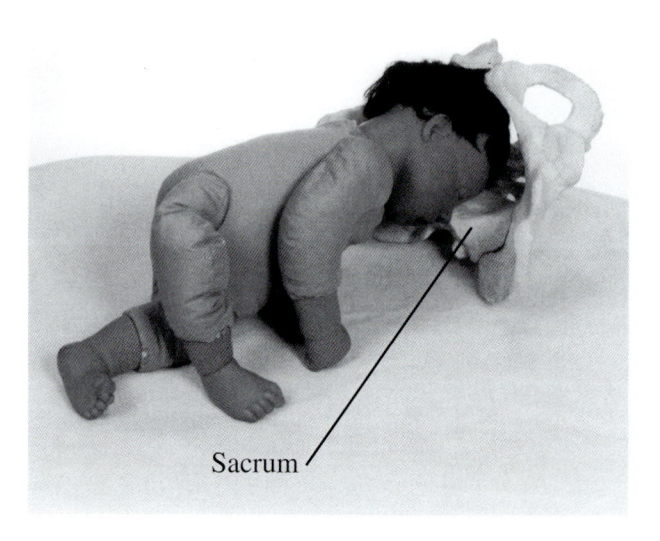

Figure 11: The baby turns his head and shoulders so that his face is nestled in the curve of his mother's sacrum.

STEP 4: Seek Relief for the Discomforts of Pregnancy and Birth

The temporal plates, the bones housing the middle ear and Eustachian tube (**Figure 12**), are made up of three membranous segments, which are capable of folding in on themselves. As the muscles force them to fold together, the baby's neck muscles will tighten on the left. This will cause the head to rotate 45 degrees as the muscles turn the head toward one shoulder. In the ideal circumstance, your baby will turn his face toward the curved portion of your sacrum and the back of his head will line up under your pubic bone.

Your baby can now slide even further into the birth canal without putting pressure on the many sensitive nerves exiting the inside of your sacrum. Once he has moved past two bony points inside your pelvis called the ischial spines, he will continue to turn another 45 degrees so he can line his head up with the widest diameter of the vaginal opening. The muscles surrounding your rectum will now rest against his forehead and give you the sensation of extreme rectal pressure.

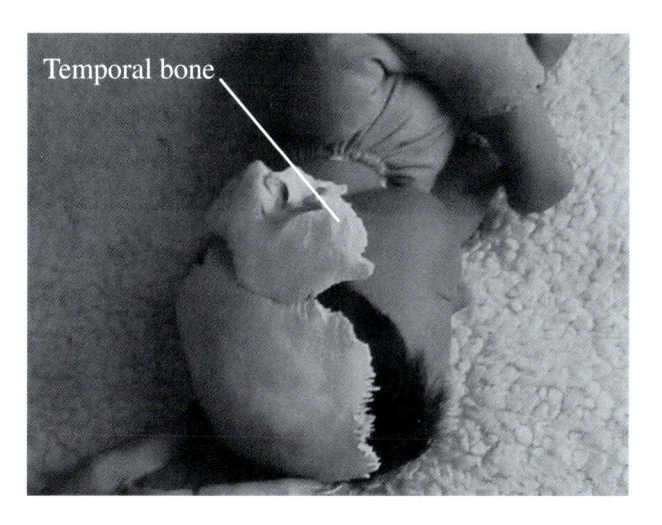

Crowning occurs when the top of your baby's head can be seen at the vaginal opening. As he slides through the opening, pressure from the anal gutter will force his head backward into extension, so he can maneuver under your pubic bone. When his head extends, your baby's sacrum will be forced to extend as well (due to the dural attachment into the coccyx). Extension will pull his sacrum forward and force his pelvis to become more compact. This will also force him to extend his knees. He can now push off with his feet against the top of the uterus and squeeze his body through the cervix.

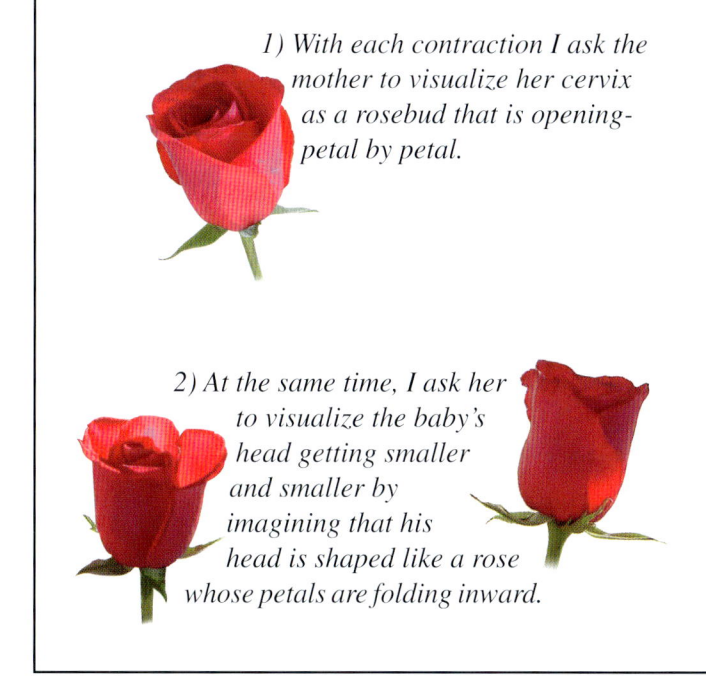

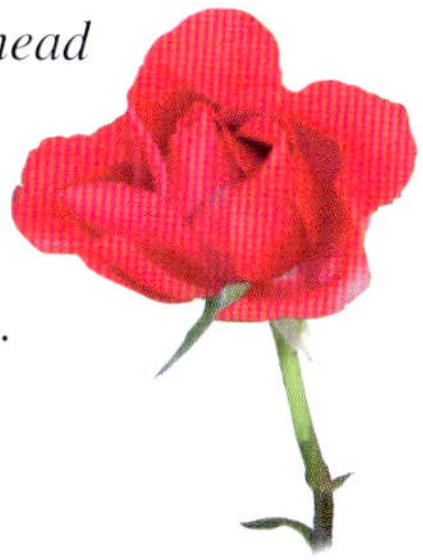

> I'm going to sleep now, Mom. God says I have to rest and prepare for the journey. Will you play Mozart for me? I get so sleepy when I hear Mozart. While I rest, could you eat something? I'm kind of hungry.

Figure 12: The three segments of the temporal plate will fold over themselves and ride over the adjacent parietal plate.

---

1) With each contraction I ask the mother to visualize her cervix as a rosebud that is opening- petal by petal.

2) At the same time, I ask her to visualize the baby's head getting smaller and smaller by imagining that his head is shaped like a rose whose petals are folding inward.

3) Eventually, the baby's head looks like a rosebud that is slipping through the open cervix which now resembles a rose in bloom.

…What your mind sees, your body feels. Fill your mind with thoughts of pain and you will feel pain. Fill your mind with beautiful visions of roses and you are more likely to stay relaxed.

Active Labor

I can hear you, Mom, and I like the sounds you are making. When you hug me really tight and say O-O-O- ... I feel a vibration all around my body.

Ouch! I think my shoulder just hit something really hard. Whew, that's better. I'm turning around so I can look toward your back and my shoulder doesn't hurt anymore. My face isn't squished anymore either. I'm sliding, mom, I'm sliding.

Wow! My head is pushed up against something that's making me look up. Gee, your body is wrapped so tightly all around me now that it feels like we're one person. Do you know that when my body hits something hard you move just right to help me turn away from it? And, when I feel like I can't slide anymore, you start hugging me tighter than ever before and it helps.

Something really warm is surging through my body! Do you feel it? Is that the rocket fuel God was telling me about? I sense a new power coming into my body. It's coming from you. Together, we can do this, Mom! We can do it!   Here I come. . .

Once his head is out of the canal, your baby must roll his shoulders around so they, too, can line up with the wide diameter of the vaginal opening. He will achieve this incredible feat with your help. Just as your muscles turned his head so he could maneuver past the ischial spines, they will turn his shoulders so they can fit past these two bony points in your pelvis. As his shoulders roll to line up with the vaginal opening, his constricted neck muscles will slowly turn his head back toward his chest—putting him back into the position he held prior to labor.

The final stage of restitution (when the baby turns his head back around to line up his chin with his chest) should not be manually forced upon a baby; only the baby knows which way to turn and how much torsion is necessary to roll his shoulders. A baby's head could accidentally be forced toward his spine, if the attendant isn't careful.

Once your baby has his shoulders lined up properly, he will slide himself out of the birth canal. Your uterus will help by applying a compressive force (like a loving shove) against his body. This force is so powerful and involuntary that it is almost impossible to stop even when asked to do so.

As your baby exits the birth canal, he will respond to the sudden insult of lights, air, sound, movement and touch. Using sound, he will intuitively cry out to increase the pressure in his cranium and force cranial fluid and blood back into the ventricles and blood vessels of the cranium. By normalizing pressure within the cranium, he will also activate the craniosacral system. The flexed sphenobasilar joint between the sphenoid (the butterfly shaped bone that directs the pattern of the face and occiput (the round

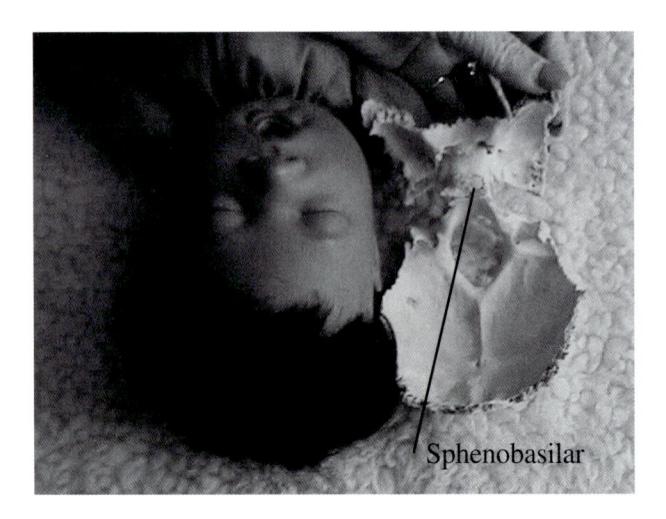

Figure 13: Superior view of the sphenobasilar joint.

bone that directs the pattern of the head) springs into motion **(Figure 13)**.

Your baby should cry out in short, low frequency bursts of sound that resemble quick bursts of exhalation. If his cry sounds like a high-pitched

STEP 4: Seek Relief for the Discomforts of Pregnancy and Birth

scream, it is a sign of physical and/or emotional stress and pain. If he continues to cry beyond the first few moments of life, he should be evaluated as soon as possible by a chiropractor and a craniosacral therapist.

During labor, will you waltz with your baby or exhaust yourself with the rigors of "slam dancing" for hours on end? The answer to this question depends on the tone of your body, the balance within your musculoskeletal system, and your psychological state of mind. With proper tone, balance, and a positive mental attitude, you and your baby have a better chance of dancing through the birth process without intervention or interference. You need only time and patience.

What happened? Where am I? What is that thing you put on my head?"

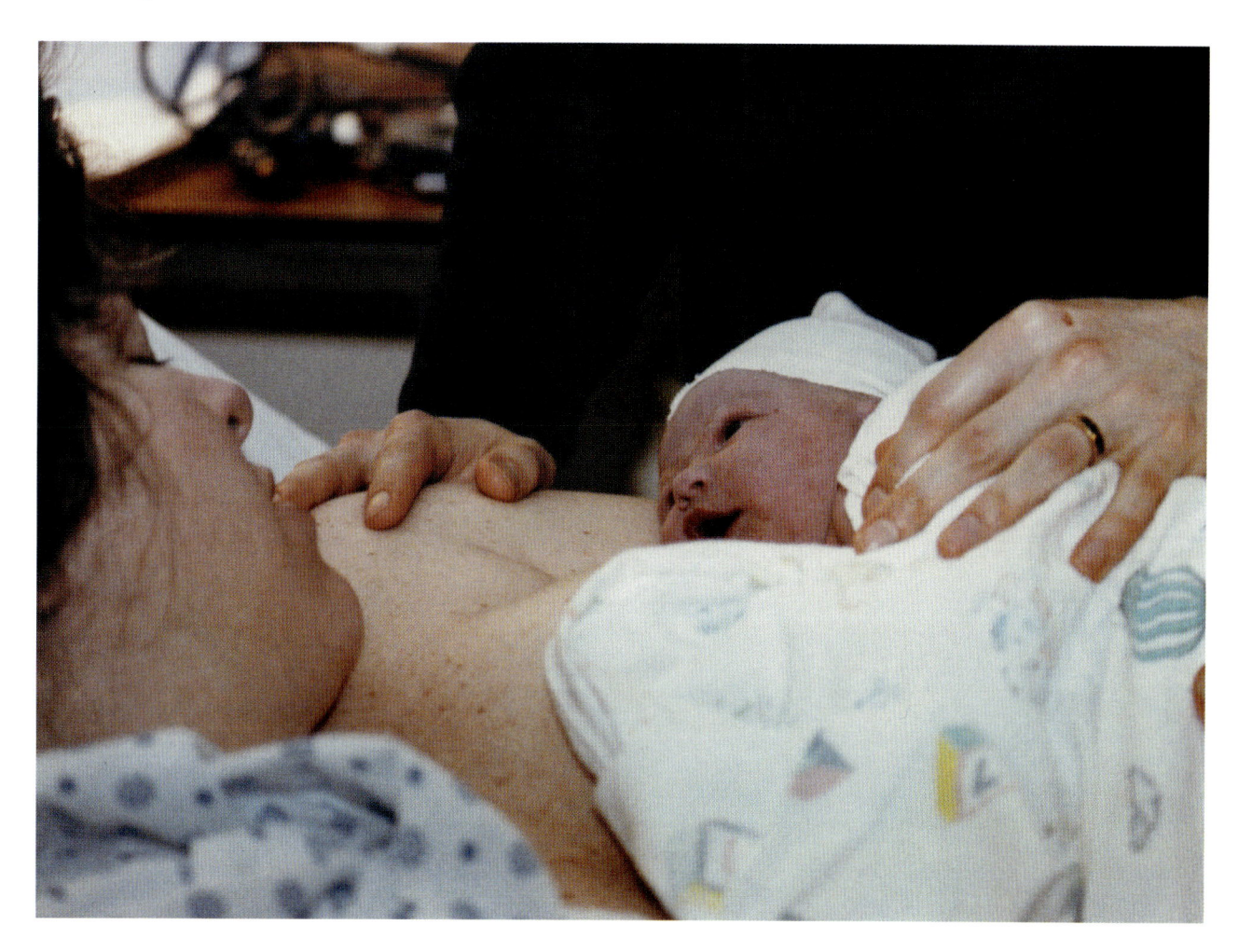

Oh! Hi, Mom!
There you are. I've been waiting to see you for a long time.

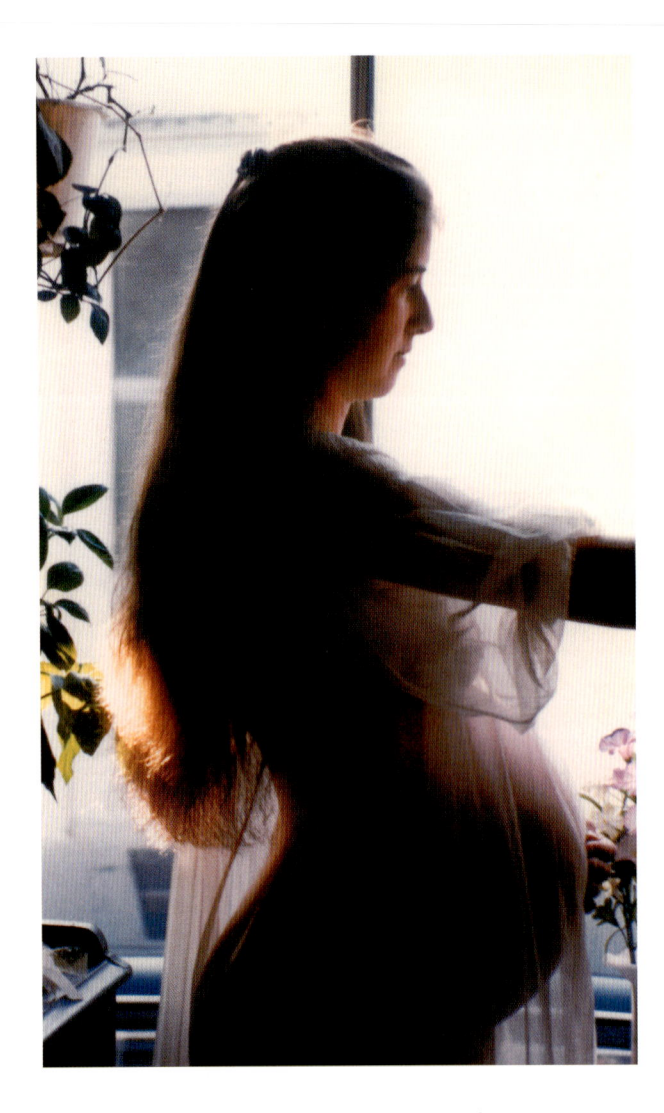

Back-Labor: A Simple Solution to a Painful Situation

Most of the births I have attended involved my own patients, so I have had the privilege of witnessing hundreds of babies born under peaceful, compassionate circumstances. But not all births I have attended go smoothly. I have also watched in agony as a mother struggled unsuccessfully to help her baby get into position for delivery. It is one of the hardest challenges I have in my career—wanting to ease a mother's pain and not being able to.

After more than sixteen years of performing doula support for my patients, I have learned how to help most women who suffer from in-utero constraint and back-labor. I have also spent the last ten years teaching other chiropractors how to help pregnant women and babies who are suffering from the most common causes of pain and dysfunction. Now, I would like to share with you a few techniques that your partner or birth attendant may perform if you have any unusual pain during pregnancy or delivery. These simple procedures will make a significant difference in how you're able to help your baby maneuver the pathway through the birth canal.

No amount of care can insure an easy delivery for everyone and, in some cases, complications crop up during childbirth that no one can resolve. When your pelvis is out of alignment, or there is an imbalance in the pelvic floor muscles, your baby may not line up correctly. His arms may be tucked under his chin preventing him from tucking his head forward during the descent. He may have one of his legs twisted backwards. This will hinder his ability to flex his sacrum and to rotate his body properly. If this happens, his body may apply pressure to the sensitive structures within your pelvis, resulting in unusual pain and discomfort. Distortion in your pelvic floor muscles may also result in your baby turning his head 45 degrees in the wrong direction.

If your baby is forced to turn his face forward toward your pubic bone, the back of his head will apply pressure to the exquisitely sensitive nerves exiting your sacrum **(Figure 14)**.

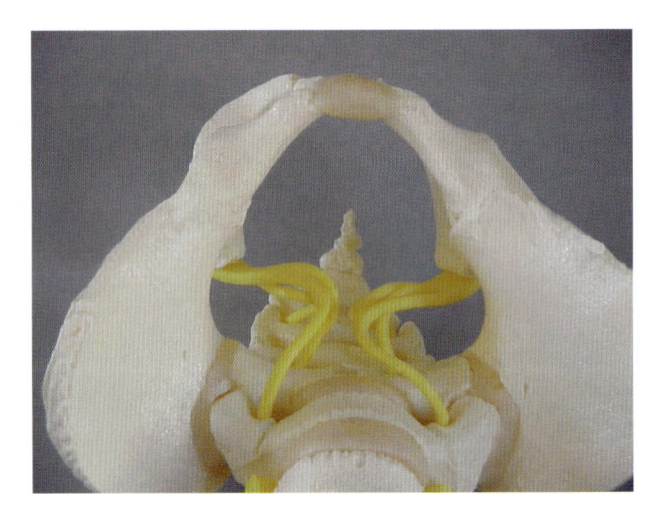

Figure 14: Parasympathetic nerves exiting the sacral foramen.

The intense nerve pain inhibits a woman from focusing and working *with* her contractions and is a clear signal that the baby is turning occiput posterior. They are often referred to as "sunnyside up" **(Figure 15)**. When a woman is having back-labor, she will instinctively contract the pelvic musculature in an attempt to pull the baby up and away from the nerves. During a contraction, she usually forces a labor companion to shove his fists against her sacrum in an attempt to dull the intensity of the pain.

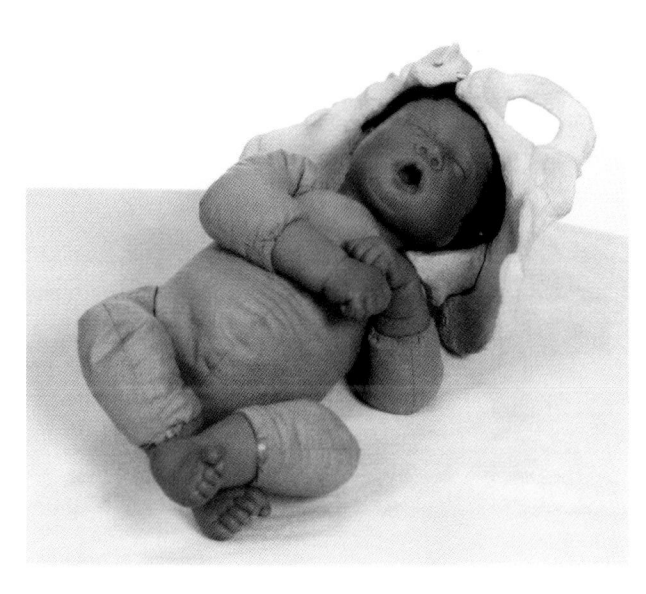

STEP 4: Seek Relief for the Discomforts of Pregnancy and Birth

Figure 15: Occiput posterior position which will result in severe back-labor.

This type of labor will result in abnormal pressure being applied to the baby's head and face. His head will be forced into extension, which compresses his bones into the brainstem instead of using the spine to protect the spinal cord. His cranial plates will be forced to mold in a distorted position that may negatively affect the function of his craniosacral system and the alignment of the spinal vertebra.

Prolonged, painful labors are not genetic, although it appears that way in many families. Women often report that their mother and all their sisters had long, difficult labors, so they expect a long labor as well. Others report every woman in their family having rapid, easy births, so they expect this.

I, too, believed there was a genetic "predisposition" to the type of labor a woman had until I helped at the homebirth of a baby who was delivering *sunnyside-up*. It was at this birth that I finally realized that this complication could be due to a physical imbalance in the mother's body. That imbalance could cause a baby to rotate the wrong way, thus distorting the structures within the his/her craniosacral system.

Here is the story of the birth I was referring to. Bruce and Marie are both chiropractors. Since Marie received routine spinal care, they felt confident that their baby's birth would proceed quickly and smoothly. Dr. Marie was not a patient of mine, but I gladly accepted when the family invited me to attend their homebirth and provide chiropractic/doula support.

Marie's Birth Story

Marie was surrounded by her birth team, which consisted of two naturopathic obstetricians, Marie's mother, her husband, Bruce, and myself. One person was applying a hot pack while another was applying pressure to her sacrum. Marie had her arms around Bruce and used controlled breathing to help her endure one more painful contraction. She didn't cry, or scream, but we knew the pain was intense. It had been approximately 20 hours since we arrived—fully expecting Marie to deliver without difficulty. No one had counted on the severity of pain in her back, or the fact that the baby just couldn't move through her pelvis (I wish I had known then, what I know now).

The two birth attendants were constantly monitoring vital signs for both Marie and her baby. Thankfully, they were always normal. Marie's mother silently anguished over Marie's struggle to manage the pain, while marveling at her constant strength and composure. She tried to ease Marie's pain by applying hot ginger packs to her low back and sacrum. Though nothing we did seemed to help, Marie never gave in to the unrelenting pain.

The birth team was physically and emotionally exhausted, so we took turns going downstairs and resting. At one point, I awoke from a ten-minute power nap and was startled by one of the doctors resting on the opposite couch. He had a look of despair on his face. I asked him what he thought we should do next. He surprised me by saying, "If we could do that craniosacral stuff, I bet we could get the baby out." I jumped up excitedly and said, "I can do that!"

We charged upstairs and asked Marie to lie down on the bed, on her back. I positioned myself against the headboard as I reached down and began to evaluate the motion of her cranial bones. Suddenly, Marie's head began to turn slowly to her left shoulder. Her head turned as far as it could possibly go. I felt the dura mater continue to rotate inside of her cranium. Several minutes passed with Marie's head rotated as far as her muscles would allow. I continued to maintain my contact at the base of her skull. Throughout the session, Marie appeared totally relaxed and comfortable because the contractions had suddenly subsided.

I supported her head in this abnormally stretched position and turned to her mother who sat beside the bed. I asked her if Marie was facing up instead of down (occiput posterior) when she was born. Marie's mother cried out, "Are you kidding? All of my eight children were face-up. I labored like this with every single one of them. All of my other daughters have had labors like this, too."

I turned to Dr. Stowell as a light bulb went off for both of us. Marie's mother had a distorted pelvis. Therefore, her children were forced into a distorted position as they exited the birth canal. That distortion affected their muscles, the fascia covering the muscles, and their bones. When the girls grew up and went into labor, another generation of babies had to twist their bodies to accommodate a distorted pelvis. (Do you see a cycle developing?)

Marie delivered her baby approximately ten minutes after the cranial release allowed her sacrum to shift. You can't imagine how happy we were to see that little baby enter the world! What a happy day!

A few weeks later, Marie's mother watched in agony as another daughter endured back-labor with dystocia (labor stopped). She, too, couldn't get her baby out. This was in a different city, so Marie's mom could do nothing but cry as her daughter was rushed into surgery. She now knew there was something that could be done to help her daughter, but no one was around that could do it.

A few years later, I treated Marie throughout her second pregnancy by adding craniosacral therapy to her chiropractic prenatal care. When active labor began, I went to Marie's home to provide doula support. When I arrived, I found her lying on her side O-O-O-ing through contractions. I climbed on the bed and maneuvered myself into a position where I could work on Marie's cranium without disturbing her. After freeing any restrictions I found in her dural membranes, Marie got up and went to the bathroom. She delivered her baby a few minutes later by squatting on the soft blankets at the foot of her bed. Marie's mother was again at her side. I smiled as she voiced her amazement at how easy and rapid this delivery was in comparison to the first one.

Marie has had two more homebirths. Unfortunately, I missed both births because the babies arrived in the quiet darkness of night before I could get there. I think the midwife was also late for the last one.

Back-labor indicates an alteration in the normal childbirth process—it is not a normal sensation associated with birth. In fact, after having a birth with this complication, many women anticipate the same degree of pain with subsequent deliveries and are often unaware that they are in active labor. Childbirth without back-labor is an entirely different experience. Until I learned how to use body mechanics to turn a baby around, the only way I could decrease a mother's pain was by pressing my fists against her sacrum for hours on end, applying hot packs, and encouraging her to "push past the pain."

You don't have to have a craniosacral therapist at your child's birth to resolve back-labor. Anyone can use the following techniques to help you relax your muscles and free your baby—allowing him to turn his face toward your sacrum. When he does turn, there is an immediate decrease in pain, and in some cases, a speedy delivery.

If the following three conditions are present, this technique will not work.

1) He has his cord wrapped tightly around his body restricting his movements.
2) His extremities are trapped in a distorted position restricting his ability to flex his body.
3) If he is induced before he has flexed and molded his cranium. The force of the artificially induced contractions may restrict him from flexing his neck properly. (Like being on a roller coaster that starts while you have your head turned sideways.)

Give a copy of the following instructions to your doula or partner. Have them help you at the first sign of back pain. This maneuver is also effective when dilation stalls. In these cases, your baby may be only partially turned. You may feel only slight pressure in your back; his position may be off just enough to slow the progression of dilation, but not enough to press on your sacral nerves. Try this before you resort to more invasive procedures.

STEP 4: Seek Relief for the Discomforts of Pregnancy and Birth

The Four Easy Steps to Reduce Back-Labor:

Step 1: Help the mother lie on her side (whichever side is most comfortable), with her bottom leg straight and her head resting on a pillow. Encourage her to move to the edge of the bed while you stand in front of her. You should be securing her body in position by spreading your feet about two feet apart, so you can place her belly between your thighs (**Figure 16**). The mother will feel secure in her position on the edge of the bed if she is resting directly against your legs.

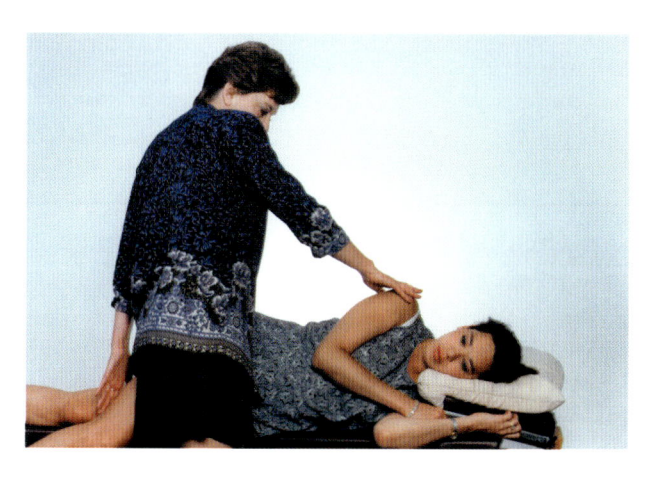

Figure 16: This is the position a mother would get into when being treated for back-labor.

Step 2: Position the mother so her hips and shoulders are straight up and down and perfectly perpendicular to her spine. It is imperative that she does not rotate her shoulders or hips, as this may increase torsion in her diaphragms and tighten the muscles that are trapping the baby.

Step 3: Help the mother drop her top leg off the side of the bed. Allow her leg to hang downward for several minutes, while you continue to support her body so she will not roll forward. Place your hands on top of her pelvis, and hook your thumbs into the bony crest in front. Press lightly downward to hold her in position (**Figure 17**). Your downward pressure, combined with the weight of her leg hanging off the table, will flare the sacroiliac joints, free the sacrum and decrease the tone of the pelvic floor muscles. The baby may now be free to wiggle his head and turn his face away from the pubic bone into a more comfortable position—for both of them.

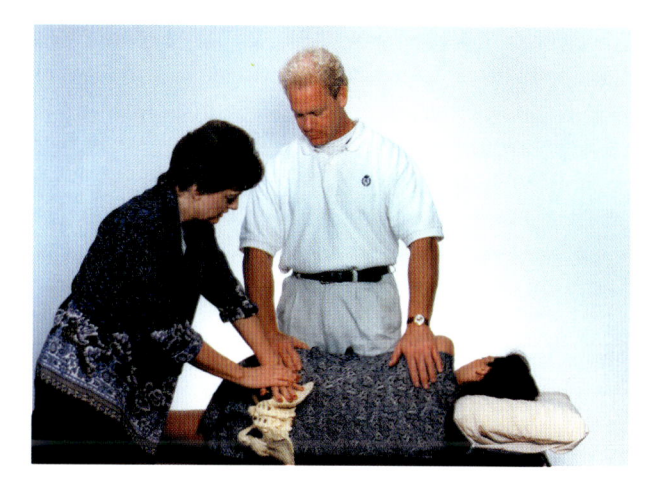

Figure 17: The mother drops her leg off the side of the bed to decrease the tone of the pelvic floor muscles.

Step 4: After a few minutes, ask the mother to roll over to her other side and repeat the procedure. You will know the baby has moved if there is an immediate change in the intensity of the back-labor, or if the mother exhibits a sudden increase in the frequency of labor contractions.

Should this technique fail to free the baby, there is another method that I have found to be clinically effective in dislodging a baby who has become engaged in an awkward position, causing hip pain, abnormal dilation (dystocia) and/or back pain during pregnancy or labor. Use this highly effective position whenever a baby is causing the mother to experience any type of pain during pregnancy, whenever dilation is stalled during a strong active phase of labor, or when she experiences back-labor that does not resolve with the side-lying position.

To perform this second technique, have the mother get on her knees on the end of an adjusting table or hospital bed. Next, ask her to lean forward onto a chair placed at the foot of the bed. As she rests her head on her forearms, slowly raise the bed to elevate her hips above her head. This maneuver will float the water toward her lungs. Her baby will float down toward her lungs, as well. Hopefully, this downward shift will dislodge the baby enough for him to quickly rotate his face away from the pubic bone.

Before inverting the mother, I ask her to visualize the baby moving as she tells him to tuck his chin, to pull his arms down onto his chest and to pull his legs forward. After about 30 seconds, the bed is lowered and the mother rises back up. The baby drops quickly back down against the pelvic floor in a better position. Labor usually continues with a reduction in back pain and a rapid delivery.

If you are at home, this technique (see below) works great if you kneel at the top of a few stairs. By walking your hands down the stairs and resting your head on your forearms, you can assume the same inverted position. After a minute or so, walk your hands back up to the top step, raise up and your baby will drop back down against your cervix. The change in fluid dynamics may have an added bonus of floating an umbilical cord up that may be wrapped around your baby—hindering his descent. I can't tell you how many of my patients successfully used this maneuver to float their babies out of the pelvis and who felt an immediate reduction of the pain in their hips or back as the baby changed his position.

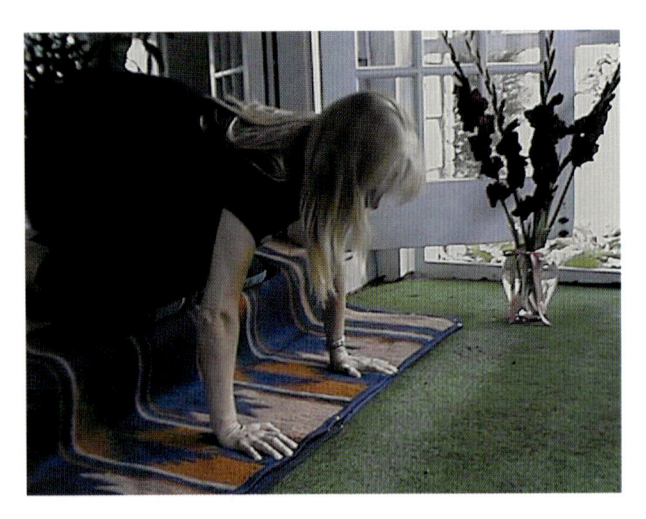

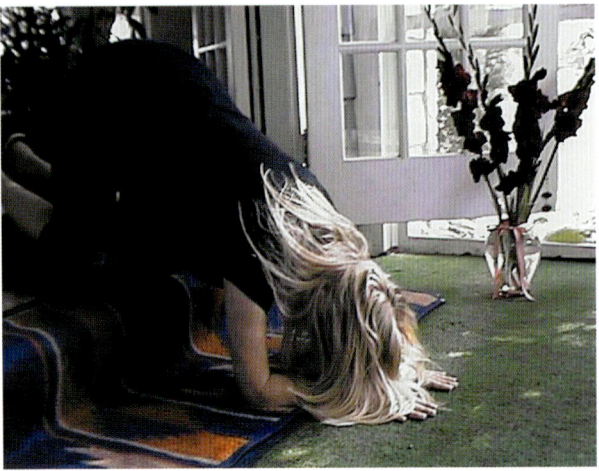

While chiropractic care and craniosacral therapy can reduce the incidence of back-labor in most cases, there is no way to completely avoid pain in ALL cases. Women who have come into my practice with a history of back-labor or dystocia (failure-to-progress) during a previous birth, generally report several common historical findings. If the problem is not addressed during their next pregnancy, these have become red flags for possible complications.

The first red flag (and most prevalent historical finding) is a history of a car accident, either before or during pregnancy (an accident in which the woman was wearing a lap belt and harness).

There is no question that seat belts save lives, but our current single harness design can cause a severe torsion within the respiratory and pelvic floor muscles, especially if a person's car is struck on the side opposite of where the person is sitting. Torsion within the diaphragms occurs because the lap belt restricts any movement of the pelvis while the harness supports only one shoulder—allowing the unrestrained shoulder to twist violently forward while rotating toward the restrained shoulder.

In women, torsion of this nature may go unnoticed until childbirth. When the abdomen is extended by the expansion of the uterus, stretching of the abdominal muscles increases tension within the transverse respiratory and pelvic diaphragms. This makes it difficult for the baby to line up properly or dilate the cervix evenly.

The second red flag is a history of sports related activities that may result in twisted trunk movements and injury. Examples would be: falls while skiing, horseback riding, cycling, and kick boxing. Again, all of these injuries will result in muscular torsion and an increase in muscular tension.

The third red flag is an occupation that forces the mother to twist her upper torso repeatedly. This occurs with clerks who use a register that is off to the side, computer stations that have a monitor off to the side, and chiropractors who twist their bodies while performing a side posture adjustment.

Any woman who has a history positive for one of these red flags may suffer from back-labor or dystocia. If you have any of these red flags in your history, I strongly advise you to add both chiropractic care and craniosacral therapy to your prenatal program. You should also practice the two techniques I have described. If you do, your partner will feel confident helping you at the first sign of back pain.

If you identify with one of these red flags, remind yourself that patience is a virtue during childbirth. You may need more time to help your baby maneuver your tight and possibly twisted pelvic floor muscles.

STEP 4: Seek Relief for the Discomforts of Pregnancy and Birth

The Cascade Effect of Managed Childbirth

Research has shown that the duration of labor and delivery can be reduced by actively managing childbirth (i.e., hormonal gels to soften the cervix, stripping of the membranes, breaking of the water sac, pitocin induction and augmentation—which requires constant electronic fetal monitoring, manual dilation of the cervix, fundal pressure, vaginal stretching, forceps, vacuum extraction, episiotomy, and planned cesarean deliveries).

No mother wants her unborn child to suffer. No doctor wants his patient to suffer. Medical management of labor and requests for drugs evolve from our human desire to bring order into chaos and to block the pain of childbirth. When a birth attendant insists on taking a managed approach to childbirth, they feel they are saving a baby who may never come out on its own, or they simply want to help a mother get through an uncomfortable situation faster. Mothers who request an epidural at the first sign of labor believe that a *relaxed mother* equates to a *relaxed baby*. They have no way of knowing that requesting the use of epidural anesthesia may equate to asking an unborn child to ride the rapids of a violent river without a guide or a life jacket. Neither the doctor taking over, nor the mother giving in, realizes how the long-term effects of managed childbirth can change a child's life forever.

It is not the purpose of this book to share with you the documented evidence that supports the concern about managed childbirth, but I would like to appeal to the heart of everyone working in the birth arena.

Doctors, nurses, and midwives perform some of the most important work on the planet. No one else has the power to influence the future as they do. No one else runs the risk of altering the human potential as dramatically as they do. And, few people are required to deal with the same degree of stress in the workplace. On the other hand, they have the fortunate opportunity to see the miracle of birth on a daily basis.

But, we must keep in mind that their work ends as soon as the mother delivers the baby and leaves the hospital. Members of the medical team are not given the opportunity to see the long-term effects of a managed verses a natural childbirth. The baby is alive. That is enough. If they could spend a few days in the offices of other healthcare professionals who treat children on a daily basis, they would think twice before deciding to manage the outcome of a child's birth. They would discover that the cascade of interventions used during labor often lead to a cascade of problems that leave parents bewildered, emotionally bankrupt and physically exhausted; the list goes on and on: colic, chronic ear infections, seizures, delayed development, autism, ADD, ADHD, Bi-polar Conduct Disorder, genetic abnormalities, and a multitude of *Syndromes*.

Mothers, childbirth is intense. By nature, as the baby moves down into the pelvis, you should experience a gradual and timely increase in the sensation of discomfort and pain. When you do, your brain receives that information and begins to respond appropriately by secreting endorphins (natural painkillers). The endorphins flood not only your body, but your baby's as well. Your baby is enduring the physical effects of being forced through an extremely tight space and he needs all the help he can get. He needs you—emotionally and physically. If you begin to ride the rapids, and cascade down the river of intervention, you baby will need you more than ever.

Become an informed parent right from the beginning. Know that induced contractions cannot be compared to the controlled contractions of nature. Know that pitocin induction and epidurals require that you remain connected to the electronic fetal monitor (EFM). Be aware that the continuous use of EFM may alter your baby's genetic material (especially the eggs of a female fetus). Consider what your baby may be feeling as he endures the violent forces of an induced labor, while denied the benefits of maternal endorphins. Is that really how you want your baby to be introduced into the world? Are you truly prepared to deal with the long-term, often subtle, consequences?[1]

I am not saying there isn't a place for pitocin augmentation or pain medication. For instance, an exhausted mother who has been laboring unsuccessfully for several days can sometimes be helped with augmentation and pain relief. Just a touch of additional hormones and short acting pain medication can help her complete the delivery. However, experience has shown me that an informed mother can often avoid intervention if she receives chiropractic care, incorporates a doula, and hires a patient, compassionate birth attendant who incorporates the techniques taught in this book.

During labor and delivery, if you do everything you can to prevent managed childbirth, but still find

---

1 See Appendix A and B for research articles that voice concern about the overuse of routine ultrasound and epidural analgesia.

yourself on the river and out of control, take your baby to a chiropractor (ideally one that is also trained in craniosacral therapy), as soon as possible. Early warning signs of underlying birth trauma include nursing difficulties, a hyperactive gag reflex, sleep problems (too much or too little), excessive crying, esophageal reflux, difficulty swallowing, colic, tight neck muscles, or any unexplainable problem they are exhibiting. The treatment for babies is so subtle you may not be aware the doctor is doing anything at all. Trust me, in most cases, you will see the dramatic effects almost immediately.

By the way, your pediatrician or specialist may ease your concerns about your child's discomfort by saying, "Let's just wait and see what develops." This is a good idea, from their perspective, since the options for medical treatment generally involve invasive techniques (i.e., drugs and surgery). Chiropractors look at your child differently. To us, tiny bones are ossifying, blood flow is being restricted, and the brain is being starved of nutrient exchange from restrictions within the craniosacral system. We can't afford to "wait and see," and luckily, all of our options for treatment are gentle and non-invasive. Birth trauma issues can be addressed at any age in life, but it is better to catch it early, before the effects begin to tax the body's innate ability to adapt.

Recommendations for a Safer Birth

Unless a baby's life is in obvious danger, give him the freedom to work his way into the world at his own pace. Allow him to start and stop labor as he maneuvers the pathway. If his water breaks before the onset of contractions, give him time to get into position and activate labor on his own. Keep in mind that it could take him three to five days to get molded and in position. Vital signs should be monitored regularly, but internal examinations that can introduce bacteria into the canal should be avoided. (A mother who remains at home during early labor will be subjected only to the bacteria she is resistant to, while avoiding the unfamiliar pathogens in the hospital.)

If the water doesn't break spontaneously, keep it intact for protection and reduction of pain. Learn to respect human physiology. Work with a baby and not against him. Remember, he, too, is going through an emotional, physical, and spiritual transformation.

Last of all, remember that a baby was created from the most powerful egg released and from the strongest sperm in the bunch. He has conquered all of the obstacles to life and knows what he has to do. Trust him and trust in the power of Innate.

There are six things to remember when you're in labor...

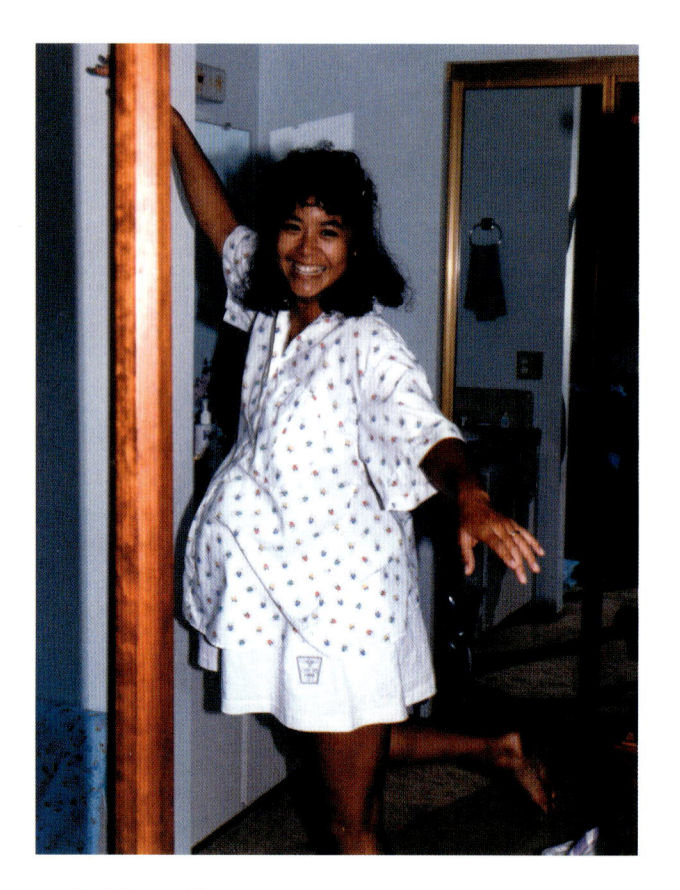

1. Have Fun.

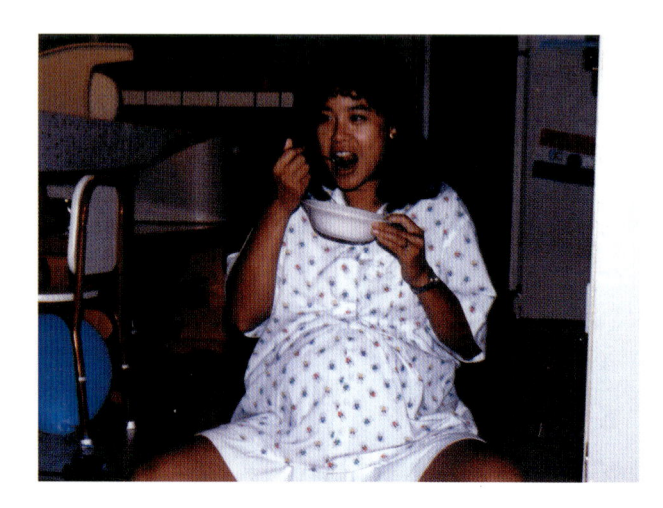

2. Eat something substantial.

STEP 4: Seek Relief for the Discomforts of Pregnancy and Birth

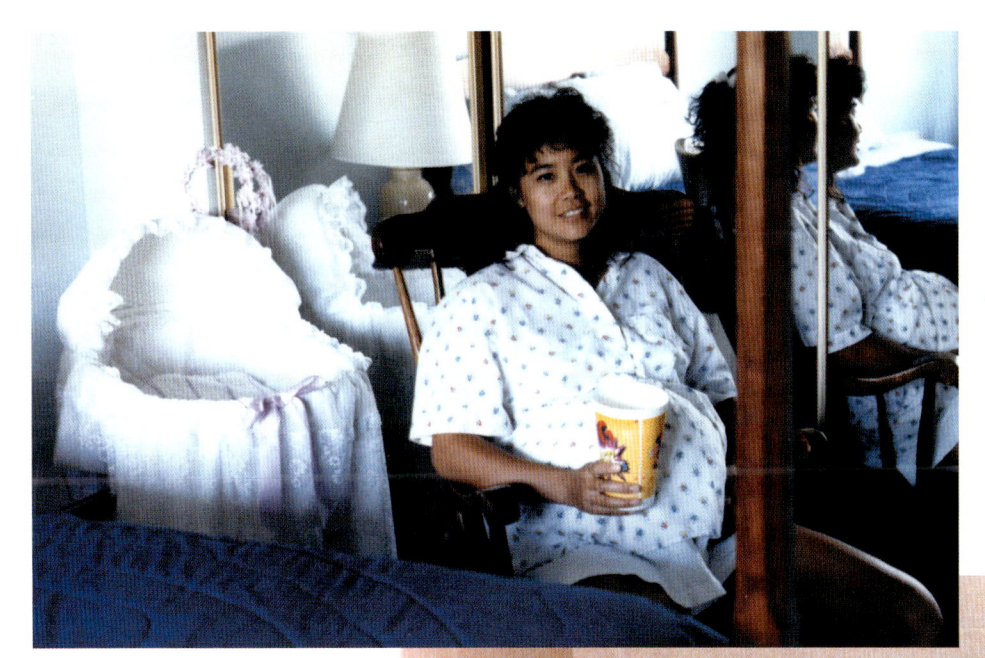

3. Drink water or juice after every contraction.

4. Soak in a warm bath to relax your muscles and float the baby.

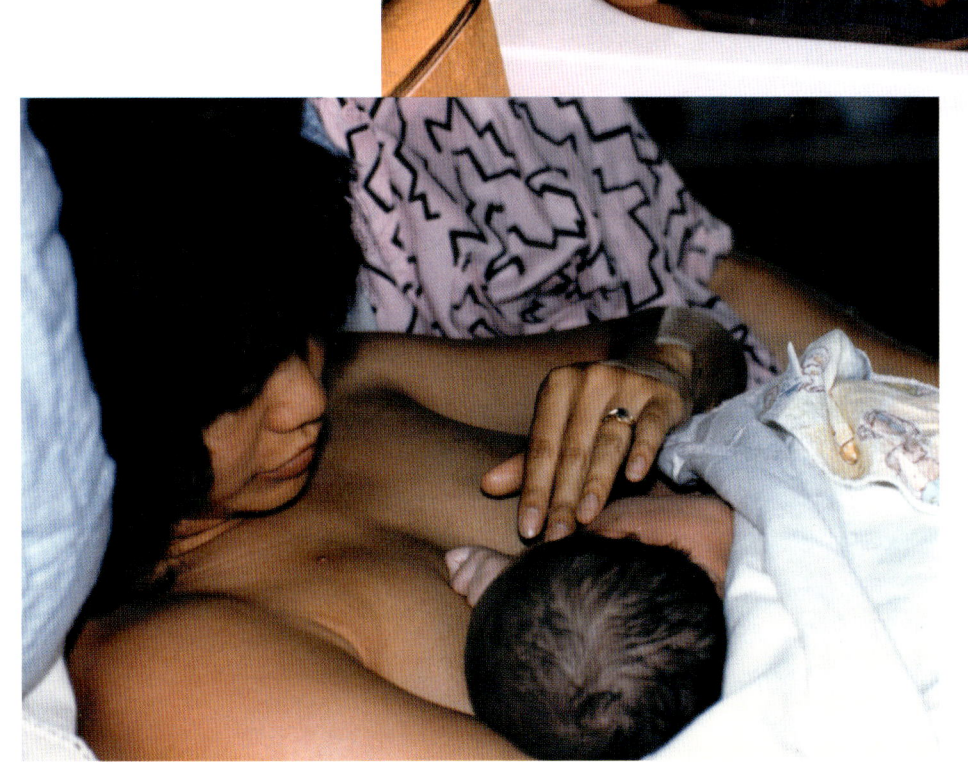

5. When the going gets rough—

visualize your reward.

135

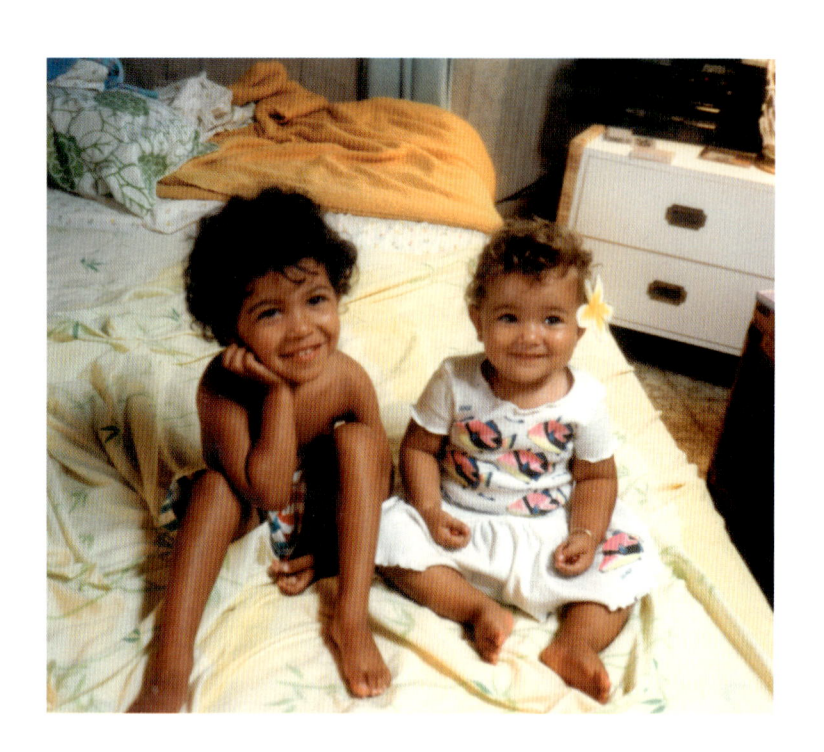

And when it's all said and done, take pride in your accomplishment. Bringing a child into the world has its ups and downs, but nothing compares to the love and joy that will flood your body when you hold your baby for the first time; when he takes his first steps; when she makes it to the potty chair all by herself; when he performs in his first play; when she graduates from college; when a grandchild is placed in your arms...

STEP 4: Seek Relief for the Discomforts of Pregnancy and Birth

There is no greater gift than loving a child.

Hands Of Love

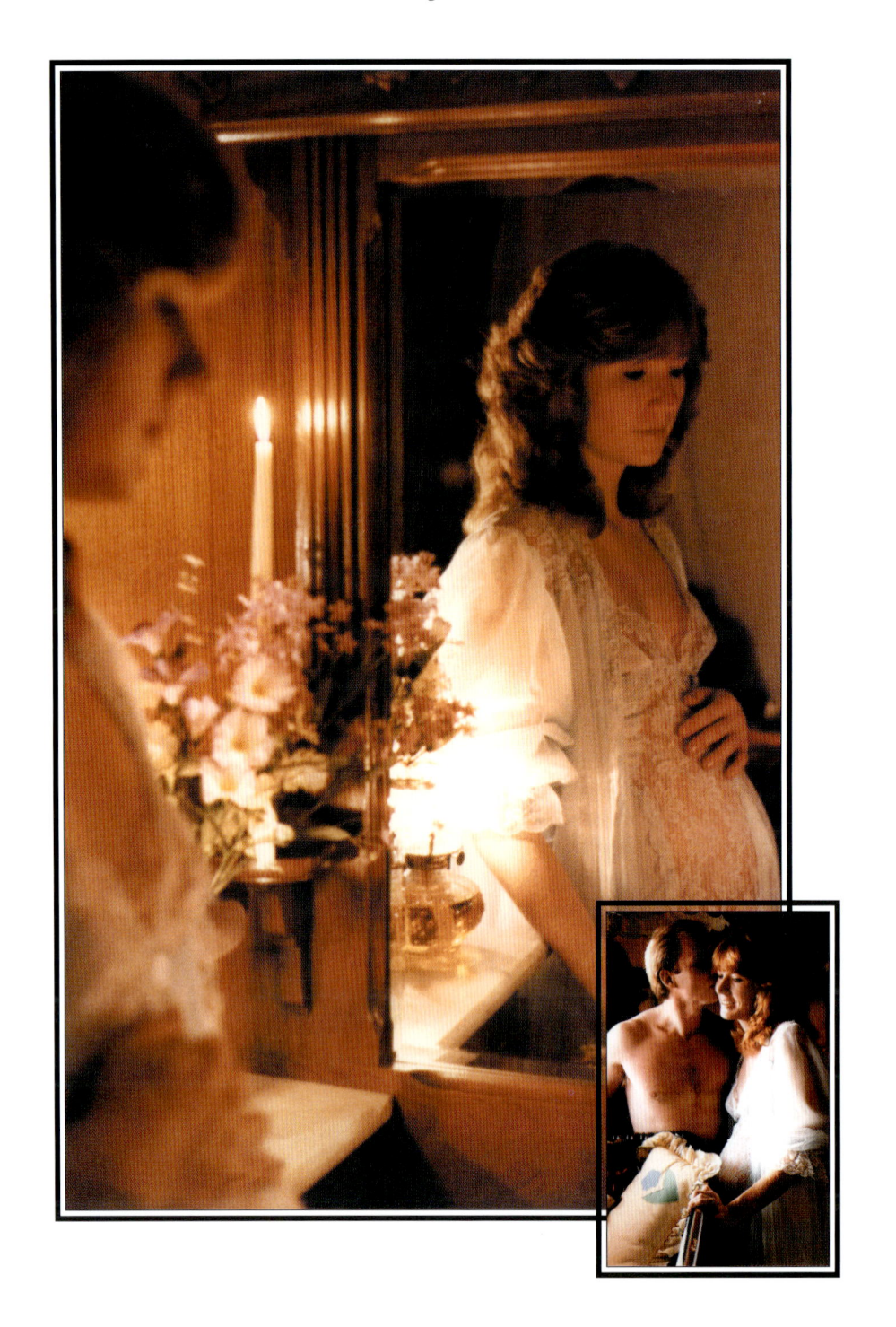

𝓑abies are at the mercy of their in-utero environment. If unseen forces cause your baby to defy gravity and turn away from the path out of the womb, look within yourself for a solution. If the problem cannot be solved, create an alternative birth scenario that preserves an atmosphere of love and compassion.

# STEP 5
Be Prepared in the Event of a Cesarean Delivery

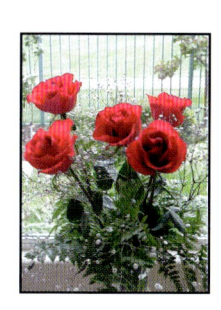

Suppose your dream is to have a perfectly natural low-tech birth for your baby. You've read several books on pregnancy, written the perfect birth plan, attended an excellent birthing class, and now you're shocked to learn that your baby is lying in a breech position and you must face a surgical delivery. You're devastated. Your heart aches for the baby who will not be handed to you after he has made his way into the world. You cry for your body because it will not physically feel the ritual of birth after so many months of preparation. You worry about the risk that major surgery holds for you and the baby.

What do you do? Do you still have options? Must you surrender all of your plans and dreams for a natural birth and accept that the birth is now entirely in the hands of a surgeon? Is there some way you can still have a birth experience that will allow you and your baby to meet and bond in the manner that is so crucial to the development of your emotional relationship?

When a fullterm baby is found to be lying in the breech position, many birth attendants perform an external version[1]. This will usually occur in an operating room so the baby can be surgically delivered if there are any complications during the procedure. Babies commonly turn back into the breech position within a few days so if the procedure is successful, a mother is scheduled for an induction. If a doctor feels an external version would be too risky, due to the position of the placenta, an immediate cesarean delivery is scheduled.

Recently, there has been a resurgence of birth attendants allowing mothers to attempt a vaginal delivery with their breech baby. For many people this sounds like a positive move for the birth attendants. After all, babies are designed to experience the trip through the birth canal. It stimulates the sensory receptors and activates the central nervous system; it squeezes the lungs and prepares them to take that first breath of air. The final exit through the vaginal opening is also responsible for the activation of the craniosacral rhythmic impulse[2]. All of these things considered, it seems like a move in the right direction. But I believe, from a craniosacral point of view, it is unwise for a mother and her baby to go through a long and difficult vaginal delivery if the baby is lying in any position other than head down against the cervix.

If the baby were allowed to slowly exit without any interference from the outside world, it might be fine. But, chances are that a well-meaning birth attendant will pull on the emerging body; the cervix will then close around the baby's neck. The upward force on the baby's jaw will then reverse the normal molding pattern and cause a flaring of the cranial bones. This can result in serious long-term consequences for the baby. A vaginal delivery is not worth the risk of serious long-term problems. Of course, the same damage may occur in a surgical delivery if the surgeon utilizes a forceful technique when removing the baby. That's why a parent would be wise to discuss the procedure her surgeon typically uses to remove a baby who is lying in the breech position.

Here are the stories of two patients of mine who found out, late in their pregnancies, that their babies were in the breech position. Both had adopted the

---

1 An external version is the medical technique that actively manipulates the baby into a head down position. The technique requires the use of medication to paralyze the uterus and ultrasound sonography.
2 The craniosacral rhythmic impulse is a motion that is distinctly different from the physiological motions related to breathing and cardiovascular activity. It is responsible for the movement of the cranial fluid that bathes the brain and spinal cord, as well as, the inherent movement of the fascial system of the body.

humanistic-assisted model, and both mothers were devastated when they were scheduled for cesarean deliveries. Delivering ten years apart, they both took whatever measures they could to work within the technocratic environment and achieve the humanistic birth they had planned for their babies. You will find their stories inspirational and helpful if you, too, find that your baby must be delivered surgically.

Becky's Birth Story

When they found out they were pregnant, Becky and Jim immediately signed up for a Bradley birth class (they didn't want to waste any time).

During the second trimester, Becky had an ultrasound sonogram and discovered they were going to have a girl. She was lying in the breech position at the time, but Becky's doctor assured her that it wasn't a problem at this stage of pregnancy.

Becky had an uncomplicated pregnancy—from a medical point of view. During the third trimester, she began chiropractic care with me because of a tipped uterus, and because she had been involved in a motor vehicle accident prior to the pregnancy. Becky wanted to make sure her body was ready for a delivery. She often felt the baby tipped way off to the side and would come in feeling scared due to the lack of noticeable movement. After working on her, the baby would start squirming and the uterus would shift into a vertical position. Becky always left feeling happy and relieved that the baby was able to move more freely. It was never long, though, before her little girl would move back over to her favorite spot deep on Becky's side.

Becky and Jim had chosen a family practitioner as their birth attendant. He was extremely supportive of Becky's decision to receive chiropractic care, but he often voiced his disbelief that a car accident could have any influence on the outcome of the birth. Unaware of my concern that seatbelt injuries cause pelvic torsion, he couldn't understand how a car accident could affect the function of internal structures. To his credit, he never suggested that Becky not receive chiropractic prenatal care.

Becky and Jim knew how important it was to have a birth plan if they wanted to maintain control over the delivery, so they drafted one and copied it for everyone on the birth team. I felt their letter was a particularly good example of a birth plan so, with their approval, I have included it for you to read.

Dear Staff,

We are very pleased with the opportunity to work with Dr. Kevin Haughton, and the staff at Mercy Hospital, for the upcoming birth of our first child.

We are well prepared and educated (Bradley Method) and have done everything we can to stay healthy and low risk during this pregnancy. We are looking forward to a beautiful, natural birth and would appreciate all of the kind, encouraging care that you can provide.

Since this is a very special event in our lives, we have some preferences that may be different than your standard routine. We respectfully request that a fetoscope be used instead of an ultrasound doppler. We would also ask that you do not do routine electronic ultrasound monitoring unless there are signs with the fetoscope that the baby may be in distress. We would prefer no IV and no medication be offered to us during labor unless an emergency arises. We ask that no routine episiotomy be done. My husband and I want to remain together at all times along with Carol Phillips, our labor support person.

We would appreciate our baby being handed to us immediately after birth for breast-feeding and bonding, giving us time together until routine newborn assessments are done at the bedside. We would like the placenta to be delivered naturally with no intervention (i.e., drugs).

We will, of course, be flexible on all these points if a complication does arise. Although we feel confident that everything will go normally, we trust that you will inform us if any problems come up, so we can discuss the choices to be made and come up with a new plan of action. We take our responsibility of being good parents very seriously and want to do what is best for our baby.

Thank you for your kind attention.

Jim & Becky Wontor

STEP 5: Be Prepared in the Event of a Cesarean Delivery

During each prenatal visit, I monitored the position of Becky's baby and did what I could to reduce the tension surrounding the uterus. Unfortunately, not having learned the Webster Breech Turning Protocol (a chiropractic maneuver), I was unsuccessful in helping the baby turn into position.

Just before her due date, Becky's doctor double checked the baby's position and shocked everyone when he found that she was still in a breech position. Suddenly, Becky and Jim's plans for a natural delivery were dismissed as the doctor informed them that the baby would be delivered by C-section the following Monday. It was Friday and they had only two days to deal with the shock and grief.

Becky called for my opinion. Should they go along with the plan, or find another doctor that would let them deliver the baby vaginally? Becky cried and told me how she had skipped the prenatal reading material on cesareans because she felt "that was not going to happen to her." They had attended the class on surgical deliveries and understood enough to know that surgery was not the open the zipper and lift the baby gently out of the mother's tummy procedure that many people blindly believe. She also knew it was not the best way to enter the world, so they had dismissed the information as irrelevant—she was going to have a natural birth.

Becky cried and voiced her fears and disappointments. I listened and heard the voice of regret in my own mind. Had I done something wrong? Had I missed something that could have helped the baby turn? Was there something I could do even now? I was delivered breech myself. I let my history of poor health flash through my mind and I realized I couldn't give her an unbiased opinion.

When she finished talking, Becky asked once more for my opinion. I had to tell her I honestly did not believe it was safe to have a vaginal breech delivery. I knew *professionally* the negative impact a vaginal birth would have on the delicate structures of the cranium and I knew *personally* what impact it had on me when I was born breech. Becky needed more than a yes or no answer, so I explained why I felt so strongly about it.

I told Becky my mother's doctor didn't know I was breech when he induced her. After 26 hours of excruciating pain, my mother begged for help and the doctor agreed to put her out. She has no idea how they pulled me out of the birth canal. The doctor came into her room later and laughed saying, "It's a good thing you gave up, because she would never have come out on her own in that position." According to my mother, I cried for days in the hospital after my delivery. The doctors eventually told her that my body was internally bruised from the delivery. While growing up, I endured chronic headaches in which no medical cause was ever found. I had trouble in school with memory and struggled to maintain slightly above-average grades.

After having my first child at age twenty, the headaches increased in frequency and severity. I developed digestive disorders, menstrual dysfunction, and chronic back pain. I eventually agreed to a hysterectomy at age twenty-eight. That was the final straw in my long history of illness. The surgery left me with back pain that was so severe I could barely function.

The year before my surgery I had taken my daughter, Angel, to a chiropractor and had witnessed her miraculous recovery from the long-term illness she had as a result of her forcep-assisted birth. I finally decided I needed chiropractic care as well. My recovery was also quick and permanent. I learned that the cause of all my health and learning problems stemmed from misalignments in my pelvis and neck area—a direct result of my own delivery. Once the interference was removed, I had a new lease on life—and a new mission.

I told Becky it was impossible for me to encourage her to have a vaginal breech delivery and suggested that she seek out the opinion of others who were not biased. I also encouraged her to go within and ask her baby what she wanted. I stressed that no matter what decision she came to I would still help her give the baby a compassionate birth experience. I let her know I would support any decision she made. I also promised I would treat her baby as soon as possible after birth to correct any abnormal molding.

After a weekend of crying, reading, and talking, Jim and Becky decided to follow her doctor's recommendation that she deliver by cesarean. Monday morning, Becky's mom and I joined Becky and Jim at the hospital. Their doctor knew in advance I would be there; he was happy to work with us to make this the best experience possible—under the circumstance. Becky and Jim were now happy and excited about the decision they had made. They were back in control and that helped immensely. We could not be assured until the very last minute if the anesthesiologist would let Jim and I both go into the delivery room; we put that in the hands of God and did what we could to prepare for the surgery.

Hands Of Love

The medical staff was wonderful and consistently demonstrated a reverence for the concerns and wishes of the family. They bent over backwards to help us maintain an air of peace and tranquillity around the baby. Becky's family practice doctor understood her need to have Jim and I with her in the operating room and arranged it with the surgical team.

Becky asked that I do one last diaphragm release to relax the muscles surrounding her baby. We all laughed and talked as I worked on her. A diaphragm release looks and feels like a gentle massage, so it helped Becky relax and conquer her fear of surgery. Just before it was time to walk down (yes, we all walked together to the operating room), we joined hands and formed a circle around the baby. Becky's mom said a prayer as we turned the outcome of this birth over to a much higher power.

The doctor asked Jim to stay out of the operating room while Becky was given the epidural (they were afraid he would pass out). The anesthesiologist then honored Becky's request that I stay close to keep her calm. The doctor allowed me to stand in front of Becky as the epidural was administered. As she rested her head on my shoulder, I whispered into her ear and told her where to arch her spine for easier insertion of the needle. She calmly did as I asked and never felt a thing.

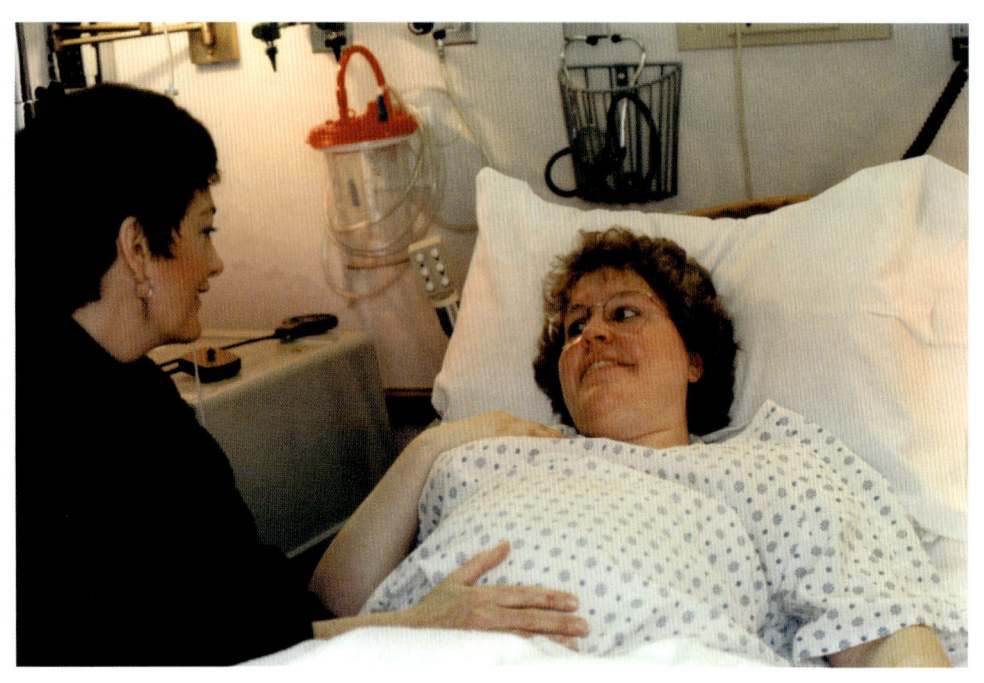

The surgeon, a very tall, muscular man, filled the room with an air of confidence and reverence for the event that was about to occur. He smiled approvingly when we asked him to let us use our music to soften the mood in the brightly-lit operating room. As Becky laid on the hard surface of the operating table, they strapped her arms out to the side and inserted an IV. I attempted to counter the effect of this restricted position by asking Becky to close her eyes and visualize herself in Hawaii. We used visualization to help her imagine she was on a warm beach making angels in the sand. We then talked softly to the baby and prepared her for the sudden and rapid exit she was about to make from her tight and confined world.

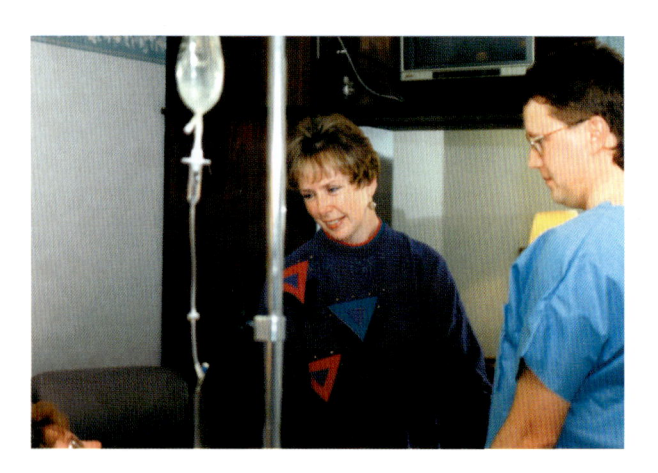

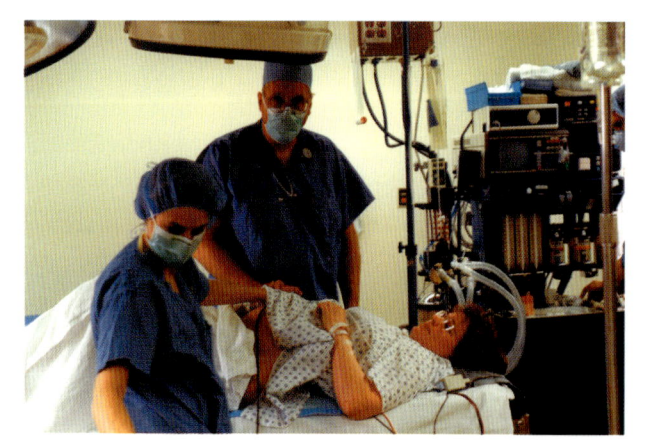

142

STEP 5: Be Prepared in the Event of a Cesarean Delivery

> Strapping of a mother's arms can result in shoulder problems after delivery. I now suggest to patients that they request that their arms not be restrained. As long as a mother agrees not to reach into the area of the sterile field, doctors have allowed them to just rest their arms on the sideboards. This eliminates both emotional and physical trauma.

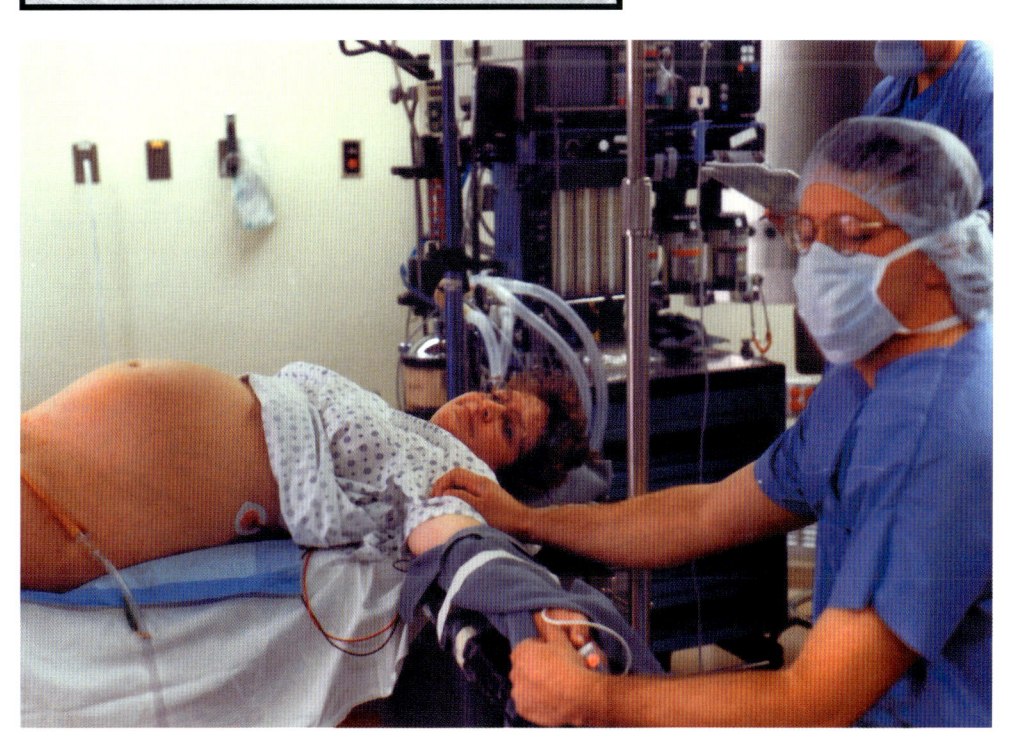

After the epidural was inserted, Jim came in and sat down next to Becky. Slipping his hand into hers, he smiled with nervous anticipation. Within minutes, Becky's little girl was pulled from the womb. Before handing the baby over to a nurse, the surgeon took a moment to hold the blood soaked newborn over the drape that blocked our view of the delivery.

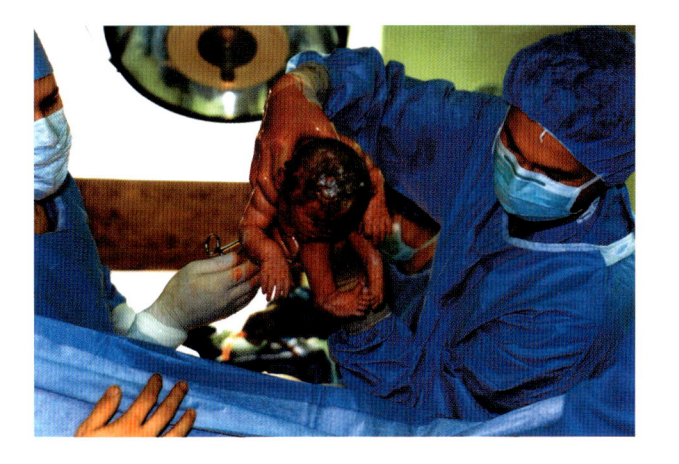

After that one quick peak, the baby was handed over to the nurse. I encouraged Jim to move quickly to the warmer and stay in close contact with his little girl. I had previously coached him on how to block the bright light from her eyes and encouraged him to touch her while the nurses worked with her. I sat down next to Becky. The curtain mercifully blocked our view of what was happening to the body she could no longer feel. Suddenly, Becky was consumed with panic.

Turning her frightened eyes toward me, Becky gasped and whispered, "Carol, I can't breathe!" I quickly stood up and looked over the curtain. I was shocked to see that the surgeon had taken her uterus out of her abdomen and placed it up on her body. With the blue drapes placed over her it appeared that the uterus was sitting on top of a table instead of Becky. I gasped as I watched the doctor lean his entire body weight onto the uterus as he squeezed it between his hands. I had often watched women gasp in pain as the nurses showed them how to massage the uterus to reduce the risk of postnatal hemorrhage, but this was too graphic—even for me.

I don't think the doctor had any idea that he was also compressing Becky's respiratory diaphragm. I sat down and told her was what happening. I encouraged her to relax and breathe slowly. I did my best to keep her calm by assuring her that the pressure would resolve shortly. I wish I'd had the courage to speak out and tell the doctor what he was doing, but I have always felt that it was in the best interest of the patient to avoid saying anything that might cause the birth attendants to become angry. There is a time and a place to discuss questionable procedures; I suspected that was neither the time—nor the place.

Several minutes later, Becky's little girl was bundled and handed to Jim. Before going to the nursery, Jim took time to bring their baby over to Becky for a quick look. Becky strained to see her baby.

Hands Of Love

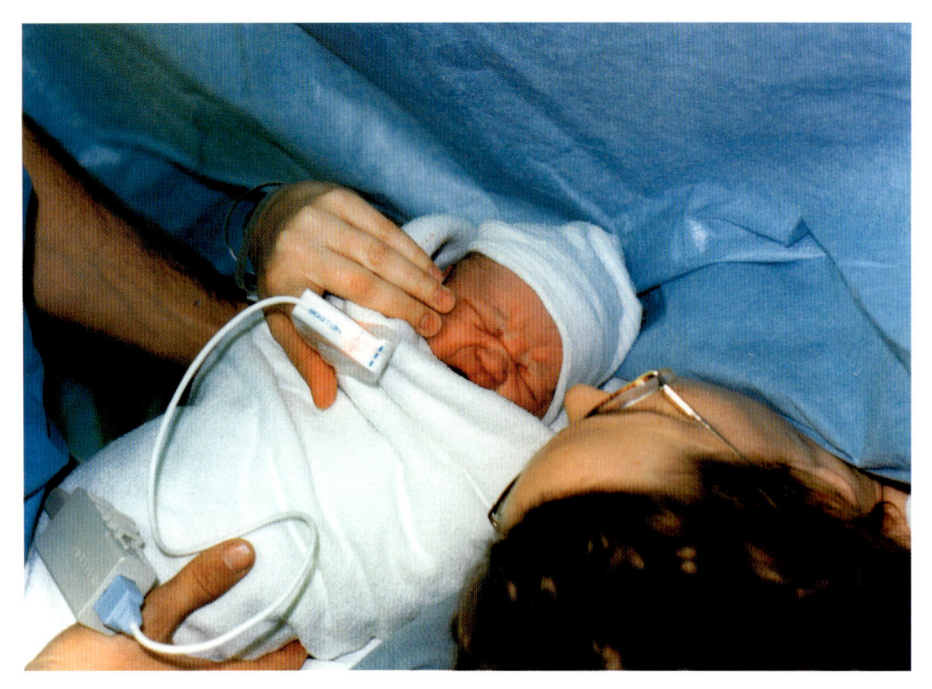

Her tiny face was so squished up that Becky was unable to make eye contact with her. Becky, herself, was in so much pain she didn't have the mental strength to focus on her newborn. Becky's mom was waiting in the hallway for news of her grandchild's birth, so Jim took the baby to meet her before going to the nursery. I agreed to stay close to Becky.

In recovery, Becky continued to gasp as she endured excruciating pain in her right shoulder area. The surgeon came in and explained that, for some unknown reason, air sometimes gets trapped in the lung cavity after surgery (I was too timid to tell him he pushed the air up there). He explained there is no way to remove it and Becky would have to wait for it to be reabsorbed naturally. She was then given pain medication that made her too groggy to care or wonder about the baby. After Becky's mother came into recovery, I left and went to the nursery to take pictures of Jim and their little girl.

When I arrived at the nursery there was no sign of Jim or the baby. I looked all around, but they were nowhere in sight. I went back to the nurse's station and asked if they knew where Jim was. They assured me that he was in the nursery with the baby. They suggested I look for the bonding room. I went on a search and sure enough—there they were. Jim was sitting in a dimly lit room that was no bigger than a tiny bathroom. The narrow room had a beautiful love seat, an end table, and a lamp.

I found Jim sitting on the loveseat with his baby nestled in his arms. She was lying quietly, but her eyes were still squeezed tightly shut. Before taking pictures, I knelt down and suggested that Jim put his little finger in his baby's mouth to encourage her to start sucking.

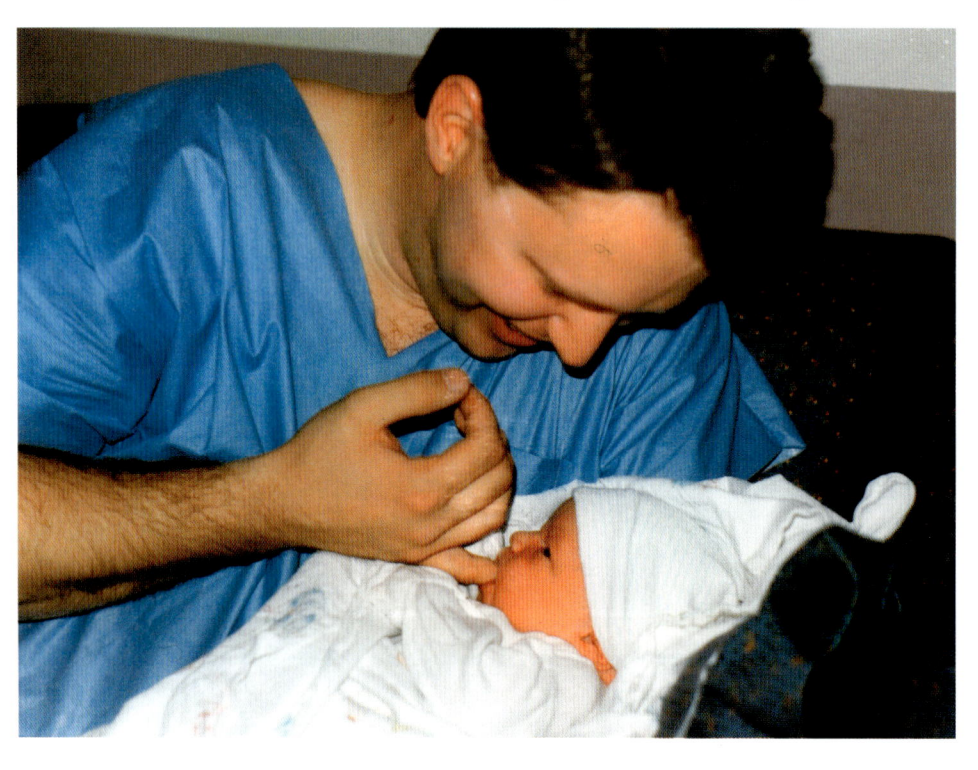

I told Jim not to apply any pressure with his finger and to allow the baby's tongue to push his finger up against the roof of her mouth. I checked her palate first to make sure there was no deviation in the cranial base. Afterwards, Jim's baby instinctively took his finger and began sucking ferociously. Within a few sucks, her face softened and she slowly opened her eyes. I grabbed the camera just as father and daughter

144

STEP 5: Be Prepared in the Event of a Cesarean Delivery

took their first long look into each other's eyes. I knew then that she would be all right. Had she started gagging, or struggling for air, when he placed his finger in her mouth, I would have been worried about problems with the position of her cranial bones and with the flow of the cranial fluid.

> If abnormal molding is severe it may negatively affect any one of the twelve cranial nerves that exit through the skull. This may alter a baby's ability to suck or swallow. Pressure against the vagus nerve (CNX), will adversely affect the function of the heart, lungs, and digestive process. This problem may be difficult for a parent to assess initially, but pain and tension may be obvious by the look on a baby's face or the tension in his hands. Sucking a parent's finger will put the baby's cranial base in motion and may help restore balance within the cranial dural membranes.

I had the privilege of watching two people bond as they looked into each other's eyes. I regretted that Becky was not able to participate in this vital activity, but I was glad that this hospital had the foresight to provide a room for babies to be alone with their dads. The soft lighting also helped the baby adjust her eyes to the bright, fluorescent world she would soon be moved into. Suddenly, I heard a soft, male voice behind me. "Hello." I looked up and saw Becky's doctor standing in the doorway. He had remained at the hospital so he could observe and assist the surgeon. He wanted to check on his new patient. I was so impressed! He smiled, shook our hands, and thanked me for a job well done. His gentle nature and supportive attitude touched my heart and brought tears to my eyes.

When we received word that Becky was ready to see her baby, Jim wrapped her up and strolled back with her toward the recovery room. Becky was groggy and still in a great deal of pain, but she wanted to have a few minutes with her little girl. Soon afterwards, Becky was moved to a regular room. The nurse set her up with morphine to self-administer. Due to the pain in her shoulder area, Becky needed a great deal of medication. Later, she told me she had no memory of the conversation we had around her bed, or the time she initially spent with her daughter. It was almost a full day before Becky was able to truly enjoy her newborn. The pain in her shoulder lasted for several days before the air finally reabsorbed.

Soon after the family returned home, I did a home visit and treated the baby. I balanced her cranial bones and adjusted her spine. I was pleased and surprised that she came through the pregnancy and birth needing only minor adjustments. It can sometimes take weeks, months, or even years to correct the effects of being in a breech position. After working on her, I felt confident this little one was going to be just fine.

As I stated earlier, if I had known how to perform the Webster technique to correctly balance Becky's sacrum and supporting structures, I might have been able to help her avoid a cesearean delivery. This technique does not require manipulation of the baby as in external version but simply balances the structures so that gravity can help turn the baby around.

The Webster Breech Turning Protocol was perfected by the late Dr. Larry Webster, the founder of the International Chiropractic Pediatric Association (ICPA), after his daughter delivered a baby who was in the breech position. Her labor and delivery was so traumatic that Dr. Webster anguished for weeks over how he could have prevented the abnormal positioning. God answered his prayers for guidance and the Breech Turning Protocol was created. Dr. Larry helped over a thousand babies turn around before he died in 1997. There are now thousands of chiropractors trained in the Webster Protocol who have experienced the same incredible results (myself included).

If your birth attendant informs you that your baby is breech, find a chiropractor trained in this procedure. It is a quick, easy adjustment that balances the sacrum and restores normal tone to the uterine ligaments. You may seek a referral by contacting the ICPA at (770) 982-9037 or by logging onto their website at www.4icpa.org

Hands Of Love

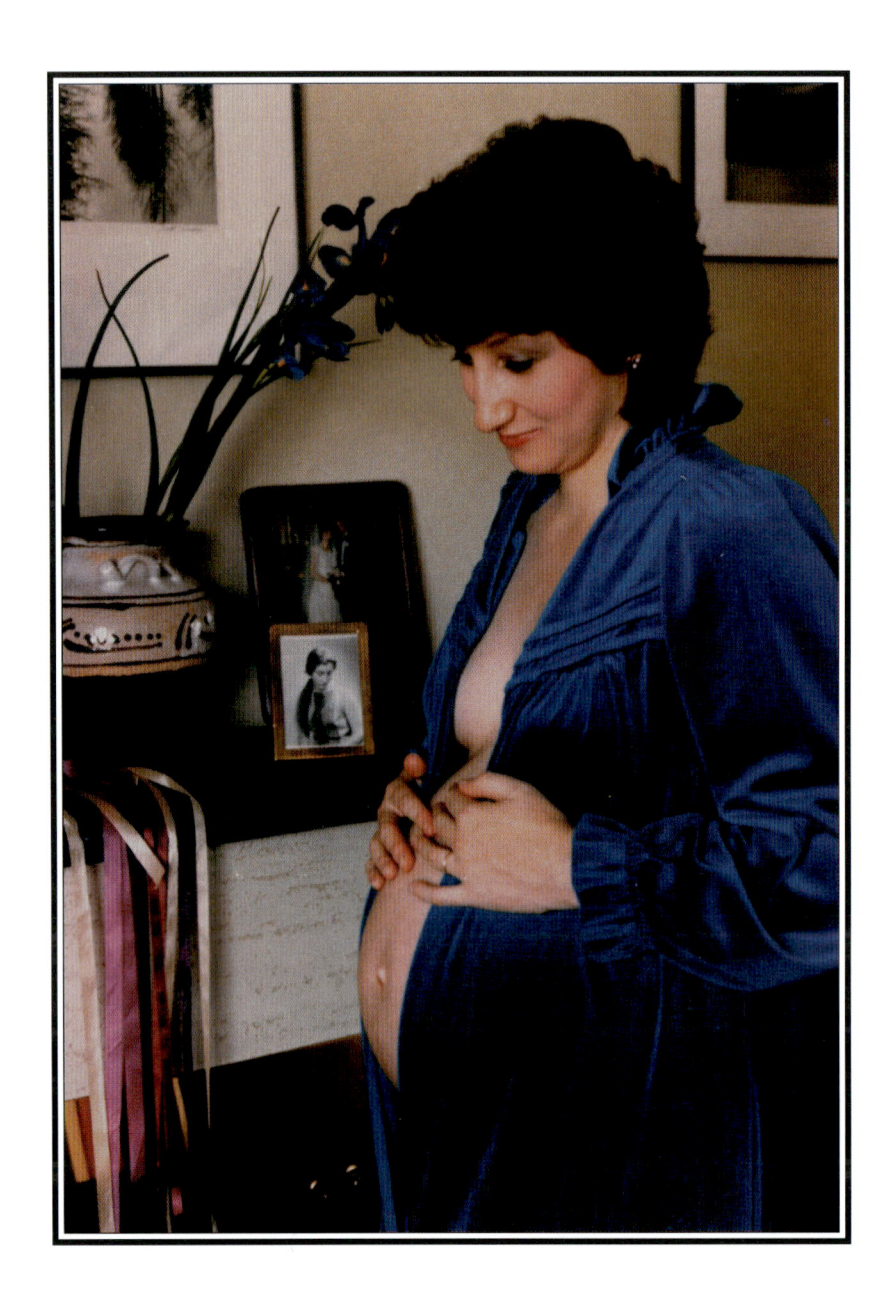

STEP 5: Be Prepared in the Event of a Cesarean Delivery

The Circle of Peace

There is a peace that dwells within me.

It flows throughout my body
out into the environment
around and about me.

I am peace.

I am strength.

I am purpose.

Thank you, Father, that this is so.
(Author Unknown)

This is an excellent affirmation for times when you feel intimated, frightened of the unknown or uncertain about your ability to endure the forces of birth. Repeat this affirmation several times while you visualize a bubble of peace flowing out the top of your head (the crown chakra). Those molecules of peace will flow down and around you as they form an invisible bubble of protection around you and your baby. Know that you have the strength to fulfill your purpose.

This next mother, Julia, was also devastated when she was told she would not be able to have a natural, vaginal delivery. Her baby was also in the breech position; his placenta was attached high on the uterine wall and his unusually short umbilical cord was wrapped tightly around his neck, causing his head to be bent and wedged against the top of the uterus.

Julia and her husband, Kyle, chose to continue using the humanistic–assisted birth model despite the need for a high-tech delivery. The medical team helped them achieve their goal of having a gentle birth experience by having the lights in the operating room turned off (forcing the staff to rely on the light above the table), by allowing the soft melody of Celtic music to fill the room, and by allowing the couple's exceptionally large birth team to surround Julia with love and reverence for the process they were witnessing.

I stood at the foot of the operating table and watched in awe at the precision in which the surgeon intricately cut through the many layers of muscle overlying Julia's uterus. I captured on video how reverently the surgeon entered the sacred space within the womb, and how slowly he eased Jared out of his snug little world without twisting or pulling on any part of his body. (I had witnessed other cesarean deliveries and often cringed at the forceful manner in which they were pulled out of the womb.)

My daughter, Angel, stood beside me softly calling the baby to us. I watched her hands flow back and forth in front of her heart. I also listened and marveled at her unbridled communication with the baby — she later told me she was energetically *holding the space for him*[1].

Julia's Birth Story

Written by Julia Matson

Almost from the moment we knew we were expecting, Kyle and I began to make arrangements for the birth of our child. Friends, who had already given birth, listened to our plans. After reading our wonderful birth plan they kept saying, "Be prepared to change those plans!" Change our plans? To me that meant nothing more than giving in to some kind of pain medication. Hoping to have a natural delivery, I had no idea how radically far from natural our birth plan would become.

From the beginning, we knew we had to have Carol with us, if not for me, then for any cranial issues our baby may have. I asked Carrie to be my doula as well, in case Carol was out of town. Then two of my friends offered to help. The next thing we knew, we had four women on our labor support team! This raised a few eyebrows, as you can imagine! But for me, every one of these women was essential—two women for me, and two for our baby. It also seemed unlikely that all four would be able to attend.

Kyle was a bit nervous about a natural birth. He has two children from a previous marriage, both born by cesarean. He didn't mind admitting that he was glad to have doula support!

For months leading up to our baby's birth, Kyle and I studied all the material we could get our hands on. We chose to see certified nurse-midwives instead of doctors. I received chiropractic care throughout my pregnancy and attended Carol's childbirth class. I saw a massage therapist every two weeks, exercised and looked into medications for labor (just in case). Kyle and I did various stretches every day to help me get ready for the big day.

Toward the end of my pregnancy, Kyle and I met with the entire birth team to discuss our birth plan. I felt ready to go!

When I was two weeks overdue, I agreed to a non-stress test. It did not go well. Each contraction made our baby's heart rate fall. Next, we were scheduled for a sonogram ultrasound, something we had avoided until now. Our hearts sank as they told us the news. "Well, first off, your baby is breech! Secondly, the cord is around his neck, tightening every time you have a contraction, and there is a shortage of amniotic fluid." There was no way they could safely try to turn him. We returned to the office where our favorite midwife, Amy,

---

1 *Angel describes* holding space *as "a means of directing a heightened level of conscious intention, with the purpose of aiding in the stabilization and balance of the molecular energy in and around the baby's body."*

STEP 5: Be Prepared in the Event of a Cesarean Delivery

told us there was really no option but to have a cesarean. To this day, I can barely type the words without damp eyes.

We were given the option of being admitted that afternoon, or early the next morning. I chose to go in the next day so I had a chance to come to grips with this overwhelming change of plans.

I called my doula team together. They were wonderfully supportive. I cried for hours even though everyone kept saying, "Thank goodness you didn't go through hours of labor before finding out!" To be honest, it was as though I was listening through a tunnel. Months of planning, and of all the different scenarios that I ran through my mind—this was not one of them! Nevertheless, we all sat around talking for hours. Kyle and I asked them if they would be there for the birth the next day and participate in whatever capacity they could. They reacted with so much enthusiasm you would have thought surgery was the plan all along! We ended the evening by drawing medicine cards (Jamie Sams' Indian Medicine Cards). We read them out loud to each other as we looked for a purpose behind our individual roles in this birth. We even drew one for the baby.

The next morning, the maternity ward was packed with new moms so Kyle and I were set up in a labor-waiting area. Hospital smells are never relaxing, so we set up our aromatherapy gadgets. Then we turned on the music we had chosen for the birth. It was early in the morning and three members of the team were able to come. They were all smiles and excitement! Kyle was doing his fair share of beaming too; he was extremely anxious to meet this new little person. Carol did a little cranial work to relax me, while Carrie and Angel prepared the camera and camcorder.

Next, we thought we would see if the doctors would let our whole team into the operating room. The nurses weren't too optimistic, but a very kind nurse-midwife brought us all scrubs, just in case the doctors approved our request. Everyone was standing around my bed in their blue scrubs when the doctors arrived. To our surprise, both the anesthesiologist and the surgeon gave us the okay. We found out later from the surgeon that the anesthesiologist had never permitted anyone other than the father to come in and here he let an entire team of people come in with a video recorder and a camera! Prayer works!

I was very nervous. Kyle was calm and loving. The staff took me in first to administer the spinal block and to prep me for surgery. They were so busy, they forgot there was a crowd, including my husband, waiting to come in! Just as they were ready to deliver the baby, I asked about my birth team; a nurse scrambled out to get them.

We were now all together, waiting to see this new little person. The medical staff turned on the music we had brought, a soothing Celtic CD, and turned out the lights in the operating room. Soft light filtered in from an adjacent area. The only bright light came from the one suspended over my abdomen.

My birth team stood at the foot of the bed. Carol videotaped, Carrie took pictures, and Angel did energy work while she sweetly coaxed our little one out, "Come on baby! Come on baby!" Kyle held my hand and occasionally peered over the drape to see what was happening. Carol told me later that the doctors worked so carefully that there appeared to be very little physical trauma. They never pulled on his arms or legs, but gently eased his folded body down onto my lap. I felt some tugging and then Dr. Junnila announced to us............. "It's a boy!"

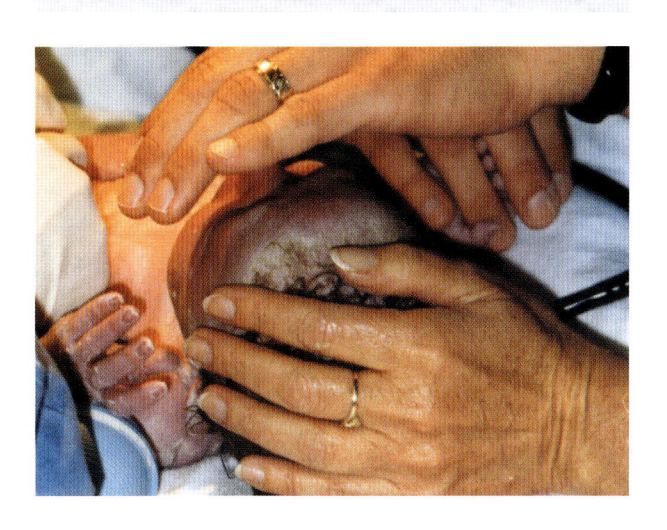

149

Kyle told me he loved me as he looked at me with a big smile on his face and shiny, wet eyes. He and Carol followed the nurse and Jared into the next room. I couldn't see them, but I was relaxed because Angel came right over and held my hand while they sewed me back together. I learned later that as soon as the nurse was finished checking Jared, Carol asked if Kyle could hold him against his chest. The nurse sounded surprised, but said they could. Kyle quickly took off his shirt, picked up Jared, and headed back into the operating room before he could be stopped.

Just moments before they arrived, I felt like I was having a heart attack! The nurses had assured me I was fine, but there was no convincing me. There was a sharp pain all down the left side of my neck and arm. Just then, Kyle brought our new baby over and laid him around my face.

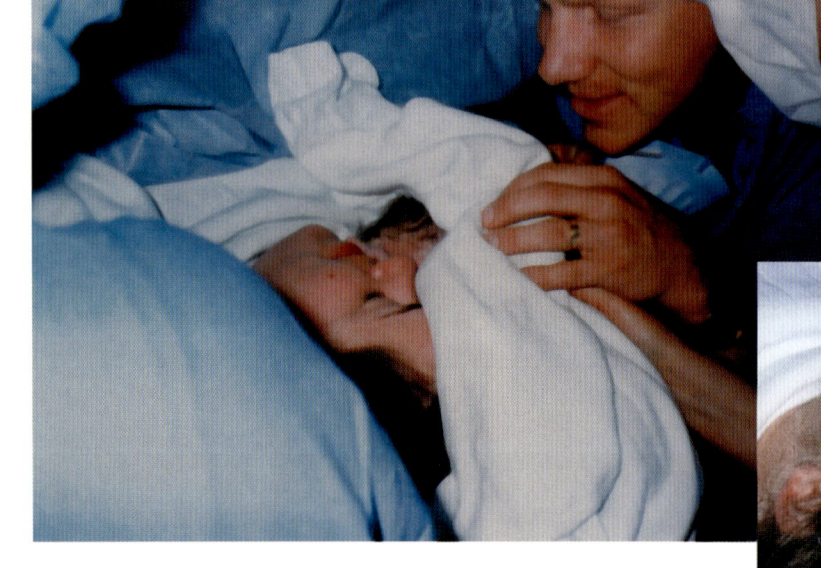

I no longer noticed the pain. Jared put his little fingers in my mouth and on my nose, while he wiggled his toes in my hair. I couldn't stop kissing him!

My head was encircled by a small mob of loving people, watching and welcoming our little wonder to this world! For the next 45 minutes, Angel worked on my shoulder, Carrie took pictures, Carol held and worked on Jared's sacrum, and Kyle just kept kissing us both. The whole time the doctors worked on suturing me, Carol and Kyle continued holding Jared around my face. The doctors and nurses kept peering at us in amazement, but no one said anything. I'm sure they wondered what Angel was doing with my shoulder (she's a doula and craniosacral therapist so she was trying to relieve my arm pain). Carol's work on Jared's sacrum and hips was so subtle, it appeared that she was just holding him in position, so no one questioned her either.

When his work was done, Dr. Junnilia came over and smiled down on us. He told us that Jared would maintain his folded up position for about three weeks. (He wasn't familiar with how quickly they straighten out when you work on them!) As they moved me to recovery, Kyle carried Jared out to my mom. She sat in a rocker with him for a few minutes before he was brought back to me.

There were many miracles the day of our son's birth. His cranial bones were distorted from the way the cord twisted

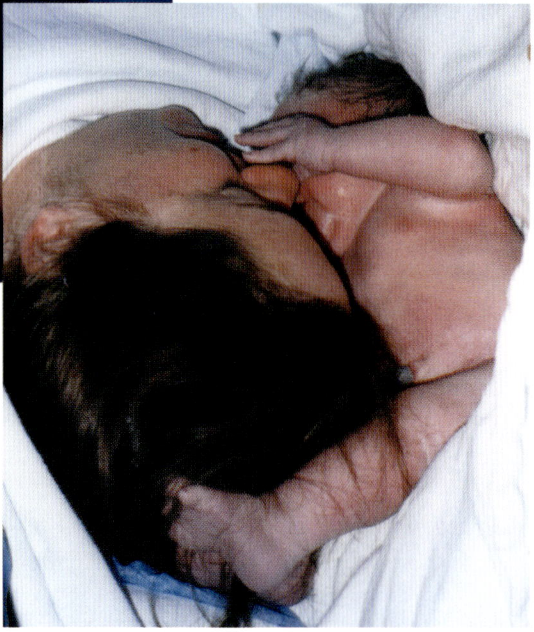

STEP 5: Be Prepared in the Event of a Cesarean Delivery

his head inside of me, but he was healthy. His birth, of course, was the most amazing miracle I have ever known, but there were many others. Since we wanted to avoid all interventions, we had a complex birth plan, but it was not ours to use. What a miracle that Kyle would have experienced two cesarean births before ours. Consequently, he was able to display strength and calmness. Another blessing was that we had three of the support team come that morning and not all four. What if four extra people were too many for the doctors to consider?

It was incredible that both doctors would let all of us be present in the low-lit operating room with soothing music, cameras, and energy work during a surgical procedure! A master plan was in place that brought Carol, a chiropractor and pediatric craniosacral specialist, into our lives so she would be able to assist our son with his many difficult cranial issues. There were more miracles of course, many we may not be aware of.

I did learn one very important thing that day. No matter how they may arrive—babies are a most wondrous blessing!

Julia and Kyle had wisely limited their exposure to routine ultrasound because there are no studies that prove ultrasound does not cause subtle long-term genetic alterations in the cell structure. They then used good judgment by agreeing to make use of this technology when Julia went two weeks overdue.

Agreeing to a non-stress test is sometimes difficult for families who want to avoid any form of intervention. In most cases, the baby is fine, but in a few rare cases, he is not. It is cases like this one that contribute to doctors recommending that all women receive routine evaluations.

In Julia's situation, she agreed to the non-stress test because she had a nurse-midwife who followed her intuition when she had a strong sense that the baby was in a breech position. Skilled hands can typically palpate a breech baby. If you push on their head—they move it. In Jared's case, his head was so restricted by the position he was in, with the cord around his neck, that he could not move it. Therefore, his head felt like a little butt. Only a sonogram could confirm her suspicions. Julia was wise to heed her recommendations.

During Julia's appointments with me, she did not have the usual structural misalignment that will result in a breech position, therefore, the Webster Breech Turning Technique wouldn't have helped. I had no idea the baby was breech. His head did not move away from my touch and it felt like a butt. If labor had occurred spontaneously, it may have resulted in an emergency cesarean instead of the one they were now able to plan for.

Having adopted the humanistic model, Julia maintained a positive attitude about her ability to have control over her birth. Thanks to the doctors who handled her delivery, she continued to feel some control over the environment in which her baby would enter the world. Her positive attitude, and wisdom in surrounding herself with a supportive birth team, helped Julia and Kyle succeed in welcoming their baby in a warm and reverent way.

I wish this family's experience could be duplicated in hospitals around the world. Cesarean deliveries would be a great deal less traumatic if other doctors made the same concessions for other planned births (i.e., dim lights, soft music, aromatherapy, and unrestricted time for bonding).

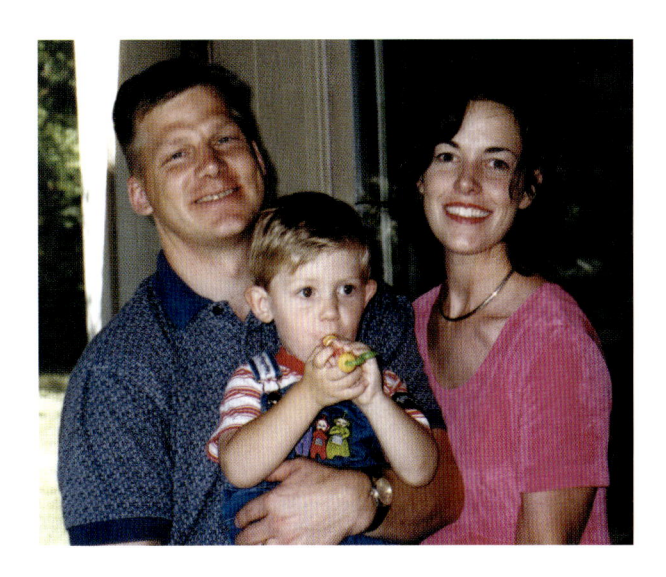

Cesarean deliveries have become so commonplace in our society that we are at risk of negating the potential emotional trauma a mother may endure when her baby is removed from the womb in this fashion. These next heartfelt words were written just a few short weeks after a mother delivered her son by cesarean delivery. Her story, like the last two, demonstrates how the compassionate response of a birth attendant can turn a potentially traumatic experience into a lesson in understanding and compromise.

Sharilyn's Birth Story
Written By Sharilyn Doyle

How do I put into words the devastation I felt when I found out that my third baby was in the breech position—when the technician said it looks like another C?

"No, it is not," I said. "I will be scheduling to have the baby turned!" The technician said nothing more to me before she left the room. While I waited for the doctor to come in, I called my husband.

I started crying when Dan answered. "Dan, you're not going to believe this! The baby is breech!" He let me cry for a few minutes, then I told him I'd call as soon as I talked to the doctor. Next, I called a girl friend for support. After crying with her, I called another friend, Susan, and asked her the name of the doctor who had successfully turned her baby when he was breech. She told me. Then she warned me that I was going to have to insist that I wanted to have the baby turned. Well, it turned out all the insisting in the world would not help.

When the doctor came into the exam room, he just said, "Well, the baby looks great."

"But the baby is breech!" I exclaimed. "Yes, that is a problem."

After this point, my recollection gets blurry. I was told it was not an option to turn the baby—due to my previous C-section. If they tried to turn the baby, the pressure and stress on the uterus would be too great. The scar could tear and rupture—risking the baby's life, and my own. He just wanted to know what day we should schedule the surgery.

The tears started and just kept coming. My emotions were growing more and more out of control. My husband had always teased me that the only reason I wanted to be pregnant again was because I had an emergency cesarean with my second baby; I didn't get to push her out. It was devastating to realize that it was happening, all over again.

The doctor was surprised at my reaction and asked me what was so wrong with a cesarean delivery. I explained that a cesarean cannot be compared to the joy of being able to deliver your own baby. He responded by saying, "Don't worry, your surgeon will help you feel at ease—he is a talker and will talk you all the way through the procedure. Afterwards, you will probably know how to perform a "C" yourself." He just didn't get it!

"That is not the point! I have watched the complete surgery on a cable channel and I have experienced the surgery first hand. It is just not the same!" He tried to make me feel better by saying that my husband would be able to hold the baby up close to me and I should be able to recover with the baby near me—sure, I thought to myself, by then he'd be all cleaned and swaddled in a blanket!

The things he was telling me in no way compared to the grand experience I had with my first baby's birth. I wanted the baby to be delivered onto my chest. I didn't want to lose any physical contact after the birth. I wanted the bonding experience to be as priceless as it was with my first birth.

My second baby was taken by cesarean. I never felt like I had worked for her. I especially never felt any sense of completion after the delivery. We did bond with time, and we have a very close loving relationship, but I can't say I will ever get over losing the experience of giving birth to her.

I had planned for a vaginal delivery with every one of my births. I had done a lot to prepare myself for a VBAC (vaginal birth after cesarean delivery). My husband and I took a special class for parents who were planning a VBAC. I made a birth plan for the nursing

STEP 5: Be Prepared in the Event of a Cesarean Delivery

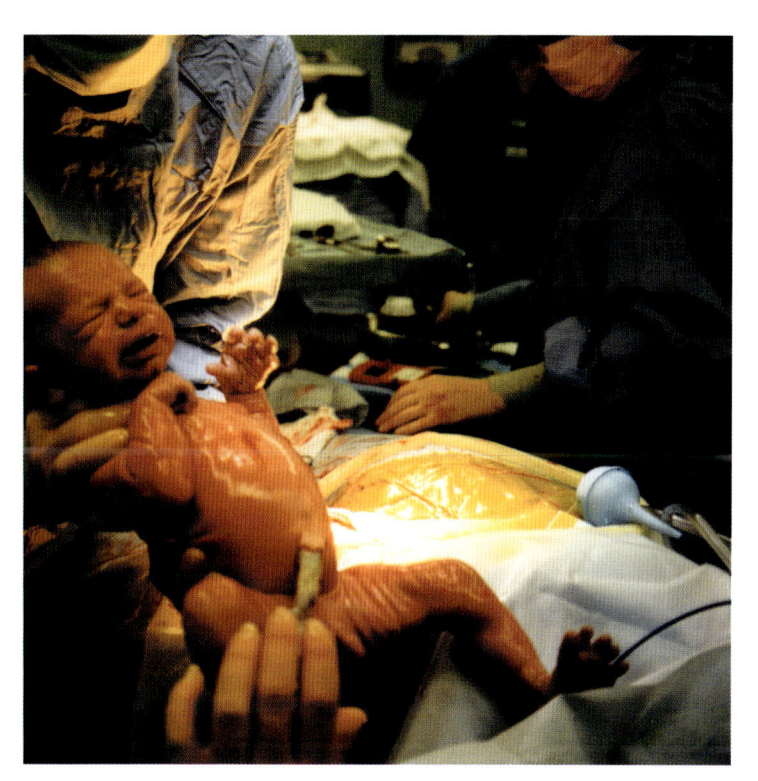

I hope these three families help you realize how important it is to plan ahead for the possibility of a cesarean delivery. Prepare for any scenario and have it written into the birth plan. A cesarean delivery doesn't have to be a traumatic event. Plan ahead. Talk to your birth attendants. Do what you can to spare yourself (and your baby) the grief and shock of separation after a cesarean delivery. And, most importantly, incorporate prenatal chiropractic care to correct any structural imbalance that would force the baby to turn into a breech position. A chiropractor who is skilled in the Webster Breech Turning Protocol may be able to prevent the *need* for a cesarean delivery.

staff so they would understand what kind of birthing experience I expected. I was even prepared to have the birth videotaped. Now, all of my dreams were being shattered, again.

Later, when I had the chance to meet the surgeon, I shared my grief (and my birthing dreams) with him. Since this wasn't an emergency cesarean, we worked together to make it a good experience. The surgeon understood how important it was for me to see my baby's birth and to touch him right away. So, he told the staff to drop the drape. I watched the delivery of my son, Nathaniel, and I was filled with joy as I reached out and touched his feet. It wasn't much, but it meant the world to me, and it helped me get through the experience of another cesarean delivery. I hope the doctor realizes how much it helped me to see Nathaniel before he was all cleaned and swaddled—and to see as well as hear his healthy cries. I hope he knows how much I cherished getting the chance to see, once again, the gift of life.

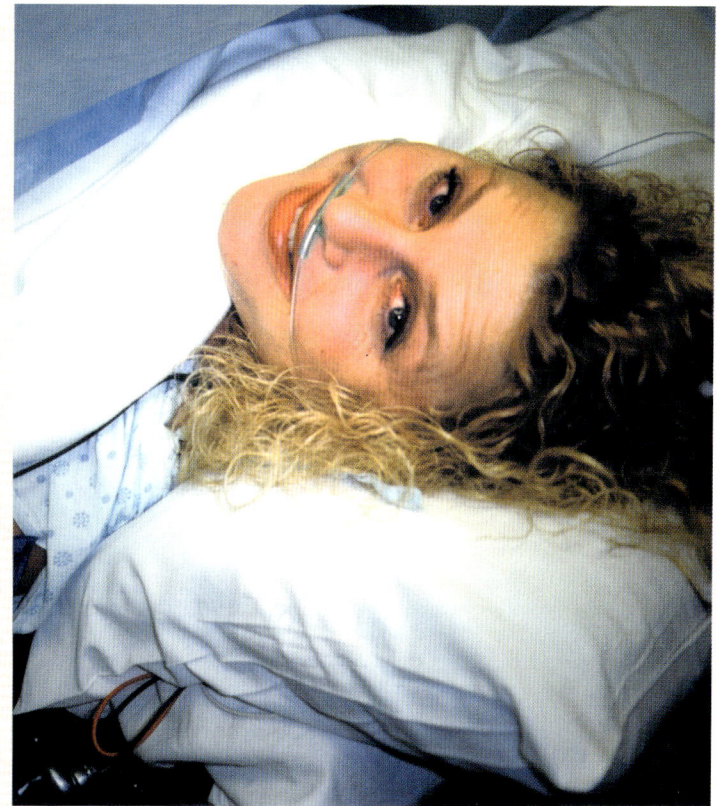

Hands Of Love

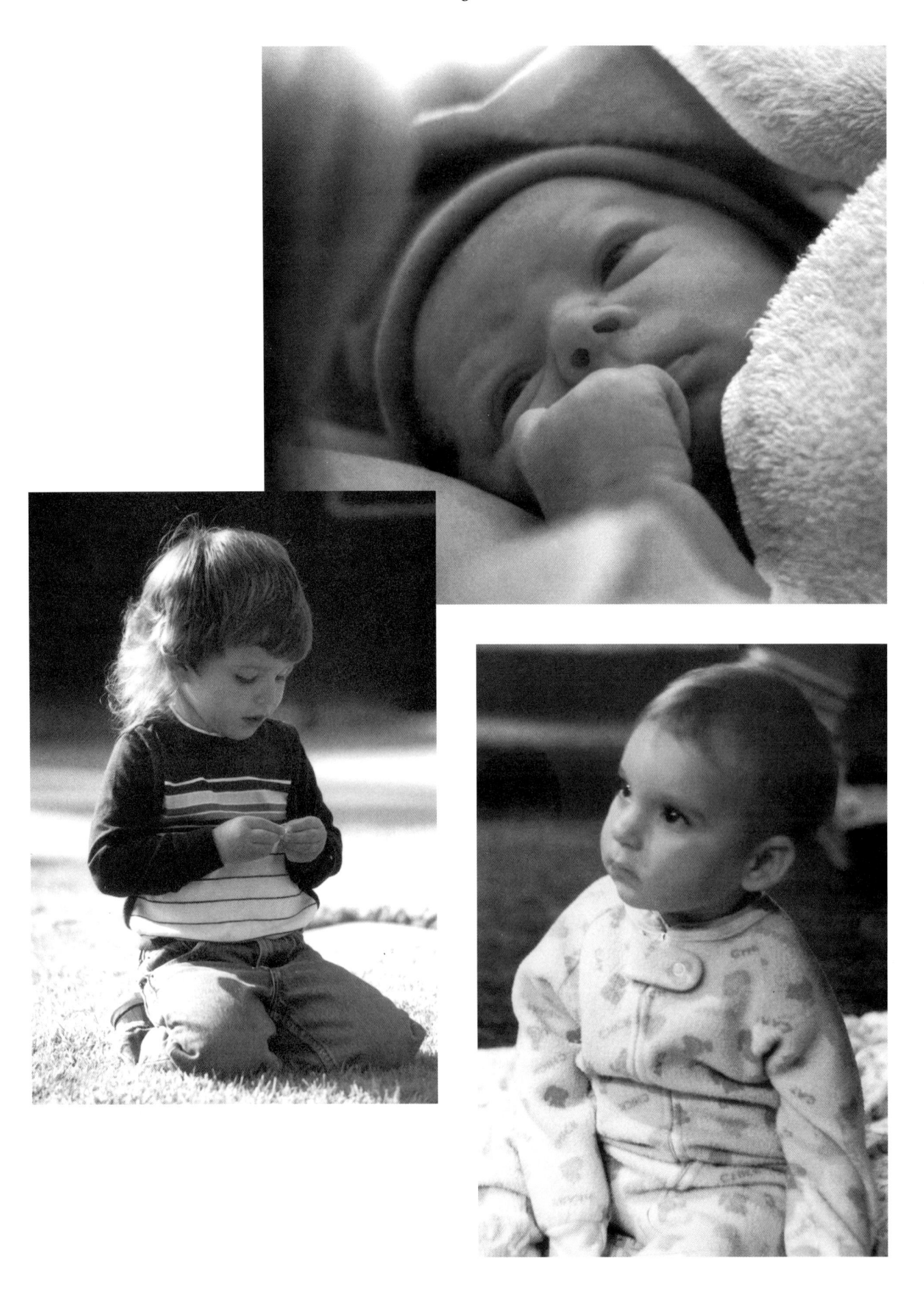

STEP 5: Be Prepared in the Event of a Cesarean Delivery

A Child of God

He is the divine child of God
With divine rights of his own
and he shall be fulfilled.

There is no factor in her life
as she moves throughout her life
that does not bring her growth.
And, with growth—changes emerge.

We accept growth.
We welcome change.
And, they therefore find fulfillment.

For within them dwells the Father
Who is always in control of their lives.

Thank you, Father, that this is so.
(Author Unknown)

Whenever I work with a child who has been challenged to endure injuries, severe illness, or a physical disability, I silently recite this affirmation (using their name and the appropriate pronoun). I also find this affirmation helpful for myself whenever I feel overwhelmed and challenged by difficult circumstances in my life; it helps to remind me that most things happen for a reason and we can always look within for the answer to our problems.

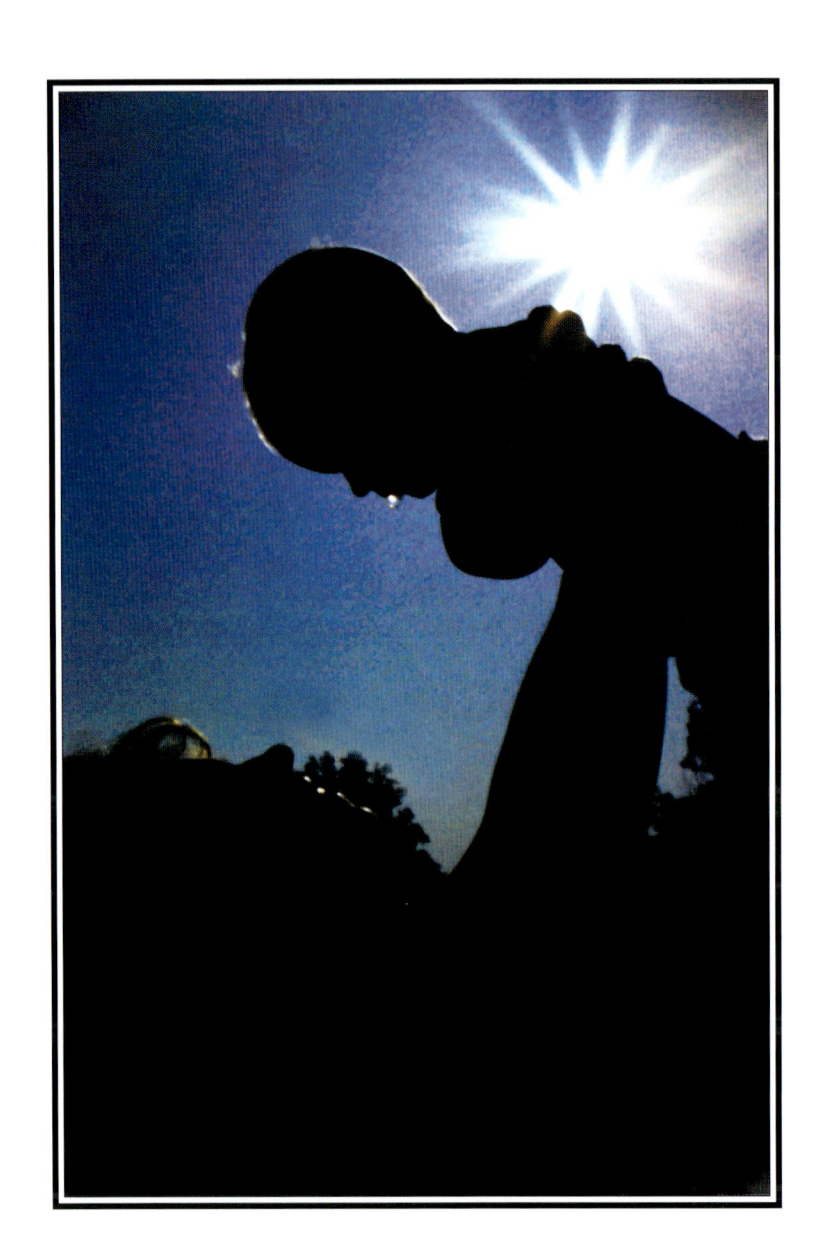

Part Three

Demonstrate Reverence for the Spirit

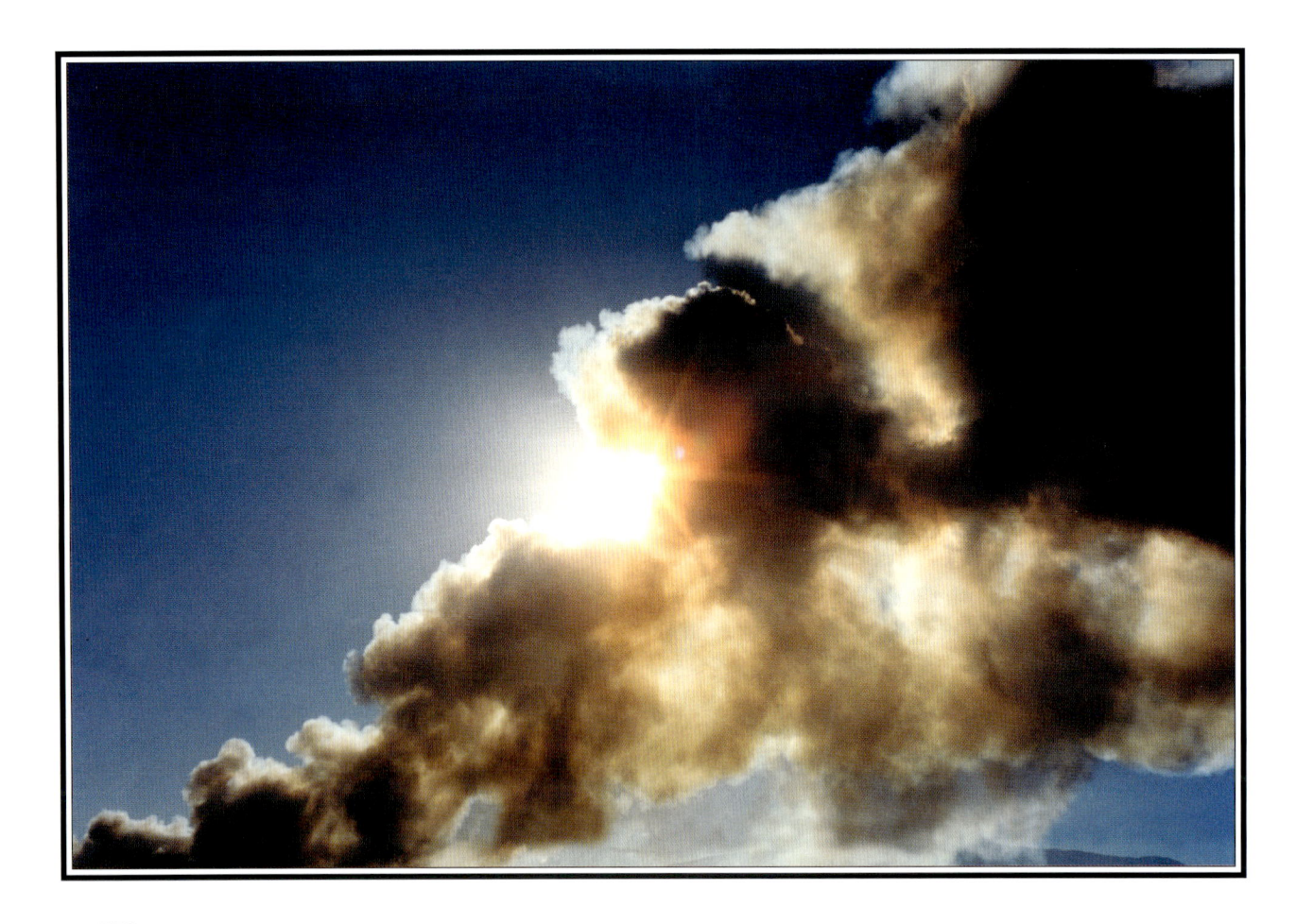

Childbirth is a spiritual experience, a mental challenge, and a test of physical endurance. If your child's birth also involves the emotional grief associated with death occurring before birth, you can spare yourself a lifetime of sorrow if you honor the physical body that remains and invoke reverence for the spirit of your heavenly child.

STEP 6
Accept the Dual Reality of Human Existence

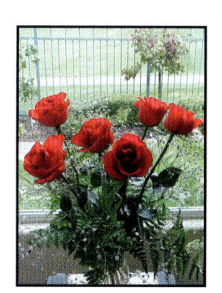

Our life began when the essence of our spirit entered the human body. Our spirit will leave the body when it no longer serves our purpose. The dual reality of the human existence dictates that we will be born and we will die. Only God knows how long the interval will be between these two points on the continuum of life. Only He knows which one will occur first.

During pregnancy, your greatest fear may be that your child will die before it has a chance to live. It is human nature to deal with that fear by pretending that it doesn't exist; what doesn't exist can't possibly happen. Or, can it? As a pregnant parent, you may not openly discuss the reality of death occurring before birth, but you acknowledge that fear with every test you agree to, and with every concerned call you make to your birth attendant. If you let that unthinkable thought drift from the dark recesses of your mind into the light of consciousness, friends, relatives, and birth attendants often discount your fears by assuring you that everything is fine. That may be kind, but not necessarily wise.

Death of a child is so uncommon that parents rarely plan for that possibility. They discuss other aspects of parenting… "Should we begin with breast feeding, or go straight to bottle feeding? Should we make her sleep in the crib, or will we have her sleep with us? If it's a boy, should we circumcise? What should we do about vaccination?"

How many parents sit down and discuss what decisions they would make if they were suddenly faced with the death of their child… "Should we insist on an immediate induction? Should I take drugs during the delivery so I won't have to feel anything? Should we insist on a cesarean and get it over with? Will they even do that? Should we have a memorial service? Where will we bury her?"

As you continue working through this pregnancy plan, be kind to yourself—and to your unborn baby. Acknowledge the fragility of the human body, plan for all possibilities, and rejoice in the endurance of the human spirit. You, and your baby, deserve to have a loving and compassionate delivery, no matter what the circumstance.

What is Spirit?

What is this entity we call the human spirit? Is it responsible for the incredible force that connects us emotionally to a child—even before he is born?

Are you looking at the spirit when you stare into the eyes of a newborn? Do we hear spirit when babies speak to us without words?

Does spirit give a child the ability to dance like a leaf floating from a tree, to run like a breeze on a warm summer day, or despite severe physical challenges create a masterpiece of art with the paintbrush he must hold with his teeth? Does a child's spirit hear us even when their body fails to respond to our caress? Does the spirit of a child remain with us until we deal with the death of a body?

For me, the answer is **yes** to all of the above. As a doula, and a parent, I believe that a child's spirit must be honored, even if it decides to leave the body that a parent and God have co-created. Sometimes, the body a child has been given is altered in some way and can no longer help him achieve his purpose in life. Sometimes, his mission is complete—before he leaves the womb. Sometimes, it's just an unfortunate accident, like the cord getting twisted up in knots. More often than not, a parent will have no way of ever truly knowing why their baby's spirit chose to leave before they had a chance to meet face to face.

During times of grief, parents can avoid a lifetime of regret, blame, and sorrow if they demonstrate reverence for the baby's spirit and honor for the only tangible object left to them—the physical body.

Hands Of Love

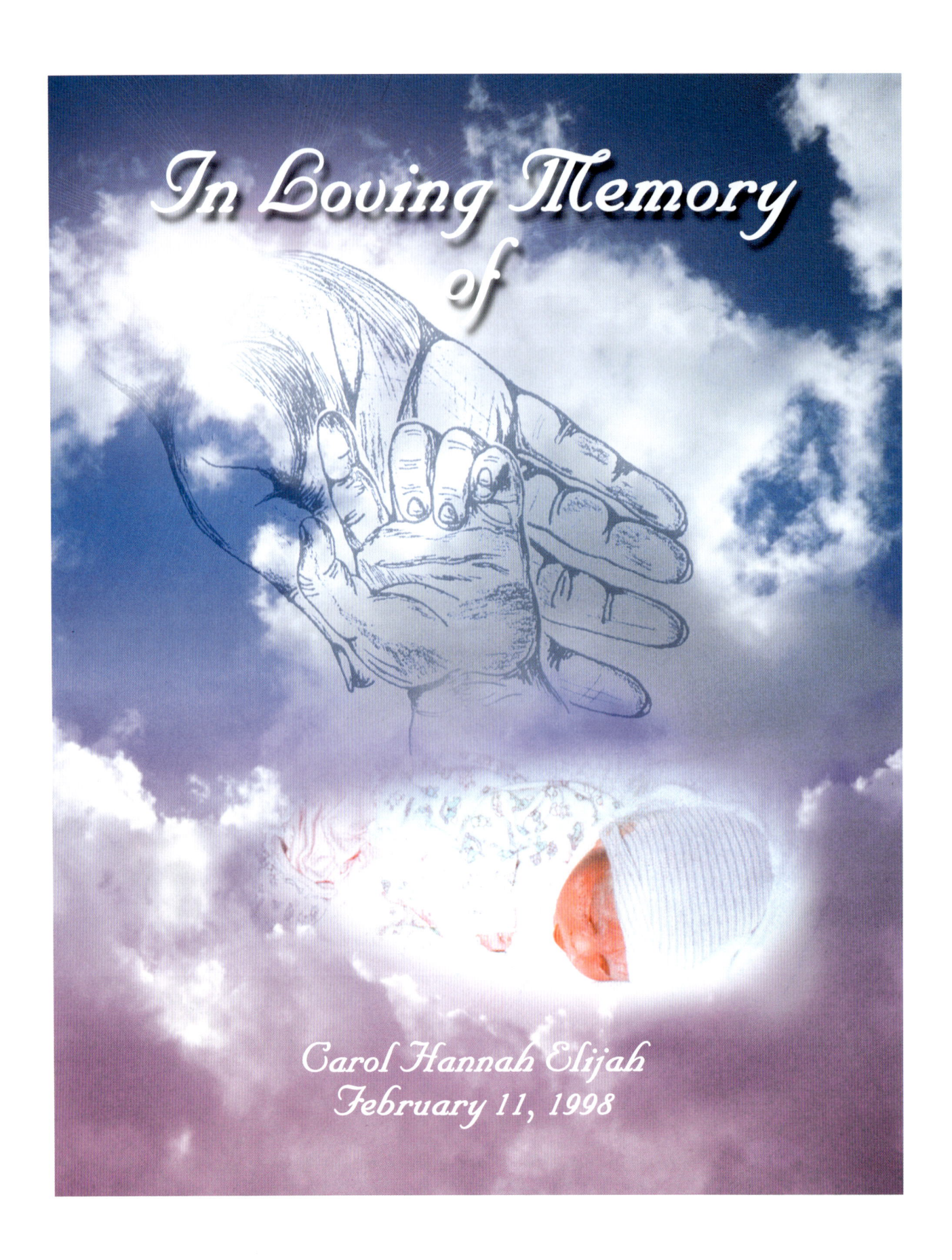

In Loving Memory of

Carol Hannah Elijah
February 11, 1998

STEP 6: Accept the Dual Reality of Human Existence

A Spirit Returns

CHERYL: Two weeks and two days. That's what I'd been saying at work in response to people who would ask when my baby was due (even though I'd started having contractions the evening before). The contractions were pretty close together, but not terribly uncomfortable. I wasn't concerned. I hadn't really felt the baby move, but I thought it was because of the contractions. After work, I stopped by a friend's house. She is a midwife so I asked her to listen for the heartbeat. She couldn't find it and was having a hard time determining the baby's position. I still wasn't worried as I assumed the baby was just not head-down anymore. I had an appointment with Carol that evening and knew she would be able to tell me more about the baby's position.

After observing a few contractions and checking me, Carol told me to take a hot bath. If I was experiencing active labor, the contractions would continue. If I was experiencing false labor, they would stop. When I told her I really hadn't felt the baby move, she suggested I drink a large glass of juice to help stimulate the baby. She also suggested I get an ultrasound if the baby didn't move soon. It was Wednesday and my next appointment with the midwife was on Friday.

I went home and took a hot bath. My daughter helped me pour water over my belly and the baby. The warm water felt good and the contractions stopped. The baby had always been most active around midnight. Since it was late and I was tired, I was sure the baby would start kicking soon and didn't drink the juice. I had decided to drink it the next morning. I went to bed and realized the baby felt different. More like a big rock. I still wasn't very concerned. I thought I couldn't feel movement because I was so close to my due date and had gained 40 pounds. I tried to get the baby to kick by poking at it, but I didn't get a response.

The next morning I realized the baby didn't kick all night, so I decided to go to the clinic right away. I called my boss to let him know I would be late. He was telling me about his sister losing her first child and not to take any chances. "Not to worry," I told him. I had just felt the baby move. I was sure it was fine. I drank my glass of orange juice, kissed my husband and told him I'd call him later.

BRIAN: When we awoke in the morning, Cheryl's contractions had eased, but she was not sure if she felt any movement. We called the midwives. They wanted her to come in and be checked right away. I couldn't understand what all the fuss was about. We had done everything possible to provide for this child. And, being a chiropractor, I felt confident we had done everything we could to provide the best environment for the birth.

Our first birth, which occurred while I was still in school, had left us with memories of a very long and difficult labor. We were determined not to repeat that first experience: 40 hours of labor, pain medication, and forceps. I really wanted this birth to be different. I stayed home with our 3-year-old, Lauren, while Cheryl went in to be checked. When she left, I gave her a kiss and said, "Call me."

CHERYL: At the doctor's office they put me in a chair and hooked me up to the fetal monitor to do a non-stress test. The nurse wanted to see how the baby was reacting to the contractions. At first, the nurse was having trouble locating a heartbeat, but she finally found one that would come and go. I felt relieved. She explained that sometimes the baby gets in a funny position, and it's hard to find the heartbeat. I was given a glass of apple juice to drink in hopes of waking the baby. The nurse left the room and said she would be back in a few minutes. I was to press a button when I felt the baby move. At the time, I was feeling really light kicks every now and then.

About an hour later, the midwife came in to check the strip. She looked confused and moved the monitor around trying to pick up the heartbeat in different places. She had me roll over on my side, but then the heartbeat would fade out. When the midwife starting taking my pulse while checking the strip, I stopped feeling relieved. I was starting to think something was wrong. I had not actually met this midwife before, so I wasn't asking her any questions. Before long, she left the room and came back with another midwife.

The second midwife had me roll over to my side while she checked my pulse. The first midwife said, "I was checking your pulse and it almost matched the strip, but not exactly." "Oh good," I told her. "For a moment I thought you were going to tell me it was my own heartbeat that the machine was tracking." The second midwife looked worried and said she wanted to do a sonogram ultrasound so they could actually look at the baby. Up until this point, we had not had any ultrasounds. We were not even allowing the use of the Doppler, but this time I agreed to the sonogram and tried not to panic as I waited for the midwife to go and get it.

I had never had a sonogram—not even with the first baby. As I watched the screen, I had no idea what it was supposed to look like. Everything just looked very still. I could see the baby's ribs, but not much else. After a few minutes, the midwife stopped, turned the machine off, took my hand and, with tears in her eyes, she said she was worried. She didn't see a heartbeat.

I asked the midwife if it was supposed to show up and she said, "Yes." However, I still wasn't worried. I figured she just didn't know what she was doing since the midwives didn't do them very often. She said she wanted me to go to the hospital to have another ultrasound performed by a specialist. Then, she asked me to call my husband. I went to her office and tried to call home, but we have caller ID and blocked certain numbers. The call wouldn't go through, so I called a neighbor and told him to please go over and get Brian and have him come to the hospital.

BRIAN: *As I drove to the hospital, I began to get an uncomfortable feeling. I noticed I was driving at excessive speeds. I parked in the parking garage as it seemed I might not be coming out anytime soon. I went to the lobby elevators and pushed the up button. I remember not having the patience to wait but I couldn't use the stairs because hospital security didn't allow it.*

As the elevator doors opened, I pushed the fourth floor button. I got off and went to the main desk at the Birth Place. The secretary knew exactly who I was, when I gave her my name. She said, "Go to the end of the hall and through the double doors. I will buzz you through. Then, go to the end of that hall and turn right. Someone will meet you."

I began to feel uneasy. How did this secretary know who I was and why did I need to be buzzed into a portion of the hospital? I went through the double doors, followed the hallway to the end, and made a right turn. My body was on pins and needles. I wanted to run. I wanted to stop. And, I felt like I was walking forever; like a convict on his last walk before the gas chamber.

I turned right. Before I could get to the end of the hall, a nurse came quickly out from behind the desk and met me half way. She directed me to the room Cheryl was in. I looked at the sign outside the door. It read, **Private Consultation Room.** *It hit me. I knew—not how or why—I just knew. I turned the knob. The door was locked. I felt relief. This was a dream. They made a mistake. This was the wrong room. I was to go somewhere else. But, then, the door opened and I saw Cheryl.*

CHERYL: *As my midwife, Janice, and I walked to the hospital, I had a million thoughts going through my mind. This was the nineties and babies don't die before they're born. During birth maybe, but certainly not before you go into labor—and, not my child. There must be some mistake. As we walked, Janice*

STEP 6: Accept the Dual Reality of Human Existence

explained we would be going to the perinatal center because the regular ultrasound place couldn't get me in for another 3 hours. That was too long to wait.

Janice held my hand while a doctor did the sonogram ultrasound. This machine was much clearer. You could see the whole baby, perfectly formed. The doctor watched the sonogram for a couple of minutes and then said, "Here's the head, here's the chest, and there is no heartbeat. I'm sorry." Janice and I were both crying as she hugged me. We went into a consultation room to wait for Brian.

While we waited, Janice asked if I had any questions. I was still too stunned to ask much. My only question was, "What happened?" My pregnancy had been very uneventful. How could the baby be dead? Janice said we might have an indication of what happened after delivery. Possibly, the cord was wrapped around her neck, or the placenta had come away from the uterine wall. Janice said the majority of time there is no indication, but we could have an autopsy done to determine the cause of death. She said, however, there could be a chance that we would never know.

I had a miscarriage the previous March, so to lose this baby was especially devastating. Brian arrived and tried to open the door; it was locked. I unlocked the door and started crying when I saw him walk in. He knew by the look on my face that something was wrong. I just blurted it out, "The baby has no heartbeat."

Cheryl's immediate reaction that day was to ask for an induction. Fortunately, the doctor denied that request because the nursing staff wasn't large enough to give them the undivided attention they deserved. Consequently, induction was scheduled for the next day. Brian was totally against an induction and did his best to try and locate me. He needed emotional support to help him discourage Cheryl from going through with an induced labor.

Brian explained to me later that he was deathly afraid of medical intervention. He remembered all too well the nightmare of watching Cheryl suffer through the first birth. Since this baby was already dead, he was afraid the medical staff would be insensitive to his desire to protect Cheryl from further emotional distress. His biggest fear was that Cheryl would die during delivery. He was also afraid she'd end up in surgery and he'd have to go through the funeral without her and doubted his ability to do that.

I was the only person Cheryl and Brian allowed in their home that day. We spent several hours together talking about the need to honor the baby's spirit. I explained that both Cheryl and the baby deserved a good birth experience. Cheryl's immediate reaction to the shock of losing her baby was tempered and she agreed to delay induction until Monday.

In the meantime, I suggested Brian put a message on their answering machine to spare Cheryl the pain of telling everyone that called about their loss.

Forcing Cheryl's body to deliver a baby that couldn't help with the delivery would increase her risk of complications, so I suggested Cheryl start taking large doses of GLA (Evening Primrose Oil). (GLA is the precursor for the hormones that soften the cervix.) Our intent was to prepare her body for labor and possibly avoid the use of pitocin.

On Monday, (due to staffing problems) the hospital delayed the induction until Tuesday. Poor Cheryl. In her mind, no one seemed to understand that she was carrying a dead baby inside of her. She just wanted the delivery over with and couldn't think about the pain or complications that induction would bring. Her emotional pain was already unbearable.

Fortunately, the time between Friday and Tuesday was spent preparing both mentally and physically for the funeral. Cheryl and Brian had time to create a birth and memorial announcement. They bought a special blanket which had a message embroidered on it that read, **Wrapped in Jesus' Love**. They bought two outfits for the baby to be buried in (they did not know the sex of the baby). They took this time to explain to Lauren that the baby was going to go back to heaven. Due to the delay, Cheryl had time to do these things and adjust to the idea that she would be delivering a baby that she couldn't bring home with her.

Prostaglandin gel was applied to Cheryl's cervix on Tuesday. She was told it would be applied several times over the next few days until her cervix was fully effaced. A few days?! Cheryl couldn't believe she would be forced to wait a few more days. Fortunately, the combination of GLA and gel helped her move quickly into active labor. By Wednesday morning, the contractions were strong and painful. Cheryl and Brian called me and asked me to meet them at the hospital. Cheryl wanted drugs and she wanted them, "Now!"

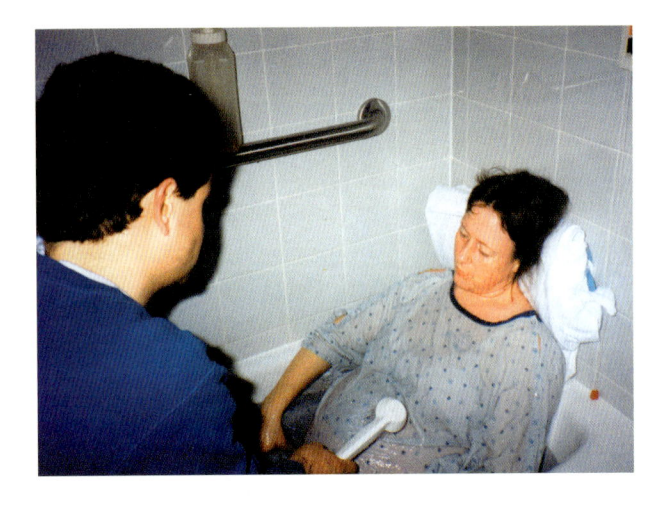

CHERYL: *When Carol arrived I was trying to dull the pain by taking a hot bath. I wanted drugs, but I was already 7-8 cm. Janice had suggested I hold off on the drugs because they could slow my labor. Carol immediately turned the lights off in the bathroom and put ice in a bucket for cold cloths. She started placing the cold cloths on my forehead and neck, while Brian continuing spraying my belly with hot water. They both continued O-O-O-ing with me and the pain was finally manageable.*

Cheryl, Brian and I worked together for some time in the tub before Janice asked her to get out and be checked; dilation was progressing normally. Cheryl moved to the rocking chair and Brian tried to keep her spirits up in spite of the circumstances.

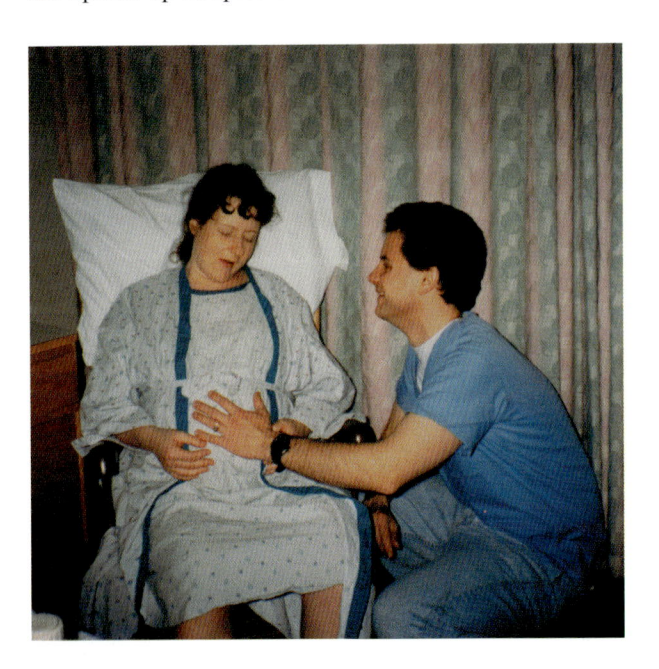

Labor had been progressing normally when the contractions suddenly stopped. I performed craniosacral therapy in an attempt to regulate the hormonal output from the pituitary gland. Cheryl suddenly had a somatoemotional release. This is a phenomenon where the body releases emotions that are locked in tissue memory. This can also occur during labor if a mother patterns her body after the baby's position. (Sounds strange, I know.)

Cheryl suddenly went into a hyperextended position with her head tipped way back. Once her tissue relaxed, she moved into a flexed position, dilated to 10 centimeters, and felt the urge to push.

I took a minute to tell Janice of the release that had just occurred and she surprised me by saying that the sonogram demonstrated that the baby was in the "*military position*"—hands and head extended up and back. Cheryl had mirrored her baby's position in-utero and then corrected it so the baby could move on down the canal.

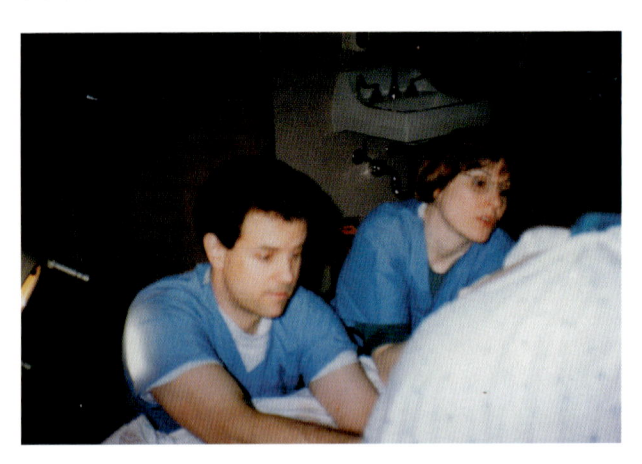

BRIAN: *Cheryl was on her hands and knees pushing. Janice knelt beside me, and we watched as the head started coming out further and further. Secretly, I had hoped that somehow, with all the miracles that were happening, somehow, some way... they were all wrong, and she was alive. As I cradled her head in my hands, I knew... I could see the deformed cranial bones; I knew she was dead. I was shocked and motionless. I wanted to cry; I wanted to scream, "Why?" I could not move. I was frozen. I was watching a miracle from God being born right in front of my own eyes. I was not wondering if it was a boy or a girl. My only thought was that I was not going to see this child grow up.*

STEP 6: Accept the Dual Reality of Human Existence

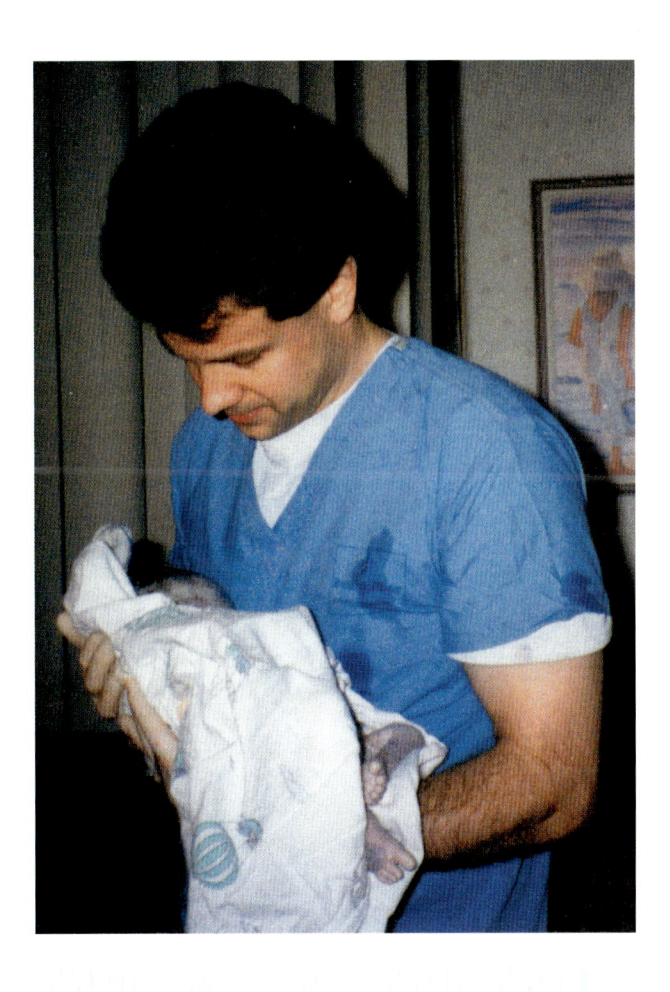

As I held my baby in my hands, I heard Janice speak from a distance. She told Cheryl we had a girl. I barely heard her. Janice wrapped a blanket around the baby, and as I held my daughter, all I could see was a beautiful child. She looked a lot like our first daughter, but I saw no life. Her spirit had left her body, but I knew she was helping us all go through this.

I placed the baby in Cheryl's arms. She and I cried as we looked at each other and then at our baby. I was at a loss for words. The baby's skin was darker than Lauren's and it was peeling off, but all I saw was a beautiful child with perfect little toes and fingers. I just kept wondering how could a child who is so beautiful, and who looks so healthy, be taken from us?

CHERYL: *As I held my little girl, I was unable to speak. It was as if the room suddenly filled with an enormous amount of love for the child I held in my arms.*

We were a tight group for several hours after the deliver. Janice, the nurse, Carole, and I helped Brian and Cheryl go through the rituals that help parents bond with their newborn. We held her, admired her little hands and feet, weighed her, had prints of her hands and feet made, and finally, dressed her. The five of us had spent several hours together without interruption. On the door, outside the room, someone had placed a beautiful picture of a leaf with a single dew drop in the center. It was a symbol to all that a child had died that night. No one entered the sanctity of the birth room. Janice and Carole bent over backwards to give this family all of the privacy and time they needed. Whatever they asked for—they received. Nurse Carole ended her time with us by taking a picture for Carol Hannah's baby book.

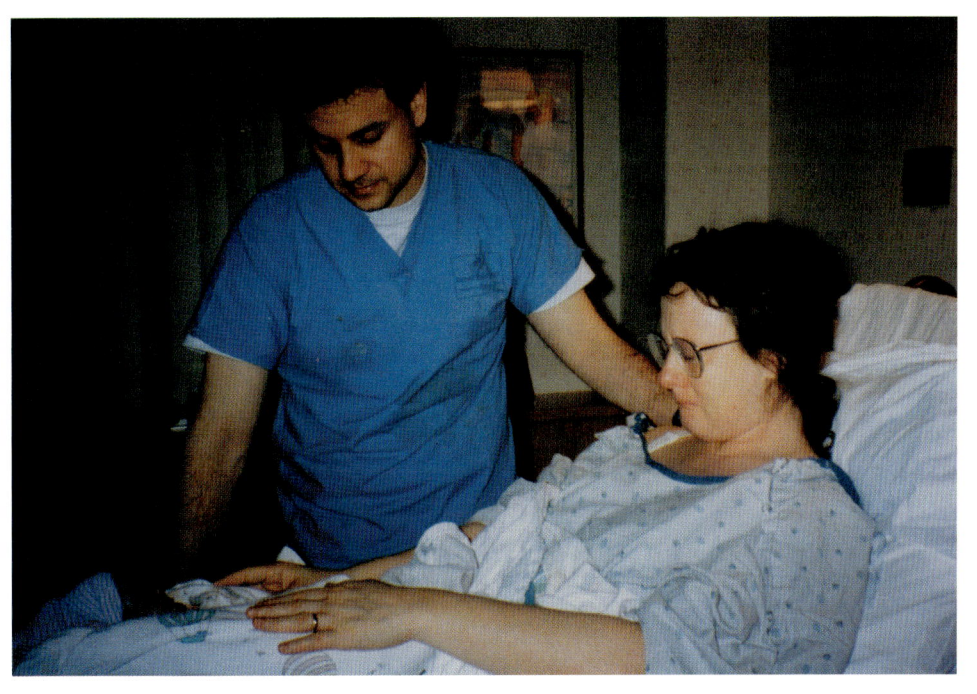

165

Hands Of Love

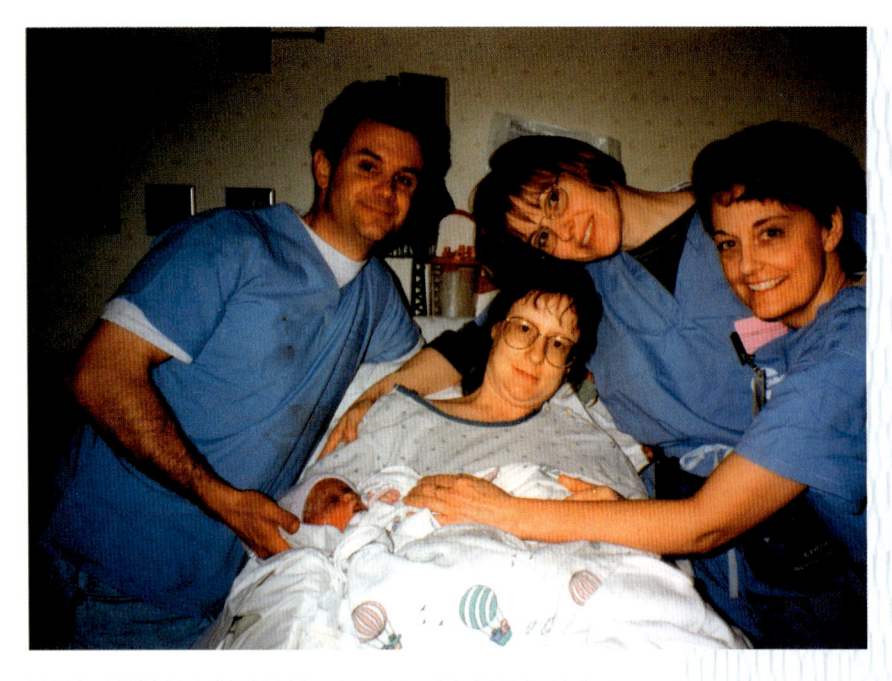

BRIAN: *It was almost midnight when the hospital priest arrived. Our priest had refused to perform the baptismal ceremony because the baby died before birth, but we still wanted it done. There was silence from everyone when the priest entered the room. He didn't know what we wanted him to do; we were afraid to ask and be turned down. Finally, Carol spoke up and asked Father if he needed a name to do a baptismal ceremony. We were so relieved when he said, "Yes, you do."*

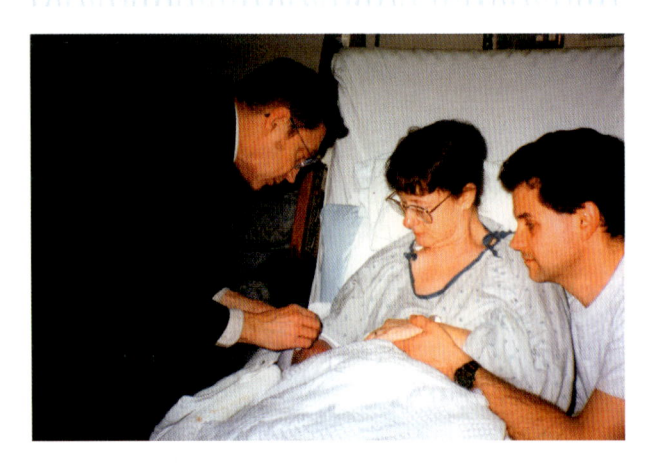

Cheryl and I had agreed on a boy's name—but no girl's name. Everyone stepped out of the room so we could discuss it. I asked Cheryl if we could name the baby after Carol. She said yes, so we named her Carol Hannah. Everyone returned and the priest gave us the baptism we felt was so necessary before we said our final good-byes.

After the baptism, the hospital staff moved Cheryl and I to a double bed so we could spend the night together.

Early the next morning, I dropped off film (taken during the birth) at the one-hour developer. I wanted to be sure the pictures turned out. If they didn't come out, that day was the last day we had to spend with our daughter—to create memories to last a lifetime.

When I went back to get the pictures, there was a proud grandfather at the counter showing off pictures of his two new grandsons. I was standing there as he and the developing staff admired his photographs.

Suddenly, a clerk handed me my package and told everyone at the counter that I had pictures of a newborn, too. The older man asked me when my child was born, which hospital, and weren't we lucky! I can't even remember paying for the pictures. I was shocked, angry, devastated and speechless. I didn't know how to handle this. Here was someone that didn't know what I had been through. How could he be so heartless? Didn't he know? Couldn't he see it on my face?

I rushed out of the store as fast as I could—I was crying before I got to the car. I broke down in the car. I couldn't stop crying. I hurt so badly. Life was not fair. I thought I did everything I could to provide for this unborn child and nothing mattered; she never had a chance.

When I arrived at the funeral, the first person I saw was Cheryl. Wearing a beautiful, long, green velvet dress, she was greeting everyone as they entered the room. I walked up and hugged her. She tried to look happy to see me, but she was unable to contain her sorrow. As we hugged, Cheryl wept against my shoulder as she told me that Brian had closed the casket before she arrived. She thought she was going to

STEP 6: Accept the Dual Reality of Human Existence

have a chance to dress Carol and say good-bye one more time. She was devastated. After hearing Cheryl's story, I told her I would go talk to Brian. I looked over to where he stood. My heart went out to him. Greeting each and every person, the tears flowed freely down his face.

I went up and hugged Brian and then told him how upset Cheryl was. He cried as he told me about the early morning events.

Brian had gone in early to make the final arrangements for the funeral. When he saw Carol lying in her little coffin she looked nothing like the baby he had held at the hospital. She looked awful to him because her face had been painted on after the autopsy. He saw no life in her body—no spirit—and decided he just couldn't let this be Cheryl's last memory of their daughter. He wrapped her in her blanket, laid her back down in the bed of satin, and placed a small teddy bear beside her, (it was the first gift he had ever given Cheryl) then sealed the casket.

I explained to Brian that Cheryl would never have closure if she did not fulfill her wish of touching Carol one last time. It was important to her. Once I said that, Brian decided he would do whatever it took to get the casket open for Cheryl. He spoke with the funeral director and the priest. After the ceremony, the Father asked everyone to wait outside while the family remained with the baby for a few minutes.

I stood with Cheryl and watched as Brian used determination and strength to open the sealed white casket. I stepped away as the two of them stood together over their baby. Cheryl gingerly fingered the blanket, the bear, and her baby's face. Tears rolled down her cheeks as she spoke silently to the little girl she would never hold again. Cheryl bent down and gave Carol Hannah a kiss before stepping back and allowing Brian to reseal the casket.

CHERYL: *The only regret I have is not taking a few pictures of Carol Hannah wrapped up in the special blanket we buried her in. I was saving it for the funeral and never had any pictures taken with her in it.*

It has been three months since her birth. I think about her all the time. What would she look like? What would Lauren think of her? What does she look like in heaven? The autopsy didn't determine the cause of death, but my blood work revealed a few health areas that I needed to work on before thinking of having another child. I'm not sure I can go through pregnancy again. I look at pregnant women and remember the innocence before I found out that babies die before birth. I'd like to have that innocence back.

My mother passed away last week. Before she died, she asked me if I was going to have another child. I told her I just didn't know. She hadn't been well enough to go to the hospital and see the baby or go to the funeral. The night before she died, I showed her Carol Hannah's photo album. I hope she's with her in heaven.

If you ever have a child that dies, no matter what the age, make sure you do the things your heart tells you that you need to do. Hold them, take photographs, and if at all possible, videotape them as well.

I have comfort in knowing that I collected as many memories of our child as I could; we brought Lauren to the hospital and let her hold her baby sister; we have videotape and pictures to show to our children when they get older.

Carol Hannah had a beautiful birth and a great send off to heaven. We received many beautiful cards and letters from our family and friends after her death. This verse was on several of the special cards we received, so we had it engraved on her gravestone.

A life so young released to heaven...

Left on earth, we wonder "Why?"

But some are sent among us briefly...

Some have spirits meant to fly.

Little Angels

When God calls little children to dwell with Him above,
We mortals sometimes question the wisdom of His love.
For no heartache compares with the death of one small child,
Who does so much to make our world seem wonderful and mild.

Perhaps God tires of calling the aged to his fold,
So He picks a tiny rosebud before it can grow old.
He knows how much we need them and so He takes but few
to make the land of Heaven more beautiful to view.

Believing this is difficult, still somehow we must try.
The saddest word mankind knows, will always be "Good bye."
So when a little child departs we who are left behind
must realize God loves children—
Little angel's are hard to find.

Author Unknown

This poem has helped many families deal with the loss of their child. It is often passed from parent to parent when they hear that a child has died. I hope the author realizes how much comfort their words have been to grieving parents.
If you would like to join other families who celebrate the life of a child who has become an angel, you may contact a family who has erected angel statutes at various sites around the country. They can be reached on their web site at www.thechristmasbox.com/statue.html

STEP 6: Accept the Dual Reality of Human Existence

One Year Later

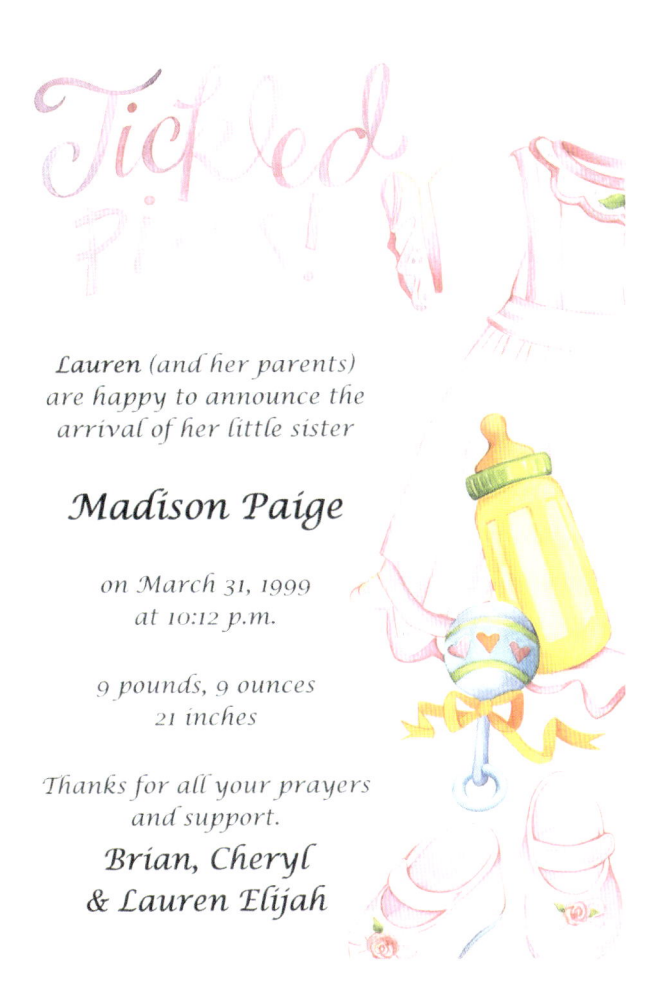

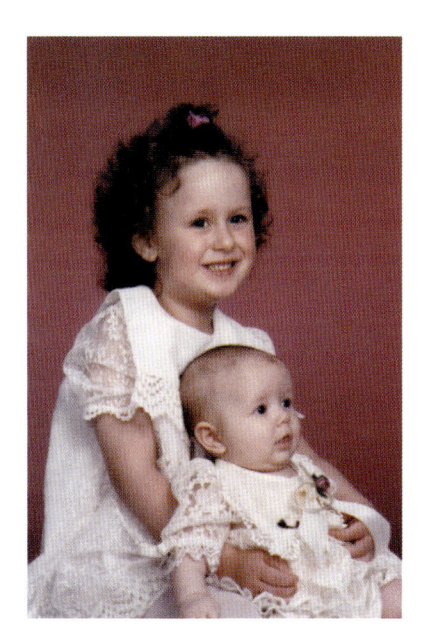

Lauren (and her parents) are happy to announce the arrival of her little sister

Madison Paige

*on March 31, 1999
at 10:12 p.m.*

*9 pounds, 9 ounces
21 inches*

Thanks for all your prayers and support.

*Brian, Cheryl
& Lauren Elijah*

CHERYL: *Tomorrow Madison will be nine months old. We named her Madison because it means: A gift from God.*

My pregnancy with Madison was very frightening. We had not planned to get pregnant so soon after Carol Hannah's death—I wasn't mentally or emotionally ready to deal with the possibility of losing another child. I felt so cheated for never having looked into Carol Hannah's eyes—for never hearing her breathe. I wanted to be sure I would eventually hold a live baby, so when I found out I was pregnant, I immediately embraced every medical precaution that could be used to assure she'd be born alive. I put my faith in medical science, but tried to maintain my faith in God as well. I found I was unable to ask Him to **spare** *this child because, by making that request, I felt I would be saying that He had caused Carol Hannah's death and I was trying hard not to believe that.*

I became more and more anxious as the due date approached. I had a non-stress ultrasound anytime the baby stopped moving. I carried a lot more fluid with this pregnancy, so it was harder to feel her kicking and playing inside of me. Therefore, I panicked and gave in to more monitoring than I would have ever considered had we not lost Carol Hannah. During my 39th week appointment, the doctor said, "Let's induce you and have a live baby." That sounded excellent to me. My husband didn't agree. He was afraid that if we induced labor the baby would die. I was afraid if we didn't—the baby would die.

We scheduled the induction three times, and all three times, the hospital had to cancel for one reason or another. We switched hospitals and scheduled another date. At this point, I was now four days past my due date and extremely anxious to see my baby. My husband's a chiropractor, so he started doing acupuncture and homeopathy to induce labor naturally. I saw Dr. Carol almost daily so she could monitor the heart rate and keep me as comfortable as possible. I was also taking large doses of GLA to help soften my cervix. Nothing seemed to be working.

Hands Of Love

Finally, the day before the scheduled induction, I had what I thought might be the early warning signs of impending labor. The next day, Brian and I rented several movies, kissed our daughter good-bye, and headed to the hospital for the induction. Suddenly, I decided I had to make one last stop at Dr. Carol's home to make sure the baby was in a good position for the birth. Both Brian and Carol believed active labor was kicking in on its own, so we ended up staying there—for two days.

Carol adjusted me. Brian did acupuncture. The contractions were mild and irregular. We walked around the block. We went out to eat. We walked some more. We talked way into the night that first day, and finally, Carol graciously suggested we sleep at her house, since our Nanny was at home in our bed.

In the morning, I awoke knowing I was truly in labor. Carol cooked us a delicious breakfast and prepared a warm relaxing bath. She filled the room with beautifully scented candles. Later, we went for another walk. In our attempt to avoid induction, we never called the hospital (or the doctor) to say we weren't coming in. When we talked to our nanny later that day, we learned the doctor was desperately trying to locate us. We called her office and assured her that we would call on our way to the hospital, but for now, we were going to eat and watch movies. I don't think she was very happy with us.

As we watched those movies, I became increasingly uncomfortable, but we kept watching because it kept me from getting worried. All of a sudden, we were putting the machine on pause every two minutes, so we could O-O-O through the contractions; it was time to go!

Brian called the doctor and asked her to meet us at the hospital. When we arrived, Brian parked in the parking garage and I walked all the way to the labor floor—even though the contractions were one right on top of another. The nurse saw me and started shouting for me to put on this tube top looking thing so they could check me. They had to let the doctor know how far along I was before she would leave for the hospital. (I couldn't help thinking how stupid it was that she wasn't there at the hospital.) It was 8:00 P.M. and I was eight centimeters dilated. They sent for the doctor.

When she arrived, the doctor checked me and said she couldn't break the water because the baby's head was off centered and stuck in my pelvis; she was afraid the cord would come through first. Everything was happening so fast that I started shaking uncontrollably. After the doctor left the room, Carol worked on relaxing the muscles surrounding the uterus. Then she had me kneel on the side of the bed and lean over to rest my arms on the seat of a chair that was facing the bed. She raised the bed up until I was in an inverted position. The nurse came in while we were doing this. She supported the chair so it wouldn't slide and watched with bewilderment. After about two minutes, Carol put the bed down and the nurse checked me. It worked. The baby had moved back up in the pelvis and was no longer stuck on my pelvic bones.

The doctor decided to do a quick ultrasound scan to make sure that the baby wasn't breech. As she scanned over the lower part of my belly, we saw Madison shaking her head back and forth as if she was saying, "No, No, No."

I was in excruciating pain. My body was shaking and I began to throw up. I'd had enough and wanted to see my child. When the doctor said the baby had moved up and out of the pelvis, I asked her to do a C-section. The doctor and nurse left the room to talk.

Carol convinced me to stand up and allow the baby to drop back down into the pelvis. As soon as my feet touched the floor, my water broke. Brian ran for the doctor, but in his panic he kept pushing on a door that needed to be pulled—he was going nowhere. Brian made enough racket they heard him at the nurses station and came running. When the doctor saw meconium in the water she screamed, "Get back in bed!"

The doctor pulled on her gloves, while the nurses put my legs in stirrups, and then, everything stopped. No contractions. No anything. I said to the doctor, "Should I push?" She said, "You're in control." Now

STEP 6: Accept the Dual Reality of Human Existence

that was an odd statement for someone who sounded like they were panicking only moments earlier.

Carol explained that the baby needed to come out ASAP because of the meconium that was in the water, so with the next contraction, I pushed as hard as I could; Madison was born about seven minutes later.

As soon as her head and shoulders came out, the doctor squeezed Madison's chest to keep her from sucking more fluid into her lungs as they rushed her to a warmer. A specialist came in and started working on her.

I listened and waited for her to cry. I wasn't convinced she was okay. I had thought once she was born I would feel this huge sense of relief. Instead, I felt sort of numb. Carol's hand was on Madison's chest; she kept talking to her while the staff sucked fluid from her lungs and stomach. Brian wouldn't leave me, so I was glad Carol stayed with the baby. At one point, the doctor looked at Carol and said, "Grandma, you're going to have to step away and let us do our job." She said, "I'm not the grandma," then kept right on telling Madison that Brian and I were right beside her and that she would be with me in just a few minutes. Carol kept assuring Madison that she was fine and would never have to do this again in this lifetime. It seemed forever, but a few minutes later, Madison was placed in my arms. We kept her in the room with us the entire time we were in the hospital. I wanted her near me so I could hear her breathe.

I still think about Carol Hannah daily. I wonder if she would have looked more like her older sister or her younger sister. What would her personality be like? I wonder if she's in Heaven with my mom. When the girls are a little older, we'll explain more about their other sister. For now, we're blessed with two healthy girls here on earth and one beautiful angel resting with God in heaven.

~≈~

171

Hands Of Love

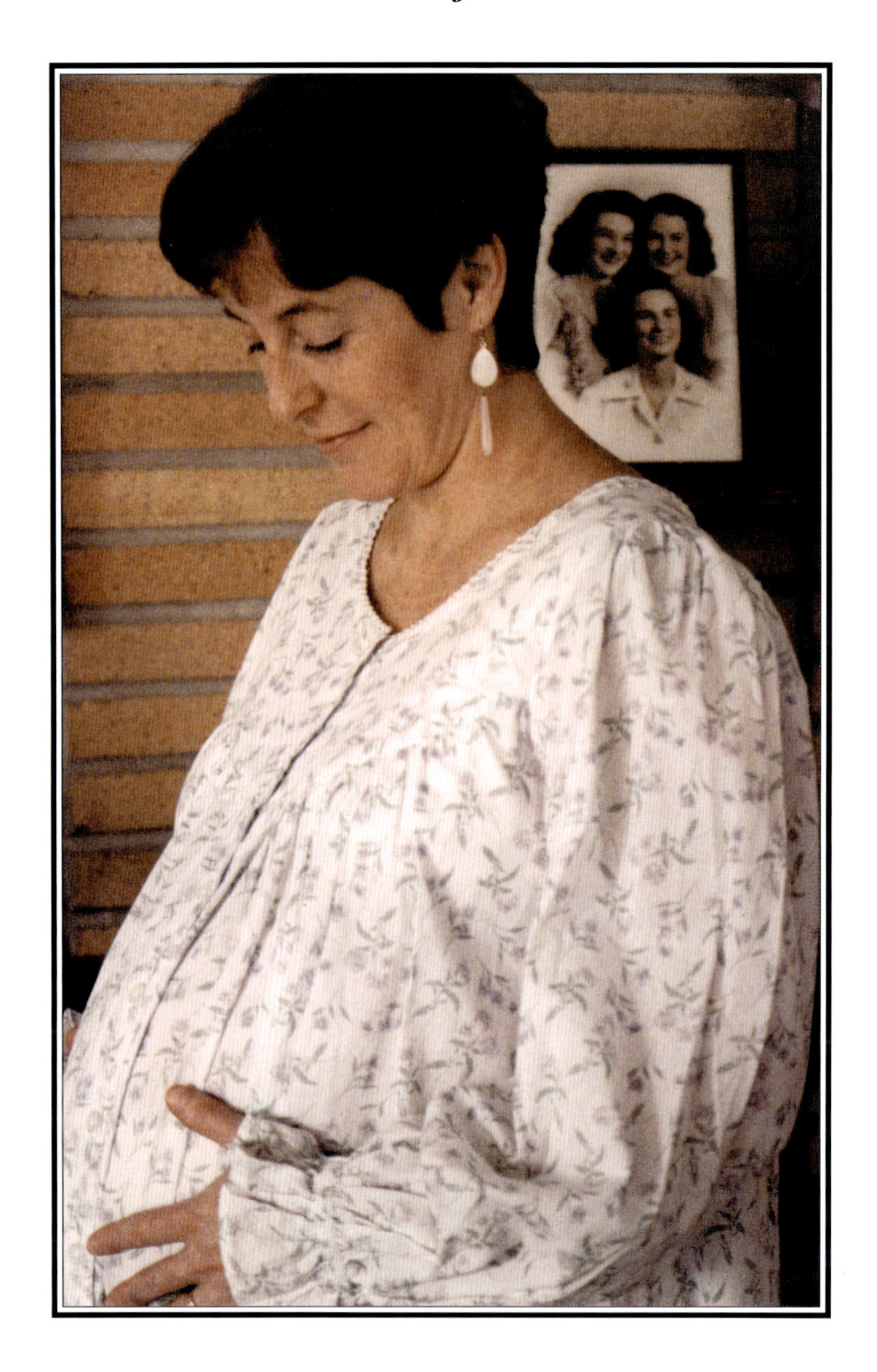

𝓜ove synchronously with your child as you begin the dance of life. Listen to her whispers, respond to her urgings and allow your body to accommodate her every need. Energetically, you are one with your child. Listen and you will know what to do.

STEP 7
Follow Your Instincts and Trust Your Inner Voice

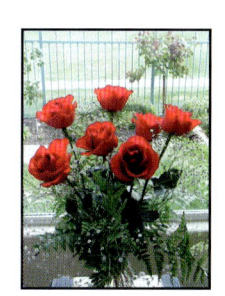

How do we prove the oneness of a mother and her unborn child? How do we know where one ends and the other begins? Are they truly a unified blend of energy and identity?

These are questions that we may never be able to answer. We may forever have to rely on clinical experience, and trust that what we feel, what we see, and what we experience must be true. In my years of work with pregnant women, I have felt and seen many things that cannot be explained scientifically, but they happened nonetheless. An example would be Jackie, a pregnant women who came into my office—two weeks overdue.

Jackie was extremely apprehensive about her impending delivery. She felt fearful and anxious. She was positive that something terrible was going to happen during childbirth. I made the mistake of discounting her feelings and said, "Don't worry, we just call that first-time jitters." "No!" she responded. "I have four other children. I know what birth is like, and I have no fear associated with it! This is different. I've had these feelings for three weeks now!"

It was embarrassing to have jumped to conclusions before getting more details. After taking a thorough history, I found no reason for her concerns. The next step was to palpate the baby's position inside the womb; that would give me a clue as to the cause of Jackie's anxiety. After getting Jackie settled, I lifted her blouse and reached forward to lay my hands over her abdomen. As soon as I touched her, my hand shot back from the intensity of emotions emanating from the baby; I, too, sensed the impending danger. I reached forward again and began to trace the outline of the baby's body—trying hard to ignore the overwhelming sense of fear that he shared with me. I found him twisted like a little pretzel with his face looking toward his back. Little arms and legs were going in all directions instead of being tucked into his chest. I had to wonder how in the world he had gotten in that position; how would he get through the birth canal?

I began my treatment by releasing the tension within Jackie's abdominal and pelvic floor muscles. The incredible tension I felt within those muscles was distorting the shape of her uterus. The baby was in a contorted position because that was the only way he could fit inside of the womb. But what caused all of this tension in the first place?

As I continued the diaphragm release, my hand was pulled down the front of one of Jackie's legs by a strong unseen energetic force. As my hand moved down to the quadricep tendon, I could feel the release of the fascia surrounding the muscles of her thigh. All of a sudden, a movie played in my mind. Jackie was running—she slipped—one leg flew out in front of her—then she landed with a thud. She looked like a cheerleader who had landed in the splits and raised her arms into a V for victory. I asked Jackie if she recalled falling in this position.

Jackie pondered over my question. Suddenly, she gasped as a spark of memory filled her mind. "Yes!" she exclaimed. "A few weeks ago, I was chasing one of my kids across wet grass when my right leg flew up in the air. The next thing I knew—I was down on the lawn with one leg stretched out in front of me and the other curled up behind me. I was immediately frightened for the baby, but as I slowly got up, I felt fine. I shook it off and took off after my child."

When Jackie left my office, the muscles attached to her pelvis were relaxed and balanced. Her pelvis aligned itself properly and the uterus moved into a vertical position. The baby changed his position and Jackie no longer felt the fear or anxiety she had come in with.

When I work with people, their bodies often relay a message to me about previous trauma. This is not as mystical as it sounds. You see, we're all electrical. When we touch, we automatically begin transferring that electrical energy. You may feel it when you walk out of an uncomicating situation and say, "There was so much tension in there, I could have cut it with a knife."

An example of energy transference is when a baby cries from hunger and her mother's milk suddenly begins to let down. Or, when a mother knows her grown child is sick and calls to check on him—even though he lives in a different country.

The electrical activity of the body works to give us sensory information and historical data. Every cell in the body has a memory receptor that records information about that cell. Trauma to a certain area is recorded and maintained until the injury has been repaired. The electrical transference of information from person to person is called *entrainment* (one nervous system drives another). In some cases, it allows the person being treated to subconsciously transfer pertinent information to the person working on them. Many skilled doctors and therapists know what to treat before they even begin working on a patient. They are not psychic, just perceptive.

I received a beautiful card from Jackie telling me that she had a perfect birth several days after the treatment. Her words of gratitude filled my heart with joy as they reminded me why I am so thankful for the career I have chosen. I could share many such birth stories with you, instead I'll tell you what I've learned from mothers in my practice.

- Trust them when they say, "Something is not right."
- Listen to them when they say they feel uncomfortable, anxious, or afraid. If they can't explain why, it is most likely a message from the baby.
- Pay attention to their dreams. The baby may be communicating with them.
- Never discount their instincts! They know things about their babies we can never know.

I learned the value of that last point through firsthand experience with one of my patients, Cindy. By listening to her instincts, I believe Cindy saved her baby's life during childbirth. Had she been in a situation with birth attendants who refused to honor her instincts, the outcome of Cindy's delivery may have been very different.

A Mother's Wisdom

Cindy called early one morning and asked me to come right over. As they squatted at the foot of their bed, she and Jeff worked through a powerful contraction (Cindy had an overwhelming compulsion to get into a tight squatting position with each contraction, so Jeff did what he could to maintain the same position). Relieved that I had finally arrived, Jeff stood up, stretched his legs, and took off to grab the vacuum. Cindy's family was scheduled to arrive for a holiday visit and he wanted to have the house spotless before they arrived… he was nesting.

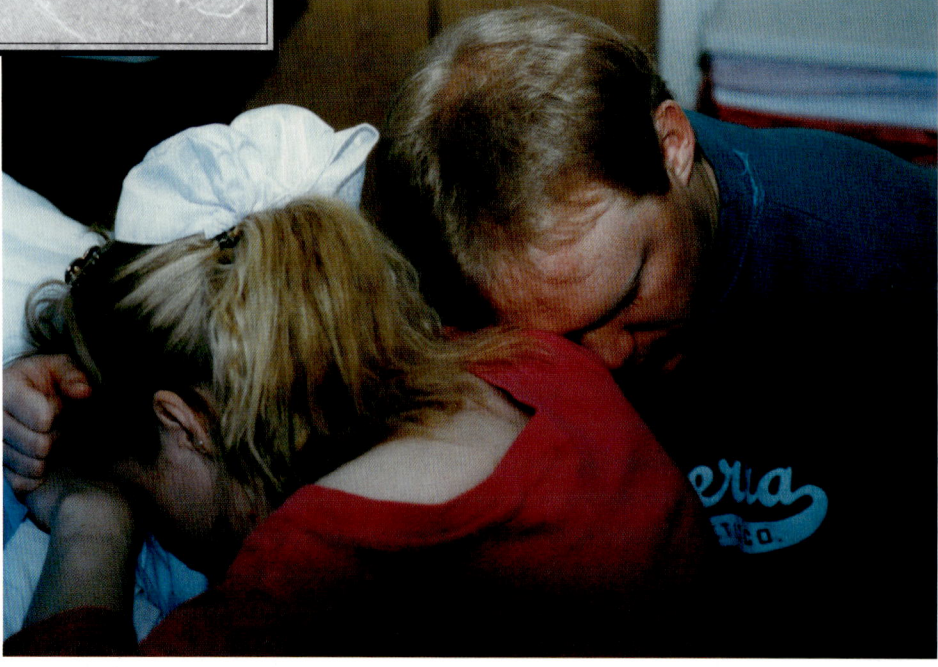

STEP 7: Follow Your Instincts and Trust Your Inner Voice

I went to work right away adjusting Cindy, but despite my best efforts to get her body perfectly balanced, she simply couldn't stand during a contraction. She tried, but her instincts made her drop to the floor each time the contraction built in intensity.

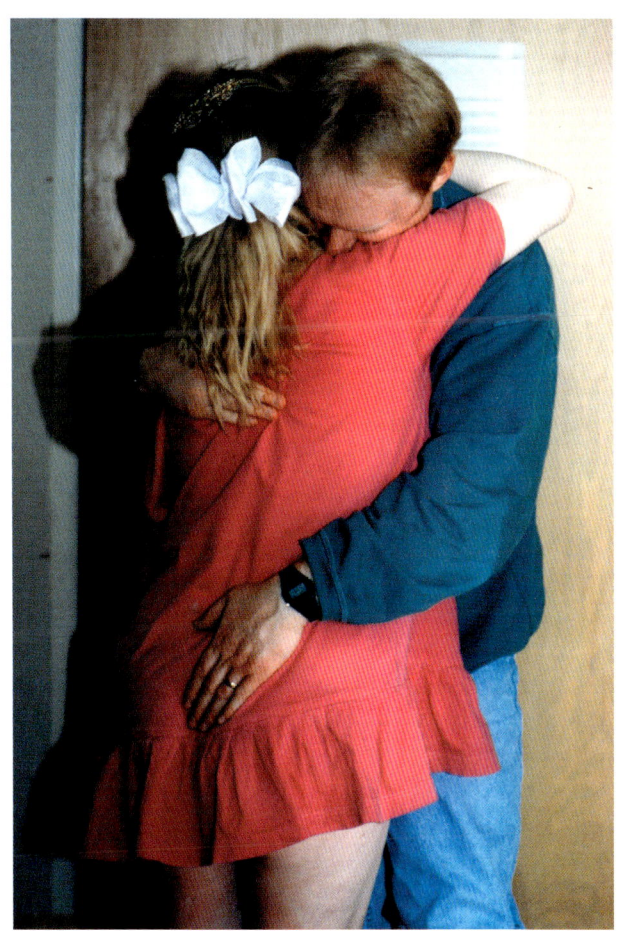

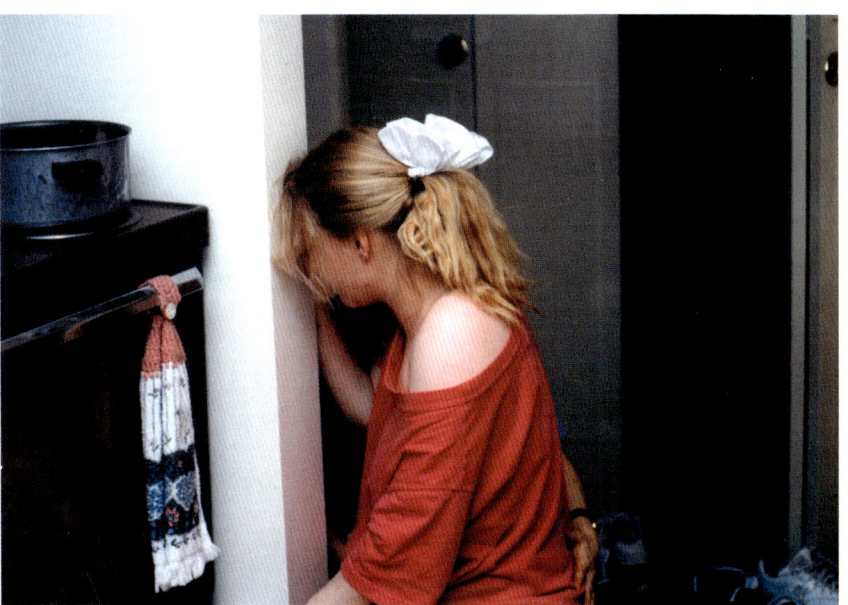

Minutes stretched to hours and my legs began to shake with exhaustion. I started to doubt my ability to continue my doula responsibilities, which included joining Cindy in her squatting position. I had to use my legs for support, as my hands were busy directing energy through the baby. Each time I struggled to get up after a contraction, I marveled at Cindy's physical strength and endurance.

As she walked between contractions, Cindy moved as if in a trance. The minute a contraction would begin it's gradual assent up the invisible mountain she was climbing, Cindy would squat back down. It took quite some time to get her to the car for the trip to the hospital; we'd take a few steps, stop, squat down, and wait. As soon as the contraction was over we would take a few more steps before the next one started.

At the hospital, Cindy had a difficult time lying on her back for the quick check with the ultrasound monitor. As soon as her initial exam was complete, Cindy took off into the halls to continue her routine of walking and squatting. Cindy's friend, Rhonda, had now joined us. She and Jeff agreed to stay with Cindy, while the midwife and I took time to sit back, put our feet up and rest. The midwife, Amy, was exhausted and suffering from a cold; she took the bed. My legs were killing me; I claimed the rocking chair so I could put my feet up on the bed. I couldn't imagine how Cindy's legs were going to feel when this was all over.

Cindy had consistent contractions throughout the day and well into the night, but the baby wasn't moving down into the canal. She was not experiencing back labor, so the baby was apparently not in a posterior position.

Around midnight, Amy suggested that Cindy consider taking some form of medication to give herself a chance to lie down and rest for a few hours. Cindy decided to have intrathecal morphine. This would allow her to continue feeling the contractions, but hopefully, she would get enough relaxation to sleep between them. After the morphine was administered into her spinal canal, Cindy was able to lie down. Jeff curled up with her in the small hospital bed. Rhonda and I went home for a few hours to get some rest and Amy retired to the nurse's quarters.

Hands Of Love

Two hours later, I shot out of bed and took off for the hospital. The nurse had said she would call as soon as Cindy woke up. She hadn't, but my instincts told me to get there right away.

When I arrived I found the nurses frantically trying to find my phone number—they had lost it. The morphine had helped Cindy's muscles relax enough to allow the baby to down on the cervix; dilation was now complete. It was time to push and Cindy was asking for me.

After we were all assembled, Cindy insisted on getting back into a squatting position. The midwife brought in a birthing stool that was shaped like a toilet without a front so Cindy could squat with support. The rest of us had to get down on the floor with her.

Just as the baby crowned—there was a tap on the door. Cindy's mother had been sleeping in the waiting room with her two-year-old niece. The little girl had suddenly woken up and wanted her mother. Cindy's sister took her daughter into her arms so that Cindy's mother could join the crowd that was assembling on the floor of that very small labor room.

Two nurses, two midwives, two doulas, her sister, her niece, her mother, and her husband all crowded around to watch Cindy deliver her baby. Cindy, on the other hand, seemed oblivious to everyone except Amy, who was squatting on the floor in front of her—cranking her neck in an attempt to look up at Cindy's perineum and the baby who was now crowning.

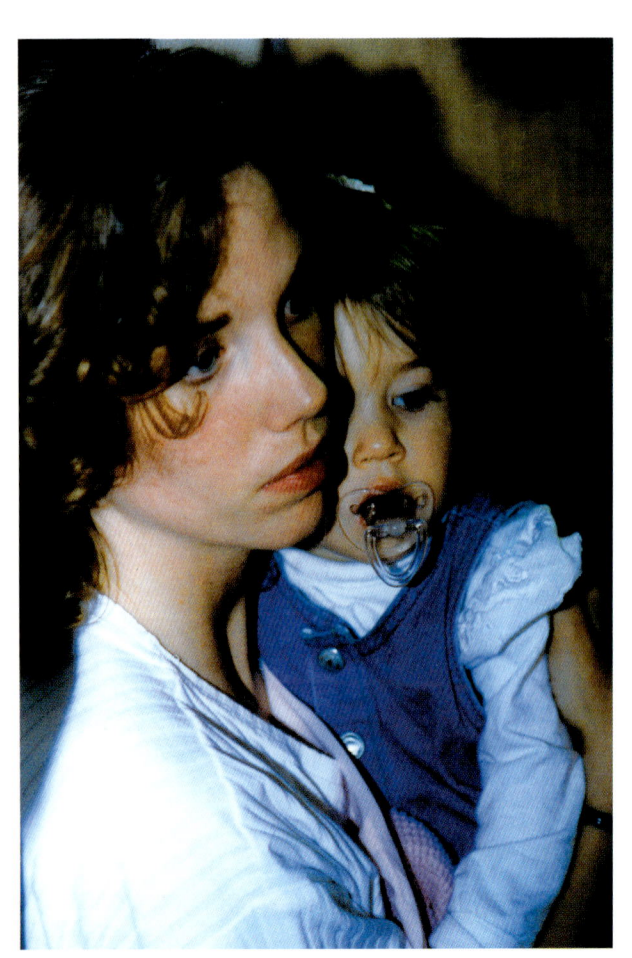

Cindy's sister joined the crowd on the floor so she and her daughter would have a better view of the birth. Cindy's niece was captivated and not at all disturbed by the scene in front of her.

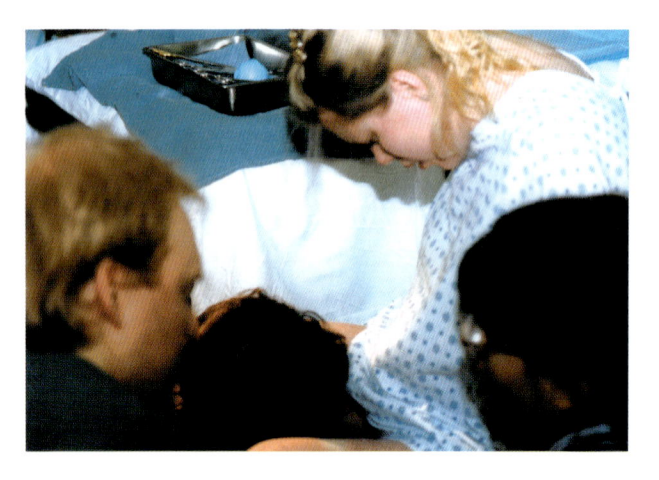

Cindy and Jeff reached down to catch their baby as the head slowly descended out of the birth canal. Suddenly, I heard, "Oh Shit!"—not what you want to hear from a midwife who is observing the delivery. A nurse was right there with scissors. The cord was wrapped three times around the baby's neck so tightly she couldn't complete her descent out of the canal. Amy couldn't loosen it; it had to be cut, immediately!

Jeff held the baby's head, while Amy worked on cutting the cord. Cindy's hands were right there ready to catch her baby's body as soon as she was free to continue her slide into the world. Both she and Jeff seemed oblivious to what was happening; they simply smiled down on their baby. There was no time to clamp the cord. Blood covered Jeff's hands, but he never showed any sign of distress.

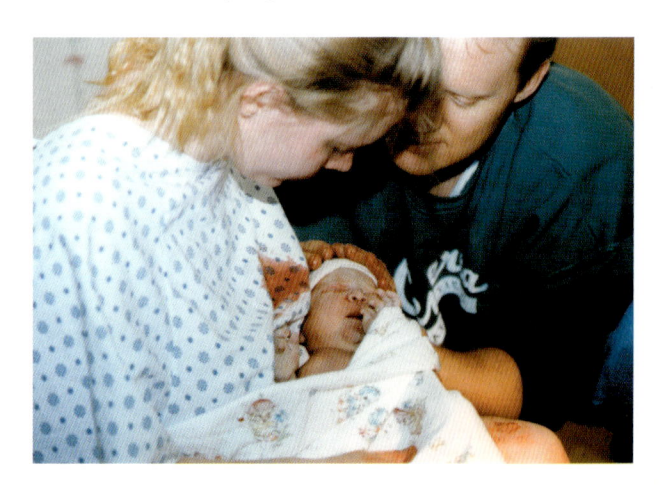

176

STEP 7: Follow Your Instincts and Trust Your Inner Voice

Cindy set the limp baby on her lap as Jeff intuitively encircled her head with his hands. Jeff was a chiropractic student—his instincts ,and his training, simply took over. He knew just what to do to bring the life force home to his baby's body. Cindy simply held her newborn and let the love flow.

Alexie, was just fine—thanks to Cindy, who followed her instinctive need to squat, and Amy, who was willing to climb down on the floor with her patient. Cindy knew intuitively that squatting shortened the birth canal and was somehow helping her baby endure the forces of labor and Amy trusted her; she did whatever she could to accommodate Cindy's desire to birth in a squatting position.

When the intrathecal morphine was used, Cindy's muscles relaxed enough to allow the uterus to ease her baby down without resistance. Unfortunately, there was a downside to the injection of morphine into Cindy's spine. The next day Cindy went home with a baby—and with a splitting headache. I went over that evening to check everyone and found Cindy still suffering from the headache. I adjusted her—but I couldn't seem to give her any relief. I had never had a patient receive morphine, or any other spinal medications, so I had no idea she was suffering from a spinal headache caused by a hole in the dura.

The next day, Cindy was unable to take care of her baby due to the intensity of her pain, so Jeff took her to the emergency room. The emergency room doctor knew immediately what was wrong. The needle used to inject the morphine had poked a hole in the dural membrane causing a spinal leak. He administered a blood patch to her spinal canal and within ten minutes—the headache began to subside.

Jeff graduated from Northwestern Chiropractic College and moved his family to Laverne, MN. He and Cindy went on to have two more children. Both were delivered fairly rapidly and without complications during delivery.

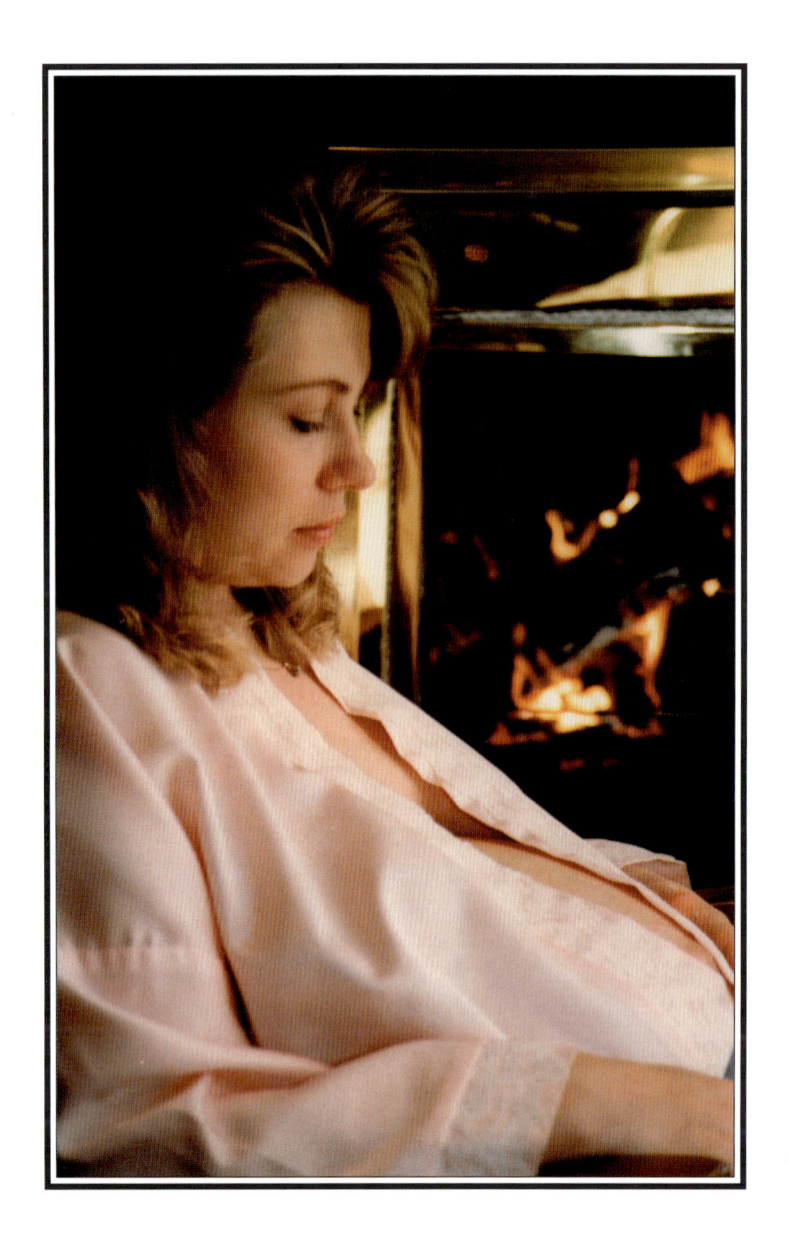

I am entering into this energy communication
From that point within me
That is the pure manifestation of God the Father.

Thank you, Father, that this is so.
(Author Unknown)

This affirmation is great for parent's who want to enhance communication with their unborn child. I use it during difficult treatment sessions to enhance my ability to tap into a patient's Innate Intelligence.

STEP 7: Follow Your Instincts and Trust Your Inner Voice

The Energy Connection

How did Cindy's baby let her know that she had a very short tight cord wrapped three times around her neck? How did Cindy get the message and know to squat with every contraction? If you work closely with unborn children as I do, you know there is something to this "energy thing."

Energy is that strong attraction you carry within your soul for your partner. It's the reason a mother knows when her children are hurt, or when her husband's had a bad day; they're connected energetically.

The human energy field is a mysterious interaction of atomic particles that make you uncomfortable around some people and perfectly at ease with others. Energy supplies us with electricity, transfers sound around the world from our cell phones, and makes it possible to see inside the womb.

Quantum theory tells us that the presence of an observer changes the behavior of subatomic particles. That is why studies have shown that having another woman in the room with a birthing mother will reduce the incidence of medical intervention. If that observer interacts with the mother in a loving and devoted manner, it will reduce the need for intervention even further. It has been my experience that an unborn baby will react quite strongly to the energy of those around him. If I say something that refers directly the unborn baby while I'm working on a mom, he will often react with a swift kick or punch. At other times, I find that babies will just play with my hand by stroking my palm.

Earlier in this book, I showed you how a mother was able to control her baby's failing heart rate simply by telling him what he needed to do. Babies not only respond to our verbal comments; they also interact energetically with other human energy fields they may come into contact with. Let me give you an example of what I mean.

I was once assisting at the birth of a baby whose parents were struggling with their relationship. The baby's mother suffered from constant emotional stress throughout the pregnancy. The baby's father worked in another city, so they were forced to live separately. The mother made every attempt throughout the pregnancy to communicate to the baby that her stress had nothing to do with him. She told him repeatedly that he was not part of the problem and that she loved him.

The baby's father arrived in town prior to the delivery and accompanied us to the hospital—having done very little to prepare himself for the delivery. During labor, I was surprised to find him sitting in the corner observing rather than helping us comfort the baby's mother. After many hours of arrested labor (failure to progress), I rested my hands over the baby and attempted to relax the mother's pelvic floor muscles. I was shocked at the degree of emotional pain I felt radiating from the baby. I worked unsuccessfully to relax the mother and assure the baby that everything was fine.

When I perform this type of energy work I often find that my body is a conduit for the transfer of emotional or physical energy from the patient's body. If there is a great deal of energy transmitted through my body (it feels like fingernails drawn down a chalkboard), I will involuntarily yawn. It is as if my lungs must help to quickly release the excess energy from my body.

The baby's father watched my strange behavior and asked if I needed a cup of coffee. (Poor guy, he had no idea what to think of me.) I responded, "No, but it sure would help if you'd come over and touch the baby." He came directly over to the side of the bed and rested his hands on the mother's tummy. Within minutes, the baby decided it was time to come on out and meet us.

A short time later, the father sat with his newborn nestled on his lap. As he looked down adoringly at his new son, I asked him what he did to make such a rapid change in the baby's progress. Without changing his gaze he said, "I told him it was okay to be a boy."

I found out later that the dad had arrived in town with a cute, tiny pair of pink tennis shoes. He bought them as a gift for the baby because he was "really hoping for a girl."

I can't tell you how many births have been delayed because the parents believed they were going to have one gender—only to find out that the baby had a different reality. In every case, the baby didn't come out until the parents made a point of saying, "It's okay if this is a girl, I just thought it was a boy—I'd be okay with a girl." Only then did they come out to play.

Be careful what you say around your unborn child. Those little ears are listening. And, little wheels are turning in their tiny well-developed brains. Explain everything to them as if they understand. Who knows—they just might.

No matter how well you plan your birth, no matter how confident you are that labor will progress exactly as planned, the only constant in life is change. As you make those final plans concerning your baby's birth, you would be wise to keep that thought in mind and construct a tiny door in the back of your mind—a door labeled **Detour**.

Childbirth Requires Patience and Reverence

It is difficult to demonstrate patience and reverence for the birth process when control remains an option. Control over delivery starts out innocently enough. Based on a general rule that is applied to every woman, a due date is often determined. A mother accepts that date and proceeds to tell everyone she knows what it is. Soon a mother begins to believe she will have the baby on that particular day. Two weeks before the scheduled "*due date*" family and friends start the onslaught of phone calls. Three – four weeks later a mother starts hearing, "Are you still there?" "You haven't had the baby yet?"

By the time a mother reaches the designated day of delivery, many women swear to me that if one more person asks them if they've had the baby yet—they'll hang up on them.

As each day passes, a mother begins to feel threatened. At each prenatal visit she is often warned that her doctor "won't **let** her go past 42 weeks." Finally, mothers usually throw up their arms and surrender. After all, "he won't **let** her go any longer!" It's not her fault that the baby needs to be induced. Even when the required non-stress tests are negative, some women who have resisted induction are told, "The baby will **never** come out without induction. The placenta will stop working, your baby will die, and it will be your fault."

Some people seem to have forgotten that the Universal Intelligence who created such a tiny human being is also controlling how and when they should exit the womb. In reality, babies can come any time they please up to four weeks past their due date. Only they know exactly how much time they need to maneuver the birth canal.

Ideally, when a baby decides it's time to start his descent, he will start and stop labor many times as he works his way into the world. Labor can progress this way for weeks before the final descent. Babies need time to mold their cranium. First time mothers need time to stretch out a multitude of muscles and activate many nerve pathways. A mother/baby couple also require an adequate amount of time to adapt to the surge of hormones that will coarse through their bodies and fill them with the power of birth.

It is believed that only first births go through this long and erratic process and that each successive birth gets quicker and quicker. I personally do not believe they get quicker simply because of physiology. My experience tells me it is because a first-time mother has never experienced the sensations of birth before. Therefore, she anticipates any sign of impending labor and runs for the hospital long before the baby is truly ready.

TV and movie births have given new mothers a false idea about birth. They often think they will suddenly have an unbearable cramp, their water will break, they will go flying through the city in a car driven by their partner at breakneck speed, and the baby will come flying out as soon as they arrive at the hospital. Now, granted, this can happen, as I showed you in Susan's birth at the beginning of this book, but that was her second birth and a very rare occurrence. First births average 15 hours of continuous active labor *after* contractions have remained consistently five minutes apart for one – two hours.

With subsequent births, a mother has removed the variable of the unknown. She often ignores the early work of labor. When symptoms become a little more noticeable, she remains busy getting the house ready for her departure. There are clothes to wash, dishes to wash, and a house to clean; they must wait for a baby-sitter to arrive. If she has a homebirth, there are plenty of ways for a mother to keep busy and ignore the signs of impending delivery.

With each successive baby, there are more and more things to prepare before a mother can get down to the business of birthing. Finally, it dawns on the mother that contractions are regular and intense. Before she knows it, she is moving into the active stage of labor and everyone thinks she had a rapid delivery. Not so!

It usually takes at least one birth to learn about the danger involved in allowing someone else to orchestrate the birth of a child. By the second time around, many women learn to trust their baby, and their bodies. When they do, women often report a reverence for the birth process and a renewed sense of power within themselves.

STEP 7: Follow Your Instincts and Trust Your Inner Voice

As a parent, try to accept that no one knows the exact day when a baby is ready to be born. No one has all the answers about childbirth and no one should intimidate a mother into making choices just for the sake of convention.

Maintain flexibility and hire only those birth attendants who will honor your wishes. If you make certain choices surrounding the birth of your baby and things do not progress as you predicted, change your choice. Start out with the best of intentions. Keep everything as simple and non-invasive as possible, then, if your inner voice tells you that you must enter that back door marked, **Detour**, listen. Trust that voice and follow your instincts.

Here is the story of a young couple whose birth taught me a great deal about patience, intuition, and the power of a mother to protect her baby.

A World of Choices

This is the story of two chiropractors that were raised to have reverence for Nature and to believe in the innate power to heal; they had never received a vaccination; they were raised without medication; and both received chiropractic care from the day they were born. Stacey and Jason hired a midwife and planned a homebirth because they wanted a private, peaceful, safe environment for the birth of their first baby.

I had been their pediatric instructor and was now Stacey's mentor during her final chiropractic externship. By the time Stacey and Jason graduated from college, I had become a friend of the family. When Stacey found out she was going to have a baby, she asked me to provide chiropractic-doula support. I agreed to try and be there even though she and Jason had moved to Fargo, North Dakota.

It was the last week of December. I had time off from my teaching and clinic responsibilities and decided to visit Stacey. The baby was due in mid–January and I thought, just maybe, I would get lucky and she would go into labor while I was there. (There we go, anticipating an early delivery—see what I mean?)

Stacey and Jason had temporarily moved in with her dad, David, who lived out in the middle of nowhere. (At least it seemed that way to me.) It snowed continuously while I was there and the average temperature was 60 below zero (windchill)—we stayed indoors watching movies and talking by the light of a flickering fire. One evening, I persuaded Stacey and Jason to let me photograph the three of them. It was a hobby I'd enjoyed for more than a decade and their carefree, joyful attitude about the pregnancy made them perfect subjects.

Just before I was due to leave, Stacey started having contractions. She wanted so badly to have the baby before I left that she called her midwife and asked her to come over. Jill lived more than an hour away, but she agreed to drive in to see if there had been any changes since Stacey's exam earlier that week. I decided to stay until Jill arrived. After all, I didn't want to have to turn right around and come back in a day or so.

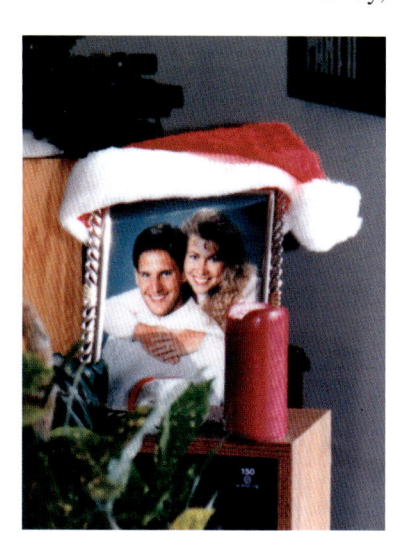

181

Jill braved the snow-covered highways and came prepared with all the equipment needed for a delivery. After examining Stacey, she reported that it looked promising. Stacey's cervix was effacing (thinning out), and dilation had begun. Taking all things into consideration, (i.e., the birth team was assembled, it was snowing heavily, and it was almost New Year's Eve) Jill and I, both, decided to stay.

Jill thought Stacey just needed a little push to get the contractions a little stronger, so Stacey decided to use a tincture of Cohosh to enhance the labor. (Cohosh can be effective in speeding up and regulating erratic contractions.) It worked; Stacey's contractions became stronger and more frequent. In fact, it worked so well that Stacey had strong, painful contractions every five minutes for the next several days… but no baby.

At first, Stacey was able to watch movies and rock through the contractions. But, it wasn't long before sitting and lying down became unbearable; walking and standing through a contraction was all that Stacey could endure. When she tired of walking, Stacey would take long, hot showers with the water beating on her back. Eventually, she could walk no more, so she tried sleeping in the rocking chair with her fists pressed against her low back.

When fatigue overwhelmed Jason, he slept on the bed beside Stacey's rocker, while Jill slept on the floor. Earlier in the labor, Jason had been so anxious for labor to begin he could barely contain his excitement. He never dreamed labor could persist for several days. He wanted to believe that Stacey would start, and finish, in a short period of time. Piece of cake. This was not a piece of cake. Now, he just wanted to get some sleep so he could study for his upcoming chiropractic state board exams.

Stacey's father, David, closed his chiropractic office and stayed home to help. He had no idea of the commitment he had entered into. None of us knew we were in for a marathon birth. As the hours wore on, we took turns walking around the house physically supporting Stacey. We hugged her and let her hang on us during each contraction. We were a team, so when sleep deprivation kicked in, we would take turns supporting Stacey. At one point, I had crashed on the bed for about ten minutes when I woke up worried about Stacey. I rushed into the den and found everyone asleep except David, who was cradling Stacey in his arms. I took over, and seconds later, I turned around to find David passed out on the couch. That is the way it went for days; time lost all relevance.

It was tough on us, but at least we were able to rest from time to time. I wish we could say the same thing for Stacey.

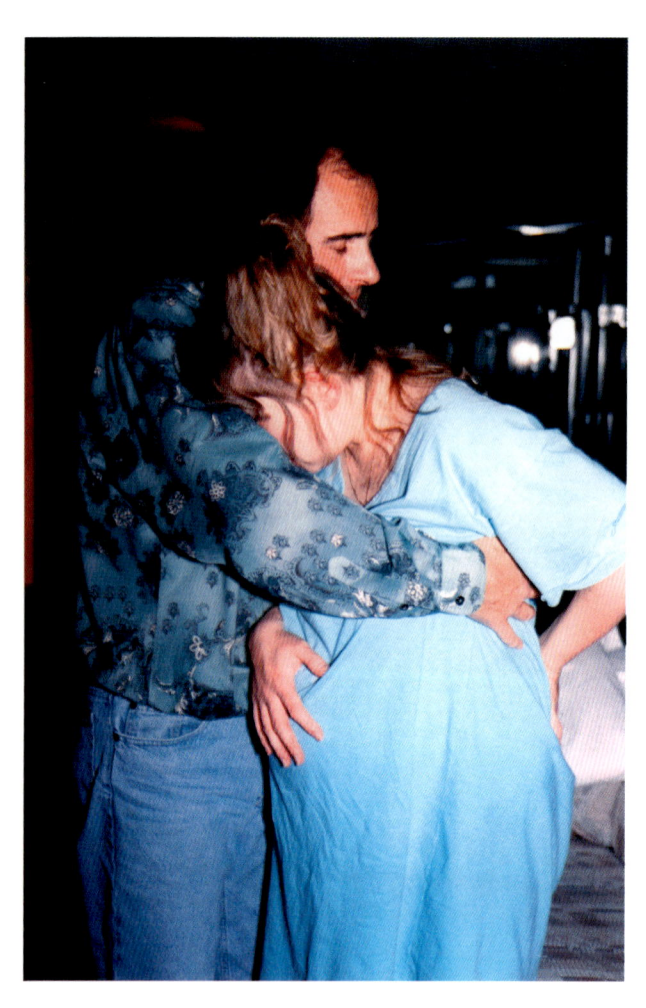

She could not sleep or escape the constant contractions. Stacey had no choice but to endure the painful, erratic flow of labor; she could not stop it once it began. The cohosh-induced contractions seemed to have forced Stacey's baby down into the canal before he was lined up properly; he was now stuck and couldn't move forward or backward.

After several days of labor (and hours of pushing), Stacey realized that standing was not helping. We decided to try a different form of gravity in an attempt to free him from his locked position in the birth canal. We threw the couch cushions on the floor to construct a makeshift pregnant adjusting area. The cushions were spaced so there was a hole for Stacey's belly. We used gravity to help us as we tried to free the little guy. It didn't work. We just couldn't help him. We tried every position we knew to do at the time, but nothing worked.

STEP 7: Follow Your Instincts and Trust Your Inner Voice

> This is exactly what I was referring to in Step 4 of this pregnancy plan. At the time of Stacey's delivery I hadn't figured out how to correct the problem. If we had placed Stacey on her side with her leg dropped off the bed, we might have been able to reduce the torque in her pelvic floor muscles. If that had not worked, we could have inverted her by having her kneel at the top of a few steps and walk her hands downward. We would have used the amniotic fluid to float him out of the pelvis, thus allowing him to correct his position.

We did not have the advantage of having a hospital bed that could be adapted to support Stacey in various positions. We had to do it.

By the third day, I was exhausted. I leaned my head into Stacey to give her back support, while I pushed my fists up against her aching sacrum. My back was killing me from being in this position for so long, so David sat behind me and tried to support my back, and ease my pain, by doing subtle energy work on me. We were all hurting and exhausted, but we couldn't desert Stacey. (Jason remained in front of her as he tried to keep her focused and relaxed.)

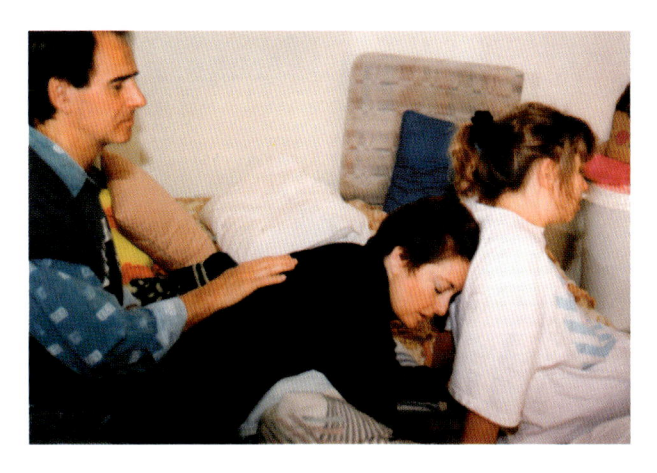

Later that evening, Stacey stood again in the hot shower trying to ease the pain. She was fully dilated and had been pushing for hours. Jill sat on the shower floor prepared to catch the baby should he suddenly turn and drop through the canal. Modesty was gone for Stacey as her consciousness dropped down into the primitive portion of her brain. Jason, David, and I stood in the bathroom feeling totally helpless—Stacey's strength and endurance was amazing.

During those three days of labor, Stacey had almost no sleep and little food. However, she was operating from a mysterious place deep within herself and she never gave in.

> Michel Odent, obstetrician and author of *The Nature of Birth and Breast-feeding*, writes clearly about the physiological aspect of birth. He explains how a woman begins labor with her consciousness in the cerebral cortex of the brain, but eventually must allow the limbic portion to take over; labor becomes an involuntary survival mechanism. Anyone who observes women throughout the entire process of labor and delivery can recognize when a woman is still functioning in the cerebral cortex (she can answer questions, talk, tell jokes, and carry on a conversation). When her consciousness drops into the limbic portion of the brain, Nature takes over and the process becomes instinctive. All five senses are heightened, inhibitions are reduced, and mothers remove their clothing. They become hot and their skin has the heightened sensory response often felt when two people make love. Birthing generates the same power that consumes a woman when she has an orgasm. Oxytocin, the same hormone that causes the uterus to contract and pull sperm up into the uterus, is also responsible for contracting the uterus with enough force to birth the child that was created from that initial union.
>
> This natural hormonal process is easy to recognize in home births, but it is rarely witnessed in the hospital, as the nature of the environment keeps the mother in the cerebral cortex for most of the labor and delivery. Bright lights, forms, questions, checking and recording of vital signs, IV's, monitors, etc., are all factors that stop Nature from taking a woman into this vital and necessary place for a truly natural delivery.

Obviously, this birth was not progressing as Jason and Stacey had planned. Their goal in creating their birth plan was to avoid anything that would hinder the progress of labor. They had carefully created a private environment in their home for the birth. Stacey had avoided the use of ultrasounds. She had avoided narcotics and analgesics, and had surrounded herself with a carefully created birth team. She had prepared her body for labor by getting adjusted. They had done everything to insure an easy delivery, but it just wasn't happening the way they expected it to!

Stacey stepped from the hot shower as Jill and I dried her off. Weak, tired, and discouraged, Stacey draped her arms over Jason and David's shoulders. They helped her walk down the short hall from the bathroom to the baby's room. We wrapped Stacey in a robe and settled her into the rocking chair. I asked everyone to leave the room to give us some time alone. It was clear that Stacey had to take a new approach. It was time to enter the door marked, **Detour**.

It was around 7:00 P.M. and the room was dark except for a light that was shining through the window. The large yard light gave the illusion of moonbeams breaking through the darkness to shine down onto the spot where Stacey sat rocking her baby—her hands resting on her tummy. It was hard to imagine there was a struggle for freedom going on inside of her. We had tried everything we knew to ease her pain, and we had failed. Then, in desperation, I realized this was the perfect environment to ask Stacey to tap into her subconscious and allow me to use visualization to help her enter a hypnotic state of mind.

I knelt in front of the rocker. I had Stacey close her eyes and go within to be with the baby. I suggested she take the baby in her arms and picture herself walking away from the house. She was to walk past the fields that had moonbeams bouncing off the snow and down the long, dark, snow-covered road that led to the highway. Behind her, the house would slowly fade into the darkness of the isolated countryside.

I kept suggesting that the farther she got from the house, the better she and the baby would feel. We visualized the illuminated house getting smaller and smaller as she walked with her baby in her arms farther and farther down the road. I kept suggesting that by the time she reached the highway—the pain would be gone.

This visualization process worked. When Stacey reached the highway in her mind, she was relaxed and at peace with the baby in her arms. I then asked Stacey what she needed to do to help the baby. Without hesitation she responded, "I need to go to the hospital!" After making that statement, Stacey opened her eyes and looked directly at me. There was no hint of doubt in them. She knew exactly what she needed to do. We both realized, she was not going to deliver at home.

Everyone was called back into the room. I told them Stacey wanted to go to the hospital. Jill did not hesitate, judge, or advise against it. She turned and went to the phone to call an OB she knew and respected. It was New Year's Eve—not the best time to ask an OB to take on a new patient he had never seen before. We were lucky; he returned her call right away.

After learning that all of Stacey's vital signs were normal, the doctor asked if she could wait a few more hours. When Jill returned to relay the message, Stacey looked at her and said, "No, I need to go now!" Again, Jill did not question or argue. She returned to the phone to call the hospital and let them know we were coming in. She then paged the doctor and told him. He agreed to meet us there as soon as he could.

Jason stood beside the rocker. He was exhausted and frustrated. Still, he couldn't bring himself to support Stacey's decision. He wanted this baby to come out as much as she did, but he wanted to stand by his previous decision that neither his wife, nor his child, would be traumatized, drugged, or operated on in any way. To go to the hospital now was to admit defeat.

Stacey looked up into his face and a look of stern determination strengthened her young delicate features. She sounded strong and sure when she said, "Jason, this is my baby and I want to go to the hospital, now!" He did not argue or complain. He simply said, "Okay," and went to get his shoes on.

David, Jill, Jason, and I scrambled to get ready. Within moments, we were all set to go and turned to help Stacey get dressed. Suddenly, we realized she was nowhere to be found. Where was she? A frantic search found her downstairs in the garage, in the back seat of the car—fully clothed.

> Never underestimate the power of a woman who has made a decision and is acting on it. Physiology is a strange and powerful thing. Change what you are thinking and you change what you can do. Take control of your mind, and you can take control of your body. Was this the same woman who needed two people to help her walk from the bathroom? How did she dress herself? How did she get down the stairs without our help?
>
> When you make the right choice—the strength will come.

STEP 7: Follow Your Instincts and Trust Your Inner Voice

In the rush to get going, Jason grabbed a baby outfit and I grabbed my camera. We didn't take time to bring the car seat, the video camera, or a diaper bag. As we drove down the dark highway from David's home in the country, everyone was silent except Stacey. A determination to deliver naturally still ran deep within her, but fear was rapidly taking over. With anguish in her voice, Stacey asked me what would happen to her at the hospital. Would they drug her? Would they take the baby through a C-section? I could only reach over the seat and pat her hand as I assured her that we would treat the baby. We would work together, all four of us, to correct any problems the baby might have after the birth.

We had done all we could. It was time to "**bring in the medics**" as old-time chiropractors often say. When we arrived at the hospital, we walked with Stacey up to Labor and Delivery. Not knowing what kind of reception we would get, we were prepared for the worst. It is rare for homebirth families to transport to the hospital. When they do, the medical staff will sometimes treat the family as if they are irresponsible, negligent, and bordering on abusive.

I said a silent prayer that this wouldn't happen. My prayers were answered. We entered the quiet, empty ward and were met by two smiling nurses. One of them took Stacey's hand and said, "We know this isn't how you intended to have your baby, but we'll try to make it as close to your wishes as possible." They helped Stacey out of her clothes and into a gown. They asked her no questions and allowed Jason to fill out the admission forms.

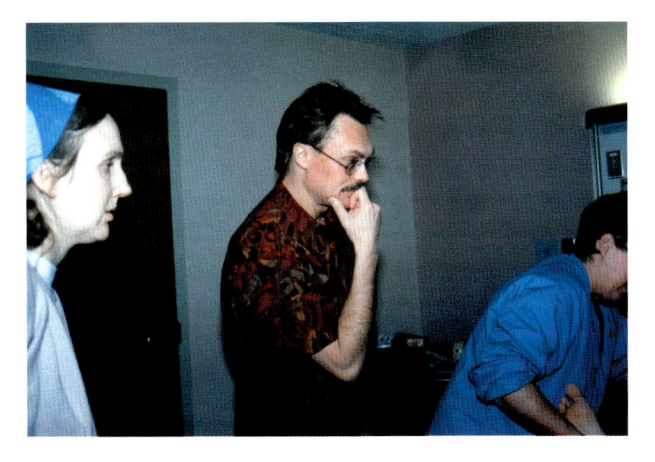

Not long after Stacey was settled in bed, the obstetrician arrived. Wearing a short–sleeved silk shirt and dress slacks, he made no attempt to change into the customary blue scrubs. Smiling warmly at all of us, the doctor shook Jill's hand before walking over to Stacey. He touched her softly and said, "Let's see if you can do this all by yourself." He checked the baseline ultrasound monitor strip for any signs of fetal distress; the baby looked fine. He checked the size and shape of Stacey's pelvis; there was plenty of room. The baby was just twisted and stuck in there. Within minutes, the doctor told Stacey that with a little help he believed she could have the baby without intervention.

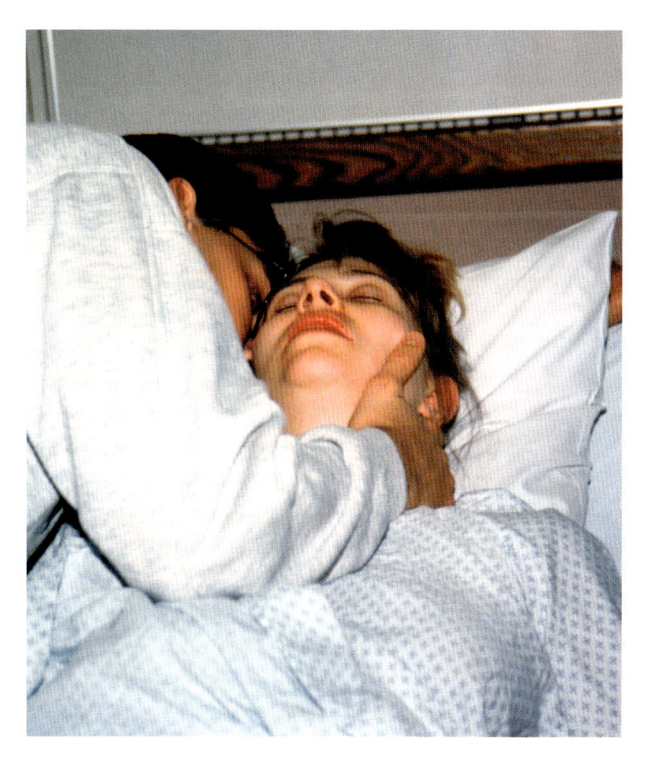

Jason then leaned over Stacey and whispered in her ear, "Give me my baby!" Stacey was willing to comply with his request, but she knew she needed help. She was perfectly willing to turn control over to this kind, gentle doctor who believed in her ability to deliver the baby.

The doctor asked Stacey to work with the nurses and push as hard as she could when he told her to. I was delighted to see that the nurses asked her to push in the manner that I find works well when the baby is slow in their descent. Jill hadn't been comfortable with this form of pushing as it increased the force of the contraction—and increased the risk of a tear. Jill wasn't equipped to suture a significant tear, so she had discouraged this form of pushing.

Stacey was told to take a deep breath and hold it to the count of ten when the next pushing urge consumed her. Jason and David were told to raise Stacey up as she tucked her chin to her chest and rounded out her spine. The nurses would push her legs into flexion to open the pelvic outlet, while the doctor pulled the vaginal wall open, hopefully freeing the

185

trapped shoulder. The doctor then asked Jill to stay close and be prepared to catch the baby.

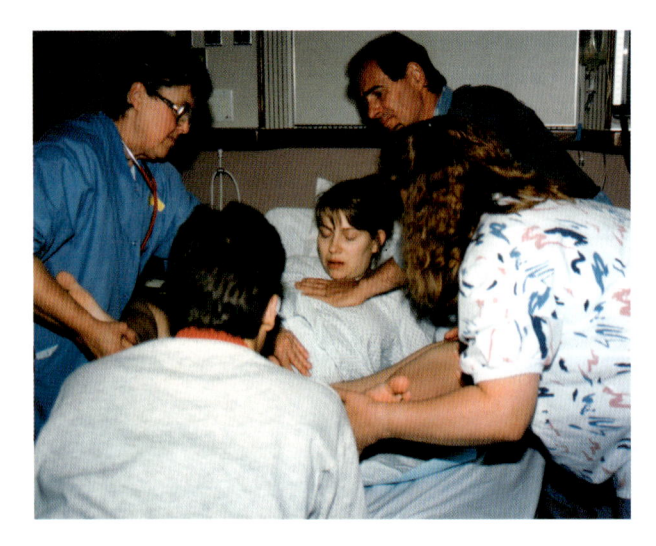

Jason gave Stacey words of encouragement as I stepped away to grab the only camera we brought. We could not finish the video we had started days before, but at least I could photograph this baby's entry into the world.

David placed his hand over Stacey's heart and the members of her newly expanded birth team took their places. The head of the bed had been elevated to support Stacey in a semi-seated position. David and Jason lifted Stacey forward as we all voiced words of encouragement. The two nurses positioned themselves on either side of the bed, preparing to take Stacey's feet and help her pull them toward her shoulders. Stacey's pelvis had to be widened to give the baby more room; this was the only way to do it.

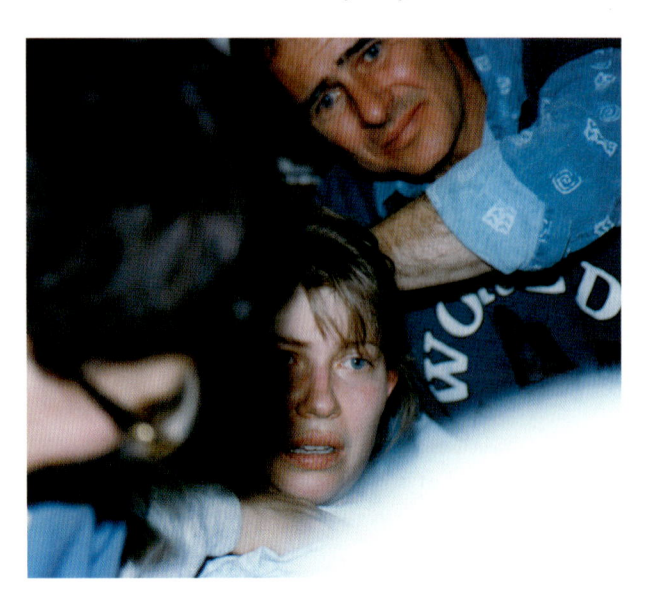

Next, a nurse again coached Stacey on how to take a big breath when the next contraction started. She encouraged her to hold that breath and bear down with her abdominal muscles, while they counted loudly to ten. Stacey was to try and do this three times. Suddenly, she stopped all further instructions as she announced, "Here it is."

Jason and David lifted Stacey's shoulders. She, then tucked her chin toward her chest in an effort to round out her spine and flex her sacrum.

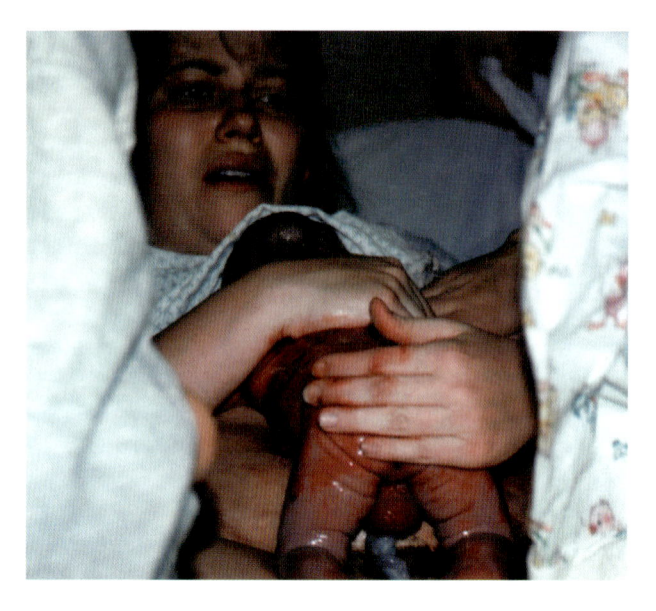

Stacey pushed with all her might. The doctor physically pulled the vaginal canal apart and, with everyone working together, Sammy's shoulder was free. Stacey's tissue tore as Sammy slipped into Jill's outstretched hands. In one swift motion, Jill caught Sammy and handed him to Stacey. One moment, her face was shrouded in doubt and despair, and just a second later, she lit up with joy and love.

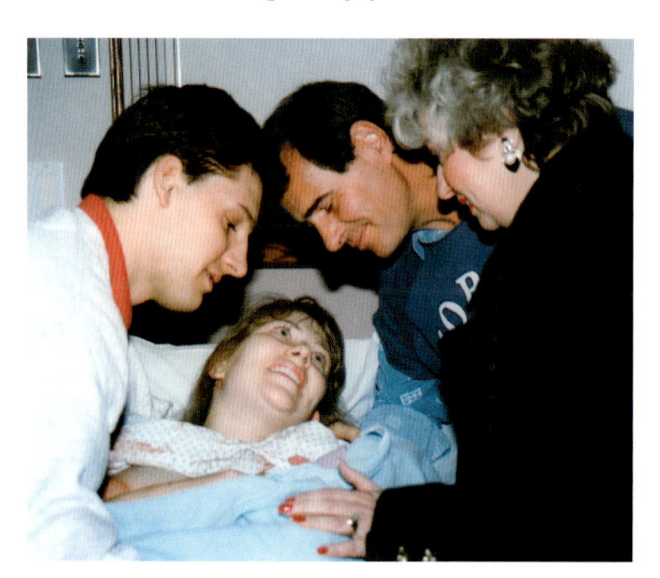

STEP 7: Follow Your Instincts and Trust Your Inner Voice

As soon as Stacey took Sammy in her arms, the nurses gently placed her legs down and stepped away. They were extremely discreet as they quickly monitored vital signs and covered both Stacey and Sammy in warm blankets. I put down the camera and reached for the phone to call Stacey's mother, Marlys. I had no sooner dialed the number when the door opened and someone whispered, "Carol, can I come in?" I turned to see who it was. It was Marlys! She had left her home as soon as she had heard we were going to the hospital. She had no idea that her grandson had just been born. Dressed and ready to leave for a New Year's Eve party, Marlys, and Stacey's stepfather, had decided to come to the hospital instead.

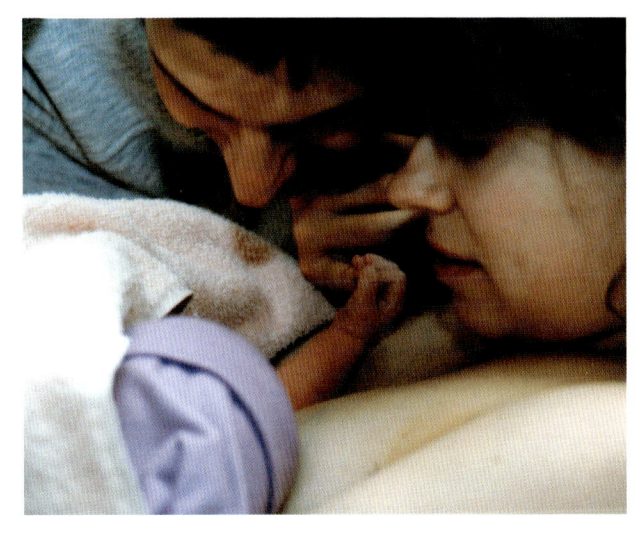

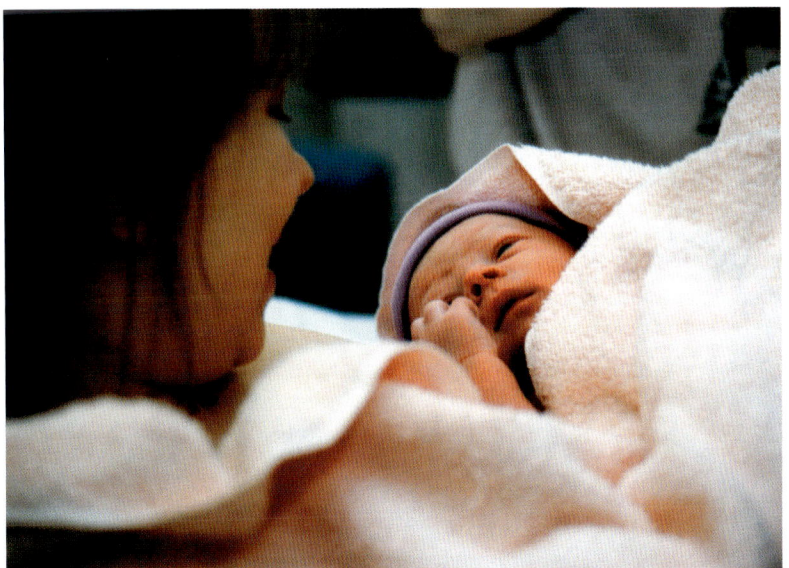

From the moment of his birth, Sammy was at peace with the world. He appeared to be oblivious to the long hours he had spent trapped in Stacey's pelvis. His cranium was molded normally. He didn't cry. His eyes, which were wide open within seconds of delivery, were locked on Stacey. He looked at her with the same adoration and amazement that she showered down upon him.

I finally turned my camera over to someone else so I could greet this child who had kept me up for so long. I bent down to say hi just as he reached out and grabbed my finger. I think he recognized me too!

I encouraged Marlys to join her family while I resumed photographing the scene before me. Jason couldn't stop kissing his wife and baby. Tears flowed down David's cheek as he placed his arm around Marlys. Stacey looked up into her parents' faces and her pain and fear washed away with their tears of joy. She was temporarily oblivious to the doctor and Jill who were waiting patiently for the cord to quit pulsing and for the placenta to disengage.

As Jason and Stacey allowed their flood of emotions to shower down on their baby, they seemed to be unaware of what was happening at the foot of the bed. The placenta had been delivered and the doctor had already begun the task of suturing Stacey's fourth degree tear through the perineum. As he worked, the doctor explained every detail of the repair to Jill and David. As a chiropractor, David was interested in assessing the damage that had occurred and Jill took advantage of this incredible learning opportunity to learn how to stitch the tissue back together.

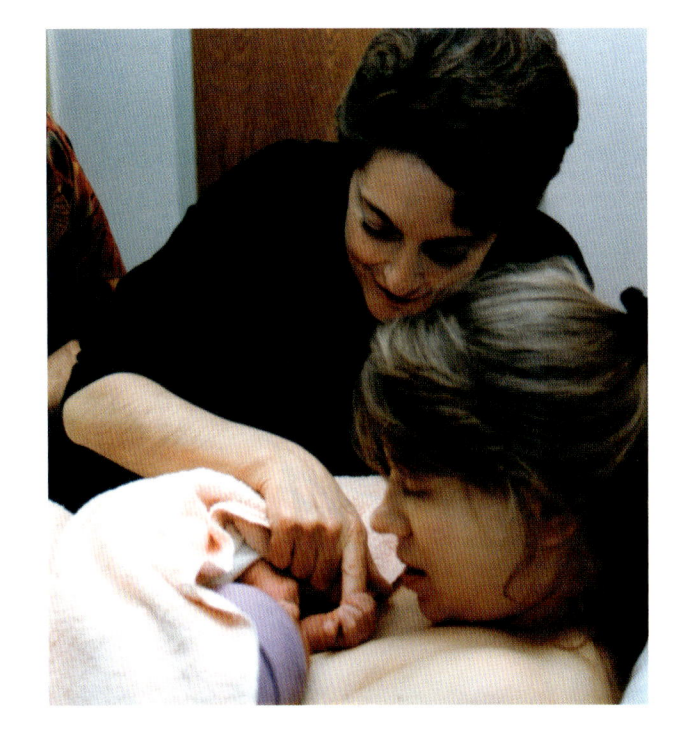

187

Hands Of Love

The nurses knew Jill would be performing a newborn exam, so they slipped away without following normal hospital protocols. There was no mention of a Vitamin K shot; he received no antibiotics in his eyes; no one asked about circumcision. Instead, the nurses went off in search of a car seat and a warm quilt to wrap him in for the ride home.

While the nurses were gone, Sammy was introduced to the other members of his family who were waiting in the hallway.

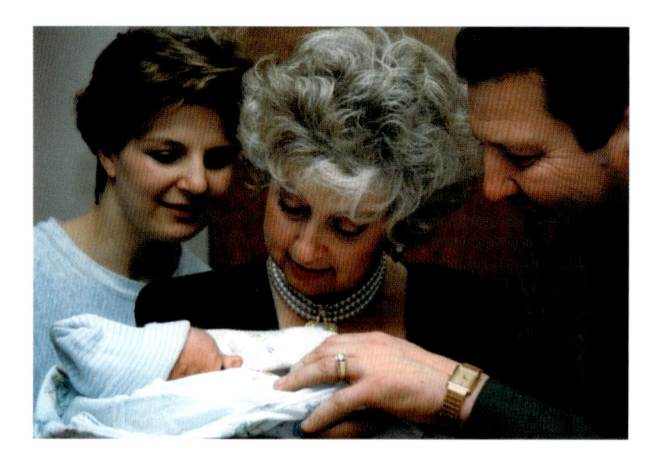

Within the hour, the doctor was finished, Jason had dressed Sammy for the trip back home, and Stacey had changed into her own clothes.

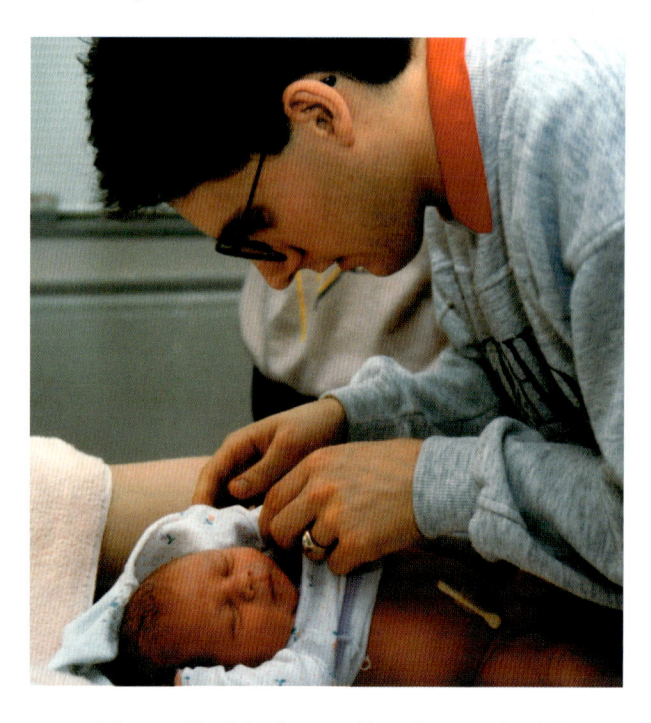

The staff wished us well as they pushed Stacey out to the waiting car in a wheelchair. Sammy was born at 8:14 P.M. on December 31st—less than an hour after Stacey decided to go to the hospital—and Stacey, Jason, and Sammy were back home in their own bed when the ball come down on Time Square.

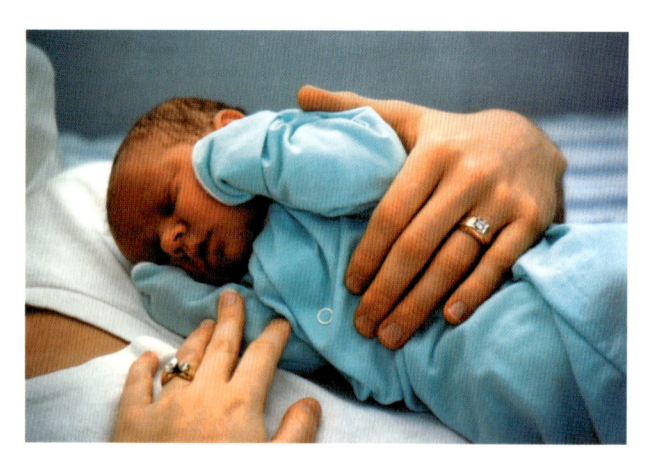

Wanting to make sure there were no complications for either Stacey or Sam, Jill came back with us and spent the night. We were all exhausted, but we enjoyed a peaceful night of sleep knowing that baby Sam was safely tucked in bed with his parents.

The next day, Jill completed her newborn exam before returning home to her family. I stayed another day and worked on Sammy. He needed chiropractic care and craniosacral therapy to undo the effects of his twisted position in-utero. We all worked together to restore balance within his body and to remove any subluxations (misalignments) within his spine. I returned home confident that Sammy was in good hands if he developed any problems from the birth.

As I drove back to Minneapolis, I went over and over in my mind all that had happened over the course of Stacey's labor. I was full of questions. Could I have done something more to free Sammy's shoulder? Did years of karate practice result in torsion and rotation of Stacey's pelvic muscles? Did Sam get stuck because Stacey took cohosh when he wasn't really ready for the descent? Why did it go so fast once we arrived at the hospital? Did I accidentally give Stacey the hypnotic suggestion to go away from the house to have the baby by telling her that the farther away she got from the house the better she'd feel?

I went over and over those questions on the four-hour trip back to Minneapolis. Somewhere along the way, several things became clear to me that quieted my thoughts. First, Stacey intuitively knew that it was not safe to deliver her baby at home. Second, Jill was not equipped to perform the extensive repair that was eventually required. And, third, had Stacey delivered at home, with the same degree of tearing, we would have had to transported her, and the baby, to a hospital under completely different circumstances—we might

STEP 7: Follow Your Instincts and Trust Your Inner Voice

not have gotten the same warm reception. I finally accepted that everything happened just as it should have and that I would never know the answer to my questions.

After Sammy's birth, Jason and Stacey started practicing in Fargo, North Dakota. Within two years, Stacey had her second baby at home. She delivered three weeks after her scheduled due date. This time, she anguished every day over when the baby would finally start labor, but she resisted helping Mother Nature. The delivery was quicker, but she still suffered from extreme back-labor.

A few years later, Stacey had a third baby at home. I was unavailable for the second birth, but the timing was right for me to attend the third one. Stacey had called as soon as she slipped into active labor. I left Minneapolis at 4:00 A.M. and arrived at their home in Fargo at 8:00 A.M. When I saw Jill's van in the driveway, I knew better than to bother knocking on the door. As I rushed into the house, I heard Stacey cry out from the bedroom, "Help me!" She was obviously having the same problem with back-labor she'd had with her other two deliveries.

I ran back to my car and grabbed my pregnancy cushions. During the next thirty minutes, I performed all of the techniques I taught you in this book and added several other specific chiropractic adjustments. Stacey was in terrible pain as I worked on her, so I worked fast. She was desperate enough to gingerly agree to walk out into the hallway with me and get into an inverted position. She rested her knees at the top of the stairs and walked her hands down several steps. She lowered her head onto her forearms and became very quiet.

The inverted position felt so good that Stacey stayed there for several minutes, despite the rush of blood that filled her head. When she raised back up, the baby dropped back down into the pelvis in a better position. With her arms draped over my shoulders, and her head resting on my chest, I walked Stacey back to the bedroom. I settled her on the bed and adjusted her pubic bone… out came the baby.

I was so thankful for a second chance to help Stacey deliver a baby. It was exciting to be able to do something constructive to successfully dislodge the baby. (It only took me a little over a decade to figure out how.)

You might think from Stacey's story that the need to "transport" is a big concern. Well, it's not. I've attended approximately 600 births and about 150 of those were planned homebirths. Of those who planned to be at home, Stacey has been the only woman we've had to transport to the hospital. As rare as it is, I included this particular birth story because it's an excellent example of birth parents who have all the right intentions, but for whatever reason, the baby needs additional assistance. In these cases, the medical field can and should be utilized for crisis care. We must give the baby every chance to control his own delivery, but we must also know when to intervene and help him out.

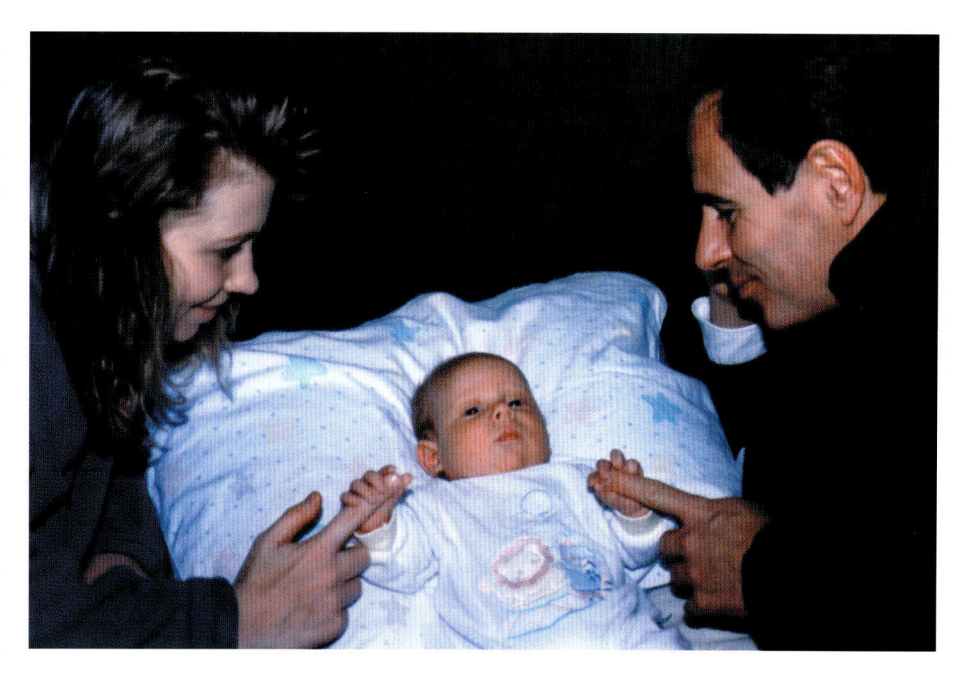

When homebirth parents decide to walk through the door marked **Detour**, an atmosphere of respect and reverence for individual preferences can help a mother overcome her fear and despair. This hospital and its incredible staff were a classic example of how we should be handling birth in the new millennium. If we work together, everyone wins—especially the baby.

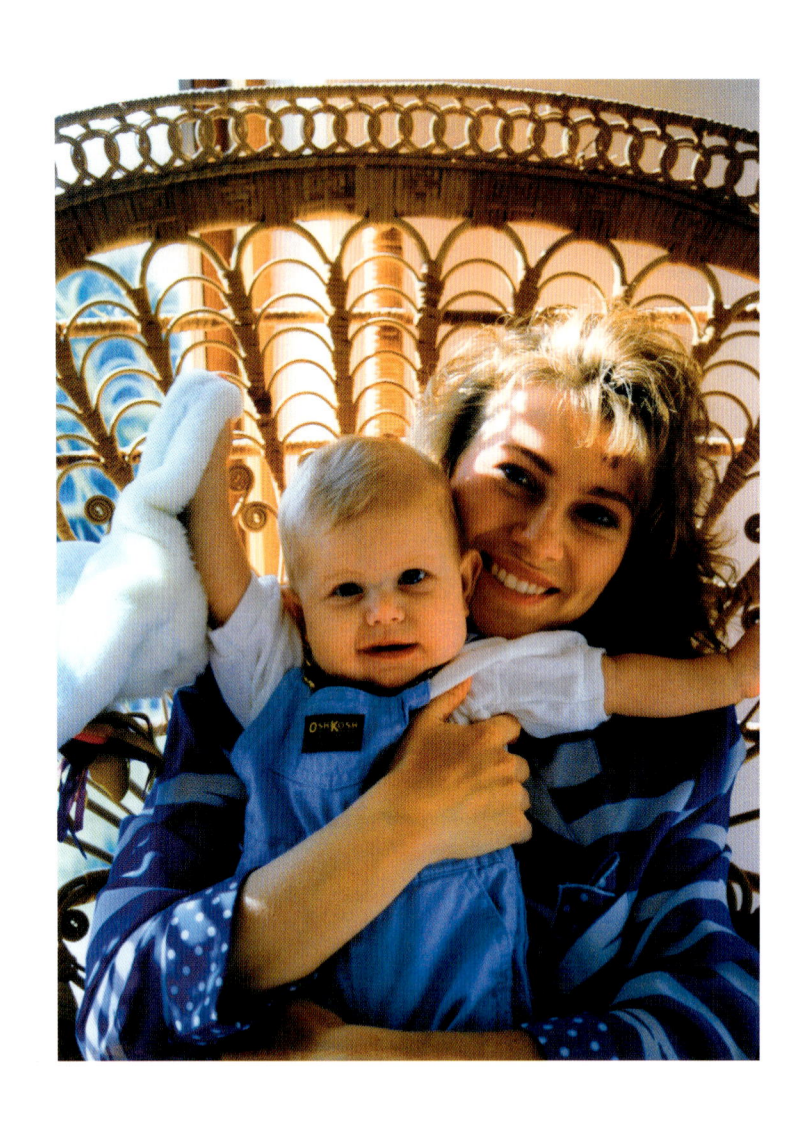

The End

Acknowledgments

I would like to thank the families who allowed me to open the albums of their life in order to bring out the richness of their stories:

Deb and Paul Machacek—Frances Reckholder and Rafael Monfort— Dr. Barb Loran and Dean LaFontaine—Dr. Steve and Heidi Sommerville—Dr. Todd Ginkle and Christy Kaehn—Carol and Leon Rettman—Dr. Meg Simans—Alison and Lee Lundy—Jeanne, Gretta, and Luke Hillstead—Jody Peterson-Lodge—Brenda and Colin Barr—Dr's Shannon and Murray Smith—Deb and Keith McLaughlin—Yvonne Perkins—Leslie Lundgren—Dr's Marie and Bruce Hoffman—Dr. Cheryl Burnett—Becky and Jim Wontor—Julia and Kyle Matson—Shari Doyle—Dr. Brian and Cheryl Elijah—Dr. Jeff and Cindy Priebe—Dr's Stacey and Jason Roth

I would also like to thank the parents, children and midwives whose photographs helped to shape the spiritual aspect of this book:
Annette Wahlgren—Dr. Brett Fischer—Dr. Jennifer Waidelich-Luke—Dr's Anne and Larry Spicer—Dr. Joan and King Elder—Dr. Dave and Lisa Lohman—Jean Chase—Lawan and Andy Jackson—Claudia Higgins—Vickie and Alleandra—Jan Hofer—Jeanne Bazille—Faith Gibson
Barbara Bumgardner is the artist who used her talents to help with the concept of the book by sketching her sleeping daughter's hand and then her own. (page 160) Thanks Barbara.

This book would not have been possible without the dedicated commitment of King Elder who volunteered his time, his talents, and his patience to help me work through the tedious task of turning this manuscript into a work of art. There are no words to express my gratitude for the many years he has devoted to this project. I can only hope that he accepts my heartfelt thanks for a job well done. My deepest gratitude also goes to my good friend, Jody Peterson Lodge, my daughter, Wendy, and my mother Rena Croft—the three people who diligently reviewed every draft of **Hands of Love** (and there were many). Their editing skills helped this book evolve from a stumbling attempt to compile stories, to the shaping and shaving of words that needed to be said, but not necessarily read. I will be thanking them forever for sticking by me as I edited and edited and re-edited every word of this book.

To Isabelle Metairion, for getting me off on the right foot, Amy Gilliland for reviewing the book and sharing knowledge from another doula's perspective, Heidi Benolkin for her enthusiastic review from a mother's perspective, to Alec Syme for adding his graphic expertise to the cover, and finally to Lori McLaughlin for stepping in at the final hour to add her expertise as a copy editor. My heartfelt thanks for the volunteered efforts of every single person who involved themselves with this project. It is our gift to the universe.

Appendix A

Ultrasound research and articles that voice concern about routine ultrasound use during pregnancy.

Haggerty LA Continuous Electronic Fetal Monitoring: contradictions between practice and research. J Obstet Gynecol Neonatal Nurs 1999 Jul-Aug;28(4):409-16

Didy GA The Physiologic and Medical Rationale for Intrapartum Fetal Monitoring. Biomed Instrum Technol 1999 Mar-Apr;33(2):143-51

Berkus MD et al. Electronic Fetal Monitoring: what's reassuring? Acta Obstet Gynecol Scan 1999 Jan;78(1):15-21

Beohm F Intrapartum Fetal Heart Rate Monitoring. Obstet Gynecol Clin North Am 1999 Dec;26(4):623-39,vi-vii

Bernardes J; Pereira AC Some Concerns About the New Research Guidelines for Interpretation of Electronic Fetal Heart Rate Monitoring. Am J Obstet Gynecol 1998 Aug;179(2):560-1

Swayze SC Electronic Fetal Monitoring: are you monitoring mother or fetus? Nursing 1998 Jan;28(1):20

Martin CB Jr Electronic Fetal Monitoring: a brief summary of its development, problems, and prospects. Eur J Obstet Gynecol Reprod Biol 1998 Jun;78(2):133-40

Lancet 1998 Jan 24; 242-247 and 326-327 (commentary)

Ewigman BG, et al. Effect of Prenatal Screening on Perinatal Outcome. New England Journal of Medicine 1993 Sept. 16: 329(12): 822-827

Pelka F. Electronic Fetal Monitoring. Mothering 1992 Fall: 71-75

Taylor KJW. A Prudent Approach to Ultrasound Imaging of the Fetus and Newborn. Birth 1990 December; 17(4): 218-222

Haire D. Fetal Effects of Ultrasound: A Growing Controversy. Journal of Nurse Midwifery 1984 July/Aug; 29(4): 241-246

Appendix B

Epidural research and articles that voice concern about the untold side effects.

Lieberman E The Risks and Benefits of Epidural Analgesia During Labor. J of Nurse-Midwifery. 1999;44(4):394-39

Graninger EM et al. Nurse-Midwives' use of and attitudes toward epidural analgesia. J Nurse Midwifery. 1998; 43(4): 250-261

Thompson TT et al. Does Epidural Analgesia Cause Dystocia? J Clinic Anesthes. 1998; 10(1): 58-65

Alexander JM et al. The course of Labour with and without Epidural Analgesia. Am J Obstet Gynecol. 1998; 178(3): 516-520

McRae-Bergeron CE et al. The Effect of Epidural Analgesia on the Second Stage of Labour. AANA J 1998; 66(2): 177-182

Thorp JA Weighing the Benefits of Epidural Analgesia During Labor. Contemporary OB/GYN. April 1997: 95-104

Lieberman E et al. Epidural Analgesia, Intrapartum Fever and Neonatal Sepsis Evaluation. Pediatrics. 1997; 99 (3) : 415-419

Thorp JA Epidural Analgesia for Labor: Effect on the Cesarean Birth Rate. Clinical Obstetrics and Gynecology. 1998;41(2):449-460

Thorp JA A Review of the Literature on Epidural Analgesia for Childbirth. Birth 1996;23(2)

Stavron C et al. Prolonged Fetal Bradycardia during Epidural Analgesia. Incidence, Timing and Significance. S Afr Med J. 1990; 77(2): 66-68

Murray AD et al. Effects of Epidural Anesthesia on Newborns and their Mothers. Child Dev. 1981; 52(1): 71-82